"IT JUST AIN'T FAIR"

D0823873

"IT JUST AIN'T FAIR"

The Ethics of Health Care for African Americans

Edited by ANNETTE DULA
and SARA GOERING

With editorial contributions from
Marian Gray Secundy and
September Williams

Foreword by Mark Siegler

PRAEGER

Westport, Connecticut
London

Library of Congress Cataloging-in-Publication Data

"It just ain't fair" : the ethics of health care for African Americans
/ edited by Annette Dula and Sara Goering ; with editorial
contributions from Marian Gray Secundy and September Williams ;
foreword by Mark Siegler.
    p.   cm.
  Includes bibliographical references and index.
  ISBN 0–275–94494–8 (alk. paper). — ISBN 0–275–95057–3 (pbk.)
    1. Afro-Americans—Medical care—United States.—Moral and ethical
aspects. 2. Health services accessibility—United States.
3. Medical ethics—United States. I. Dula, Annette. II. Goering,
Sara.
RA448.5.N4I8   1994
174'.2—dc20   93–43780

British Library Cataloguing in Publication Data is available.

Copyright © 1994 by Annette Dula and Sara Goering

All rights reserved. No portion of this book may be
reproduced, by any process or technique, without the
express written consent of the publisher.

Library of Congress Catalog Card Number: 93–43780
ISBN: 0–275–94494–8
    0–275–95057–3 (pbk.)

First published in 1994

Praeger Publishers, 88 Post Road West, Westport, CT 06881
An imprint of Greenwood Publishing Group, Inc.

Printed in the United States of America

The paper used in this book complies with the
Permanent Paper Standard issued by the National
Information Standards Organization (Z39.48–1984).

10 9 8 7 6 5 4 3 2 1

174.2
I88
1994

Copyright Acknowledgments

A version of chapter 2 in this volume appeared in Annette Dula, "Toward an
African American Perspective on Bioethics," *Journal of Health Care for the Poor
and Underserved* 2, no. 2 (1991): 259–269.

Chapter 19 in this volume is reprinted from Evelyn C. White, *Sojourner: The
Women's Forum* (Second Annual Health Supplement), Volume 16, No. 7
(March 1991): 1H–4H.

The children's lullaby which appears in chapter 4 of this volume is reprinted by
permission of the publishers from Dorothy Scarborough, *On the Trail of Negro
Folk-Songs* (Cambridge, Mass.: Harvard University Press, Copyright 1925 by
Harvard University Press; 1953 by Mary McDaniel Parker).

Contents

METHODIST COLLEGE LIBRARY
Fayetteville, N.C.

METHODIST COLLEGE LIBRARY
Fayetteville, N.C.

Acknowledgments

The seeds of this project were planted between 1988 and 1990 when I was a resident medical ethicist in community clinics associated with a large teaching hospital. Many of the ethical issues that arose in the inner-city clinic were of the same genre as those found in any hospital or clinic setting in the United States. However, I also observed other ethical issues surrounding the health care of minority populations that were not addressed by mainstream medical ethicists. These issues included African-American suspicion of the medical system, the legacy of the Tuskegee experiment, the lack of minority physicians and students, and the lack of respect by health care workers for minority populations. These lived experiences by minority populations have been the guiding force for undertaking this project. First, I would like to thank those ambulatory patients who helped me understand that the field of medical ethics had not sufficiently incorporated into its discussion ethical issues surrounding ethnic and racial disparities in health status.

The seeds of this project, however, would have remained dormant without funding from two sources: the Center for Clinical Medical Ethics (CCME) at the University of Chicago and the Rockefeller Humanities Scholars program at the Center for the Study of Ethnicity and Race in America (CSERA) at the University of Colorado at Boulder. Special acknowledgments go to these two institutions for not only providing financial support, but also stimulating intellectual environments. It was at the CCME that the seeds of this volume germinated, took form, and began to develop. While I was a fellow at the Center for Clinical Medical Ethics at Chicago, faculty and other fellows rendered critical analysis and commentary regarding the idea of African-American perspectives in medical ethics. Thanks go out to Marian Secundy and September Williams, the contributing editors of this volume, who provided valuable insights and suggestions, particularly in the early phases of the project. Mark Siegler enthusiastically embraced the project early on; he is to be commended for his contributions in helping to diversify medical ethics. James Bowman, consistently a morale builder and supporter of the project, deserves special appreciation for his encouragement and advice.

The volume was completed while I was a Rockefeller Humanities Scholar at the Center for the Study of Ethnicity and Race in America (CSERA) in Boulder, Colorado. CSERA proved to be an exciting intellectual environment for discussing issues of access, not only in regard to African Americans, but also to all ethnic groups who are ill served by the current health care system. The ethnic diversity of the faculty and their comments were constant reminders that the discrepancies in health status of African Americans are shared by all of this country's minorities. CSERA director, Evelyn Hu DeHart, was particularly supportive. I appreciate her tireless interest, which often came at a time when I wondered if such a huge project would ever be completed.

Many other people have helped in carrying out this project. In particular, the cooperation of the large number of authors in this volume contributes to the relatively sparse literature on the interrelation of access, medical ethics, and minority populations. I am particularly indebted to Barbara Farnsworth of the Center for Values and Social Policy in the Philosophy Department at the University of Colorado who introduced me to Sara Goering. Sara's dedication to this project was a major factor in its completion.

I am deeply indebted to family, friends, and the African-American community who all understand the connection between poor health and poor social conditions. For many of us, access and disparities are not academic issues; rather, they are real experiences that result from poor education, housing, employment, and racial discrimination, which in turn affect our opportunities in life.

Finally, I am most deeply indebted to Mark Gross for his encouragement and support in bringing this volume to fruition. Words cannot express my appreciation for his belief in me and in this project.

Annette Dula

Foreword

In 1990–91 a distinguished group of African-American medical ethicists assembled for a year of study at the Center for Clinical Medical Ethics (CCME) at the University of Chicago. This book, organized and edited by Dr. Annette Dula, emerged from that memorable year of intellectual ferment and creativity. The project has a history that I will recount briefly.

In 1985 the Pew Charitable Trusts and the Henry J. Kaiser Family Foundation agreed to support a leadership development program at the Center for Clinical Medical Ethics. This program would provide training for mid-level faculty, who would then return to their academic centers and develop strong regional programs in clinical medical ethics. The principal objective of this training program was to improve patient care by focusing on the ethical aspects of health care and by extending medical ethics from academic settings to community practice.

Significantly, the supporting foundations insisted that this program also emphasize the needs and concerns of minority populations. Thus, in the award letter to the University of Chicago, the Pew and Kaiser foundations stated:

We hope that you will give considerable thought to racial minorities as relates to ethics. The values and beliefs that underlie ethical standards and behaviors are likely to be different among Black and Hispanic populations compared to the white majority. Too little attention has been paid to these differences. . . . We hope that you will give consideration to the appointment of minority members to your advisory committee, to including minority faculty, to the recruitment of minority fellows from the four predominantly minority medical schools, and to the selection of fellows from institutions and regions that serve predominantly poor and minority populations.

To address these challenges, CCME invited three distinguished medical leaders with an interest in minority health care ethics to join our National

Advisory Board: Dr. Louis Sullivan, then president of Meharry Medical College; Dr. Mitchell Spellman, associate dean of the Harvard Medical School; and Dr. Edmund Pellegrino, director of the Kennedy Institute of Ethics at Georgetown University. All accepted our offer. (Unfortunately, Dr. Sullivan was required to resign from our board eighteen months later when he accepted the position of secretary of the Department of Health and Human Services.) We worked closely with these board members to develop a recruiting strategy for minority applicants.

By 1991 our effort paid off, and the training program reached a critical mass. That year, the center was fortunate in recruiting the following scholars who had a primary interest in African-American health care: Dr. Marian Secundy, the director of the ethics program at Howard University College of Medicine; Dr. Annette Dula from the Department of Family Medicine at the University of Massachusetts; Dr. September Williams from the Chicago Medical School and Cook County Hospital; and Dr. Bruce White, the director of the ethics program at Meharry Medical College. While at the center, these scholars worked closely with several of the faculty members in our ethics program, including Dr. James Bowman (who was the principal faculty mentor to this program), Dr. John Lantos, Professor Mary Mahowald, and Professor Carol Stocking.

During the 1991–92 year, the scholar-trainees and faculty developed a new curriculum to address the ethical issues of minorities and the medically underserved. We created a weekly seminar series that met for the entire year and was attended by faculty and students from throughout the University of Chicago and the Pritzker School of Medicine. This new weekly session brought together many of the individuals who later contributed to this volume, including Drs. Dula, Secundy, Bowman, Lantos, Hertz, Woods, and White. This new seminar was remarkable as the catalyst for addressing issues that had previously been largely unexamined in our ethics program. Many of the ideas brought up in the seminar reappear in this volume.

Dr. Dula's firm hand and intellectual presence are behind every crucial decision that was made in molding the current volume. In addition to co-editor Sara Goering, she was assisted at various stages in the project by Marian Gray Secundy and September Williams.

Dr. Dula's central decision was to focus on access to health care for African Americans primarily as an ethical issue rather than as an economic or public policy problem. She realized that any effort to improve access and quality of care for African Americans had a better chance of succeeding if it could be construed as an ethics issue in social justice. In retrospect, Dr. Dula made a prescient decision in choosing to employ the language of ethics to develop new social and medical policy for African Americans. Several years later, Hillary Rodham Clinton and the Health Care Task Force adopted a similar approach in their efforts to change the structure of American health care. Mrs. Clinton used the ethical principle of universal access to health care as a major force to drive health reform. For more than twenty years, since the early years of the first Nixon administration, unsuccessful efforts to reform health care had focused primarily on cost containment. To Mrs. Clinton's credit, she eschewed the primary economic approach to health reform and chose instead to focus on ethical duties and social justice as the priorities on which health reform must be based. Dr. Dula had anticipated this strategy in organizing and developing the book.

Thus, the book stands as a testament to the vision of Dr. Dula and her colleagues. It is a splendid accomplishment that will benefit not only African Americans but all Americans whose health care needs are given inadequate attention in our current health care nonsystem. The timing is right. Dr. Dula and Mrs. Clinton understand the power of ethics and its remarkably widespread political appeal in a country that embraces the values of justice, freedom, and individual potential. The appearance of this book coincides with a rising crescendo favoring health care reform. It is to be hoped that this book will in fact accelerate the movement toward political reform of the health system in the name of ethics.

The Center for Clinical Medical Ethics is proud to be affiliated with this vitally important four-year project. I also want to thank Rebecca Rimel, the executive director of the Pew Charitable Trusts, and Dr. Alvin R. Tarlov, the former president of the Henry J. Kaiser Family Foundation, for nurturing and encouraging our Center's work on ethical issues for minorities and the underserved. This project validates the insight of the leaders of the Pew and Kaiser foundations. They proved correct in their view that ethical issues that affect minorities and the underserved have not received adequate attention in mainstream medical ethics. Such attention is critically important to improve the health care and health of African Americans and other underserved populations.

Mark Siegler

1   Introduction

Annette Dula and Sara Goering

Annette's 36-year-old niece, Carolyn, has just been released from the hospital after having a hysterectomy. She exhibits many of the classic risk factors for ill health seen among poor African-American women. She is overweight; she is diabetic; she is a single divorced parent bringing up two teenagers, as well as her 11-year-old nephew. She has a minimum-wage job at a state hospital for the retarded. Carolyn was paying almost $300 a month for health insurance for the four of them. Three-fourths of her low salary went to payments for health insurance and the mortgage on the mobile home she had purchased seven years ago (at an interest rate of 15%). This left little money for other needs like decent food or paying bills on time. She received food stamps valued at $37 a month.

Complications from the surgery prevented Carolyn from returning to her job for three months. Since she did not receive a salary for two of these months, she was unable to continue making co-payments for health insurance. Carolyn lost her health insurance for six months, which meant there was no coverage for followup appointments. She also lost her trailer and was duly notified of her forthcoming eviction. When Annette told Carolyn that she was a member of the Clinton Health Task Force, Carolyn's response was, "When you go to Washington, please tell them that it just ain't fair! Tell 'em that it ain't fair that as soon as I got sick and needed health insurance, they took it away from me!"

Annette's Uncle Boy is a lay preacher in western North Carolina. Recently, he and his wife Aunt Irma, along with two busloads of church members, went to Disney World in Orlando, Florida, for a short outing. Uncle Boy woke up on his first day in Orlando with "crushing chest pain." After twelve hours, he went to the emergency room and was diagnosed with acute anterior myocardial infarction. When he was stable enough to return to North Carolina with Aunt Irma, they picked up his medical records and were at first confused and then angry to find that the information had been grossly botched. The medical records stated that Uncle Boy was an "alcohol abuser." The family joke had it that Uncle Boy had only tasted alcohol once (except for the wine on Communion Sundays) in his life. That was when he was 15 years old, and "he was so drunk, that it lasted him a lifetime." As they continued to read the medical records, they found other unpardonable mistakes. Uncle Boy's ethnicity had been recorded as "Indian." Uncle Boy is, of course, African American. The records described his mother—Annette's grandmother—as "alive and well at 91 years of age." She had been dead for twelve years. Back in North Carolina, Uncle Boy and Aunt Irma had a great story that they shared with anyone who would listen. Aunt Irma was quick to say, "*I* gave the doctors the correct information, the Reverend here was really too sick to talk." Uncle Boy looked at it philosophically,

Well it's like this. There's white folks. And there's black and brown and red and yellow folks. Now white folks done treated all us different kinds of colored folks bad. Them doctors did not care enough about me to listen and get it right. We all Niggers to the white folks. So it don't matter to them doctors whether I'm a Indian or a black man. We all into drugs and alcohol. And because my skin color is a little bit yellow-red and my hair is straight like a Indian's, they just decided I must be a alcoholic Indian. I ain't neither. I am a sick black man whose job made his health bad.

Annette's Aunt Katherine had come up from western North Carolina for Annette's graduation at Harvard. Aunt Katherine was not able to convince her husband, Uncle Bill, to come up. "In all of my 58 years, I ain't never been on a plane, and I am not about to get on one now. I don't want to take off time from the furniture factory anyhow. While you're up North, I can work and get time and a half." The same night that Aunt Katherine returned home she had to rush Uncle Bill to the emergency room where it was found that he had had a stroke. Uncle Bill never completely recovered from the stroke and was not able to finish out those seven years before he could retire. He had a hard struggle with his employer before he was able to collect worker's compensation and his pension.

Uncle Bill (and also Uncle Boy) had been working in the furniture factory since he was 13 years old. Over the years he had finished furniture by sanding, lacquering, and spraying, using toluene and other toxic substances. Though not formally educated, Uncle Bill is not naive. He asked his doctors if somehow his stroke might have been related to his many years of exposure to chemicals.

The doctors told me right to my face that all them years working in the furniture factory couldn't have done my health no good, but none of the doctors was willing to put anything on paper. If the doctors work for the company, then the company got the doctors in their backpocket. And even if they don't work for the company, then most of them is too scared to say anything 'cause they know that the furniture owners is the big bosses in town. The factories use up all us poor people, not just black people. Then they throw us out and don't want to give us no benefits. You talking about access to health care in that book. Yeah we got a little bit of access, but we got to fight like hell for it, cause the company controls it and tries to give us as little as they can get away with.

AN ISSUE OF JUSTICE FOR AFRICAN AMERICANS

The common thread that runs through these three stories is the issue of justice. As the stories illustrate, the state of health care in the United States is sadly deficient for many poor people, women, and ethnic minority groups. For many, it is a continuous struggle to achieve adequate health care, to make co-payments for that health care, to receive the same dignity and respect that the more affluent, educated, or politically informed demand and receive. This book is dedicated to people like those in Annette's family— the individual faces that have been invisible in medical ethics. The book is for those who define medical ethics as the struggle to achieve adequate health care regardless of gender, race, or ethnic origin, employment, or ability to pay. The stories show, among other things, that health care for poor African Americans addresses only acute illness. There is little or no preventive care, health education, or concern about work-related environmental problems that affect health. The implicit conception of health is the absence of disease, but these stories suggest that that is not an adequate conception.

The chapters in this book are evidence that we need to reconceive our notion of health itself; we must move from a notion of health as merely the absence of disease toward a more comprehensive definition, perhaps as a state of human existence including psychological and social as well as physiological well-being. We must move from a system in which only the privileged have access to health care to one in which all people receive preventive and curative health care—one in which the widening disparities between whites and African Americans, as well as other ethnic minorities, are reduced and ultimately eliminated. This broader concept demands justice in access to health care and the social commitment to bring about that justice. With the establishment of the Health Care Task Force in the spring of 1993, the Clinton administration acknowledged the need for reform. It remains to be seen if the task force recommendations and the implementation of the health care plan will improve the quality of health care for all people (while reducing the cost), prevent disease, and reduce disparities in health status among this nation's different groups. A partial, half-hearted step, even in the right direction, will not be enough.

THE NEED FOR DIALOGUE BETWEEN ETHICISTS AND AFRICAN AMERICANS

Although the chapters in this book show the need for serious health care reform, this book is not only a body of evidence that points to this end; it is also a bridge between medical ethicists and the grim realities faced by underserved, usually poor populations. It is an attempt to bring medical ethicists face to face with the plight of a particular underserved population—African Americans. Certainly, medical ethics has acknowledged the inequities in access and the fact that, in general, some groups are not well served by the health care system. However, the view taken in traditional medical ethics homogenizes the different groups into just one large category of underserved people. This large and growing group of the underserved has no face, features, color, sex, age, ethnic or cultural differences, or political history. To understand the morality and the real-life effects of unfair access, medical ethicists need to look at the health experiences of real people, like Carolyn, and at real populations, like African Americans. That is, they need to look at cases. Cases enrich theory and help bring it down to earth; cases humanize the theory. Generalities, like statistics, are needed because they provide us with a big picture of the problem, but they often mask the meanings and the implications for particular populations. We want to link the ethical concepts of equity and access to the particular case of African Americans, and more generally to all poor and underserved people. Therefore, this book brings together specific group experiences written by health care practitioners, with medical ethics commentary written by philosophers, medical ethicists, and others involved in discussions of ethics. It presents the particular health experiences of a historically underserved population and at the same time locates these experiences in an ethical context.

Our intent is to lay bare the gross disparities in health care access in this country (from AIDS to homelessness to maldistribution of physicians to infant mortality). We also seek to provide a basis for reforming the traditional ethical framework that in an effort to be impartial and colorblind fails to see particular groups in their unique social contexts. For example, in African-American and other poor communities, occupational and environmental hazards pose specific ethical problems (Bullard 1990; Dula et al., 1993). As Christine Cassel eloquently notes in her commentary in this book, "Most of biomedical ethics has distinguished between bedside clinical decision-making and issues of social justice and resource allocation. . . . [But] it is an illusion that these two can be so cleanly separated." Medical ethics must be concerned with more than what can only be seen in hospitals and clinics; it must also address the wider social issues that not only affect health physiologically, but that also often powerfully influence decisions about health. In Chapter 7, Stephen Thomas and Sandra Crouse Quinn point out that "Public health professionals must recognize that the belief in AIDS as a form of genocide is a legitimate attitudinal barrier rooted in the history of the Tuskegee Syphilis Study." Such an attitude may result in decisions by African Americans not to seek health care from the medical establishment and to rely only on alternative or home remedies instead. Ethicists can offer guidance to the medical profession in addressing African-American suspicion of the health care system. That is, medical ethicists need to discuss the obligations of health care providers to treat patients in ethically acceptable ways and must also assume obligations to reassure communities that, while there are good reasons for the paranoia, suspicion must not stand in the way of beneficial treatments.

INCLUDING CULTURE IN MEDICAL ETHICS

Why should African Americans, or any ethnic group for that matter, receive special attention by medical ethicists? Shouldn't medical ethics be colorblind? While there has been relatively little scholarship on this subject, articles in *African American Perspectives on Biomedical Ethics* offer insight.[1] Cheryl Sanders notes that the question is not *whether* an African-American perspective exists, but rather *why* it exists (Sanders 1992). The answer is clear—racism, "social injustice, insensitivity, and irresponsibility" on the part of both society and the medical profession have given African Americans a different perspective or outlook on life. In one of the most comprehensive discussions of this question yet written, Jorge Garcia provides a philosophical analysis for the validity of African-American perspectives. He argues, "The history and types of encounters African Americans have frequently had with white Americans in various professions and institutions (governmental, corporate and educational) will influence the perspectives we are all likely to take on questions about how health care professionals and institutions ought to behave" (Garcia 1992, pp. 31–32). As a group, African Americans have historically been excluded from full and equal participation in our society. Because they have been excluded, they have developed different perspectives regarding all aspects of their lives, from access to education, to health care, to family arrangements, to employment.

Yet acknowledging the existence of African-American perspectives (for there are perhaps many) is not enough; we must also listen to the people themselves, for who can relate the difficulties better?[2] As Edmund Pellegrino has pointed out, we must accept the nontraditionally presented ethical and practical health care stories as they come to us; "to understand another cultural perspective we must listen to that perspective as it is presented, not as we would present it, or as we would want others to present it" (Pellegrino 1992, p. vi). We cannot alter the stories we hear to fit with our conceptions of "the truth"; we must be sensitive to the different styles of delivery as well as to their content. If we listen, we learn from diversity. John Stuart Mill was right on target when he argued that if we suppress or ignore a viewpoint different from our own, we only hurt ourselves. If the new view is valuable or correct, we will have lost the chance to see that truth; if, on the other hand, it is not worthwhile, we will have lost the chance to enrich and strengthen our own convictions (Mill 1859).

At first glance, some of the chapters and commentaries may not seem to involve medical ethics. They might be seen as "only" sociology, public health, political activism, or politically correct multiculturalism. Academic discussion of African-American perspectives on biomedical ethics, however, is a recent development, and as in all new areas of academic interest, understanding is needed in the beginning stages of a new discipline. This is not to say that normal critical assessment should be withheld; rather, we should free ourselves from prejudices and biases about what constitutes "worthy medical ethics." If early attempts are incomplete, then other medical ethicists should take up the challenge and contribute to the development of the new field. Premature rejection of different perspectives "would be fatal to any transcultural dialogue and [is] an indefensible position given the de facto nature of cultural diversity in America" (Pellegrino 1992, p. viii). To ignore the voices of other cultures is to deny the multicultural makeup of our society, to overvalue the positions and biases of one particular perspective, and to thwart the potential for social justice as well as for the maturation of traditional Western medical ethics. It is well to remember that technically sophisticated medical ethics has not paid a great deal of attention to the glaring injustices of the health care system with respect to minority populations.

In what ways, then, does this book reflect distinctively African-American outlooks? Many of them were written by African Americans. They either directly or indirectly touch on issues of distrust and suspicion of the medical community, a rather common attitude in the black community; historical medical and societal abuses of African-American illnesses; illnesses that disproportionately affect African Americans; unequal access and self-help approaches for redressing that wrong; lack of respect for cultural differences; and distancing of physicians both psychologically and geographically from African Americans and other poor communities. While these conditions are not unique to African Americans, they guide the development of a philosophical explanation for a culturally sensitive medical ethics. As Garcia points out, the content of perspectives relevant to African Americans might include several elements: It would have to be antimajoritarian and antiutilitarian because blacks have suffered under majoritarian theory; it would have to take religion into account because religion has always played an important role in community and social change; it would have to be antisituationist and presumably rule-guided because African Americans do not trust decisions being made for them according to a "best interests" standard in a system that has discriminated against them with impunity, but prefer established codified procedures that protect them from racist policies; African Americans would not be bound to a neutralist position because such a position would not acknowledge that past wrongs help account for present inequalities. Finally, as pointed out before, any perspective that does not take account of African-American distrust and suspicion is clearly uninformed (Garcia 1992).

WHAT'S IN THE BOOK

Because the health gaps between people of color and whites are so large, people of color are receiving special attention in medical, social, and political literature. However, little literature exists on the ethical issues surrounding health care for racial and ethnic populations. This book integrates the practical knowledge of those working with particular underserved groups (mostly African American) with the more distant knowledge of policymakers, philosophers, ethicists, and others involved in ethical debate. The chapters display a diverse array of moral perspectives. Some refer to traditional medical ethical texts and "the canon"; others simply offer examples from their own experiences and communities; but all work toward a different, more inclusive vision of justice and ethics in medicine.

The first questions that should be considered as we work toward reform and justice must relate to politics and the place of medical ethics within a political context. Consequently, the first part, Medical Ethics in a Political Context, not only introduces the idea of African-American perspectives on biomedical ethics, but also shows some of the political underpinnings that have led to calls for a more inclusive approach to medical ethics. Furthermore, as Marian Secundy points out, unless this nation can reach a moral consensus on health care, the disparities in health will continue to widen.

The second part, Disparities in Access and Health Status: An Ethical Issue, makes clear the health care difficulties faced by many African-American and other disenfranchised peoples, from problems with infant mortality to HIV/AIDS to homelessness to inadequate rural health care. These chapters provide telling examples of the magnitude of the problems that disproportionately affect African Americans or other underserved people, although they by no means cover the full range of health problems.[3]

The third part, Ethical Responsibilities and the Medical Profession, raises a range of painful and disturbing questions—from the lack of mentoring for African-American medical students, as told by medical student Michael Hebrard, to cultural distancing on the part of physicians, to the exclusion of nonwhites from clinical trials. While this part critically assesses medical institutions, it is not an attack on all health care providers and medical professionals. Rather it serves as a reminder for those who are already aware of the problems, as an eye-opener for those who simply are not yet aware of them, and as a call for reflection and action on the part of both groups.

The closing part, A Practical Ethics for Reform: Community Empowerment, reminds us of the need for community involvement for ethical and successful health care reform. In Chapter 22 Lauren Young presents a powerful vision of caring as an ethical means of community building. Her vision extends beyond specific locations; it is a state of mind in which all individuals and populations are valued in a society committed to helping its members function fully and independently. The successful community-based models illustrated in these chapters show that including underserved populations themselves in the dialogue for health care reform is not only morally required, but also practically useful for reducing the disparities in health status for a "Healthy People 2000."

Finally, as Leonard Harris points out, "African Americans, acting from various perspectives and as agents of resistance, reshape the subject [of medical ethics] and challenge the *episteme* on which the health care system grounds itself" (Harris 1992, p. 147). That is precisely the project of this book: to facilitate a dialogue among African Americans, medical ethicists, and those working in African-American communities; and to help shape the development of medical ethics so that it no longer reflects the dominance and arrogance of any one group. We wish to encourage the growth of a community of medical ethicists whose analyses embody an ethic of caring and respect for all groups, a responsibility to condemn unjust medical practices, and a humility and an empathy regarding human suffering, which in the end transcends all cultural and racial prejudices and differences.

NOTES

1. See H. E. Flack and E. D. Pellegrino, eds., *African American Perspectives in Biomedical Ethics* (Washington, D.C.: Georgetown University Press, 1992). See also K. Brown and A. Dula, "Sociocultural Reflections on the Case of Mr. W," *The Cambridge Quarterly* 62 (1992): 256–258. For a more general comment, see J. Taylor, "Toward a Philosophy of Recovery: A Prolegomenon to Any Future African American Ethic," *APA Newsletters* 191 (Fall 1992): 14–18.

2. Not all African-American scholars agree. For example, William Banner argues that "the conduct of the science of medicine or the conduct of the science of ethics is incompatible with anything called 'ethnic perspective' " (Banner 1992, p. 191).

3. For recent coverage of some of the other problems, including cardiovascular diseases, diabetes, and alcoholism, see R. L. Braithwaite and S. E. Taylor, eds., *Health Issues in the Black Community* (San Francisco: Jossey-Bass, 1992).

PART 1
MEDICAL ETHICS IN A POLITICAL CONTEXT

2 Bioethics: The Need for a Dialogue with African Americans

Annette Dula

INTRODUCTION

Over the last twenty years, the field of bioethics has assumed major importance, as advances in medical technology and rising costs of health care have forced society to come to terms with difficult ethical choices surrounding life and death, allocation of resources, and doctor-patient relationships. Today, we find university departments and academic programs, hospital ethics committees, bioethics think tanks, and presidential task forces devoted to medical ethics policy and decision making. Furthermore, numerous conferences, journals, and books disseminate information and knowledge generated by the new profession.

Yet, the mainstream literature emerging from this influential new field rarely includes discussions of race, class, and gender. Influential ethics centers, such as the Hastings Center in Briarcliff Manor, New York, do address cultural issues but primarily from an international perspective. One reason for the dearth of critical discussion of cultural and social issues here in the United States may be the demographic makeup of bioethicists. Although feminist bioethicists are beginning to have a louder voice, the field is dominated by white, male, middle-class professionals and academics. These men decide what is important, they frame questions, and they make policy recommendations. The voices of those outside of the power circle—racial minorities, the poor, and women—have been excluded from ongoing debates on ethics and health care policy. At best, such exclusion from decision making results in paternalistic decisions made for the "good" of the powerless. At worst, it victimizes the powerless. As Renee Fox points out in her discussion of the sociology of bioethics, "relatively little attention has been paid [by bioethicists] to the fact that a disproportionately high number of the extremely premature, very low birthweight infants, many with severe congenital abnormalities, [who are] cared for in NICU [neonatal intensive care units], are babies born to poor, disadvantaged mothers, many of whom are single nonwhite teenagers" (Fox 1989, p. 231).

I intend to show that the articulation and development of professional bioethics perspectives by minority academics are necessary to expand the narrow margins of debate. Without representation by every sector of society, the powerful and powerless alike, the discipline of bioethics is missing the opportunity to be enriched by the inclusion of a broader range of perspectives. Although I use African-American perspectives as an example, these points apply to other racial and ethnic groups—Hispanics, Native Americans, and Asians—who have suffered similar health care experiences.

In the first section of this chapter, I suggest that an African-American perspective on bioethics has two bases: (1) our health and medical experiences and (2) our tradition of black activist philosophy. In the second section, through examples, I show that an unequal power relationship has led to unethical medical behavior toward blacks, especially regarding reproductive issues. In the third section, I argue that developing a professional perspective not only gives voice to the concerns of those not in the power circle, but also enriches the entire field of bioethics.

MEDICAL AND HEALTH EXPERIENCES

The health of a people and the quality of health care they receive reflect their status in society. It should come as little surprise, then, that the health experiences of African Americans differ vastly from those of white people. These differences are well documented. Compared to whites, more than twice as many black babies are born with low birthweight and over twice as many die before their first birthday (CDC 1993a). Fifty percent more blacks than whites are likely to regard themselves as being in fair or poor health (Blendon et al. 1989). Blacks are included in fewer trials of new drugs—an inequity of particular importance for AIDS patients, who are disproportionately black and Hispanic (El-Sadr and Capps 1992). The mortality rate for heart disease in black males is twice that for white males; research has shown that blacks tend to receive less aggressive treatment for this condition (Wenneker and Epstein 1989). More blacks die from cancer, which, unlike the situation in whites, is likely to be systemic by the time it is detected (Rene 1987). African Americans live five fewer years than do whites (Department of Health and Human Services 1985). Indeed, if blacks had the same death rate as whites, 59,000 black deaths a year would not occur (Miller 1987). Colin McCord and Harold P. Freeman, who reported that black men in Harlem are less likely to reach the age of 65 than are men in Bangladesh, conclude that the mortality rates of inner cities with largely black populations "justify special consideration analogous to that given to natural-disaster areas" (McCord and Freeman 1990, p. 173).

These health disparities are the result of at least three forces: institutional racism, economic inequality, and attitudinal barriers to access (Jones and Rice 1987). Institutional racism has roots in the historically unequal power relations between blacks and the medical profession, and between blacks and the larger society. It has worked effectively to keep blacks out of the profession, even though a large percentage of those who manage to enter medicine return to practice in minority communities—where the need for medical professionals is greatest. Today, institutional racism in health care is manifested in the way African Americans and poor people are treated. They experience long waits, are unable to shop for services, and often receive poor quality and discontinuous health care. Moreover, many government programs do not target African Americans as a group. As a result, benefits to racially defined populations are diffused. There is hope: Healthy People 2000 complemented by the Clinton health care proposal can go a long way to reducing these problems.

Black philosopher W.E.B. Du Bois summed up the economic plight of African Americans: "To be poor is hard, but to be a poor race in a land of dollars is the very bottom of hardships" (Du Bois 1961, p. 20). Poor people are more likely to have poor health, and a disproportionate number of poor people are black. African Americans tend to have lower paying jobs and fewer income-producing sources such as investments. Indeed, whites on average accumulate eleven times more wealth than do blacks (Jaynes and Williams 1989). Less money also leads to substandard housing—housing that may contain unacceptable levels of lead paint, asbestos insulation, or other environmental hazards. Thus, both inadequate employment and subpar housing available to poor African Americans present health problems that wealthier people are able to avoid. In addition, going to the doctor may entail finding and paying for a babysitter and transportation, and taking time off from work at the risk of being fired, all of which the poor cannot afford.

Attitudinal barriers—perceived racism, different cultural perspectives on health and sickness, and beliefs about the health care system—are a third force that brings unequal health care. Seeking medical help may not have the same priority for poor people as it has for middle-class people. One study in the *Journal of the American Medical Association* revealed that, compared to whites, blacks are less likely to be satisfied with how their physicians treat them, more dissatisfied with their hospital care, and more likely to believe that their hospital stay was too short (Blendon et al. 1989). In addition, many blacks, like people of other racial and ethnic groups, use home remedies and adhere to traditional theories of illness and healing that lie outside of the mainstream medical model (Watson 1984). Institutional racism, economic inequality, and attitudinal barriers, then, contribute to inadequate access to health care for poor and minority peoples. These factors must be seen as bioethical concerns. Bioethics cannot be exclusively medical or even ethical. Rather, it must also deal with beliefs, values, cultural traditions, and the economic, political, and social order. A number of medical sociologists have severely criticized bioethicists for ignoring cultural and societal particularities that limit access to health care (Fabrega 1990; Fox 1989; Keyserlingk 1990; Marshall 1992).

This inattention to cultural and societal aspects of health care may be attributed in part to the mainstream Western philosophy on which the field of bioethics is built. For example, renowned academic bioethicists such as Robert Veatch, Tom Beauchamp, and Alasdair MacIntyre rely on the philosophical works of Rawls, Kant, and Aristotle (Beauchamp and Childress 1989; MacIntyre 1981; Veatch 1981). In addition, until recently the mainstream Western philosophic method has been presented primarily as a thinking enterprise, rarely advocating change or societal transformation. Thus, for the most part, Western philosophers have either gingerly approached or neglected altogether to comment on such social injustices as slavery, poverty, racism, sexism, and classism. As pointed out in *Black Issues in Higher Education*, until recently mainstream philosophy was seen as above questions of history and culture (Brodie 1990).

BLACK ACTIVIST PHILOSOPHY

The second basis for an African-American perspective on bioethics is black activist philosophy. Black philosophy differs from mainstream philosophy in its emphasis on action and social justice (Boxill 1992). African-American philosophers view the world through a cultural and societal context of being an unequal partner. Many black philosophers believe that academic philosophy devoid of societal context is a luxury that black scholars can ill afford. Moreover, African-American philosophers have purposely elected to use philosophy as a tool not only for naming, defining, and analyzing social situations, but also for recommending, advocating, and sometimes harassing for political and social empowerment—a stance contrary to mainstream philosophic methods (Harris 1983). Even though all bioethicists would do well to examine the thinking of such philosophers as Alain Locke, Lucius Outlaw, Anita Allen, Leonard Harris, W.E.B. Du Bois, Bernard Boxill, Angela Davis, Cornel West, William Banner, and Jorge Garcia, references to the work of these African Americans are rarely seen in the bioethics literature.

Although the professionalization of bioethics has frequently bypassed African-American voices, there are a few notable exceptions. Mark Siegler, director of the Center for Clinical Medical Ethics at the University of Chicago, included three African-American fellows in the 1990–91 medical ethics training program; Edmund Pellegrino of the Kennedy Institute for Advanced Ethics co-sponsored three national conferences on African-American perspectives on bioethics; and Howard Brody at Michigan State University is attempting to diversify his medical ethics program. In addition, a number of current publications offer important information for bioethicists. For example, the National Research Council's *A Common Destiny: Blacks and American Society* (Jaynes and Williams 1989) provides a comprehensive analysis of the status of black Americans, including discussions on health, education, employment, and economic factors, as does the National Urban League's annual *The State of Black America*; Marlene Gerber Fried's *From Abortion to Reproductive Freedom* (Fried 1990) presents many ideas of women of color concerning abortion; and several journals (e.g., *Ethnicity and Disease*, published by the Loyola University School of Medicine, and *The Journal of Health Care for the Poor and Underserved*) call particular attention to the health experiences of poor and underserved people. Finally, literature and narrative as forms of presenting African-American perspectives on bioethics are now being explored (Dula 1994; Secundy 1992).

Clearly, bioethics and African-American philosophy overlap. Both are concerned with distributive justice and fairness, with autonomy and paternalism in unequal relationships, and with both individual and societal ills. African-American philosophy, therefore, may have much to offer bioethics in general and African-American bioethics in particular.

MAINSTREAM ISSUES RELEVANT TO AFRICAN AMERICANS

A shocking history of medical abuse against unprotected people is also grounds for African-American perspectives in bioethics. In particular, reproductive rights issues—questions of family planning, sterilization, and genetic screening—are of special interest to black women.

A critical examination of the U.S. birth control movement reveals fundamental differences in perspectives, experiences, and interests between the white women who founded the movement and African-American women who were affected by it. Within each of three phases, the goals of the movement implicitly or explicitly served to exploit and subordinate African-American as well as poor white women (Gordon 1990).

The middle of the nineteenth century marked the beginning of the first phase of the birth control movement, characterized by the rallying cry "Voluntary Motherhood!" Advocates of voluntary motherhood asserted that women ought to say "no" to their husbands' sexual demands as a means of limiting the number of their children. The irony, of course, was that, while early white feminists were refusing their husbands' sexual demands, most black women did not have the same right to say "no" to these and other white women's husbands. Indeed, African-American women were exploited as breeding wenches in order to produce stocks of enslaved people for plantation owners. August Meier and Elliott Rudwick comment on slave-rearing as a major source of profit for nearly all slaveholding farmers and planters: "Though most Southern whites were scarcely likely to admit it, the rearing of slaves for profit was a common practice. [A] slave woman's proved or anticipated fecundity was an important factor in determining her market value; fertile females were often referred to as 'good breeders' " (Meier and Rudwick 1970, p. 56).

The second phase of the birth control movement gave rise to the actual phrase "birth control," coined by Margaret Sanger in 1915 (Gordon 1990). Initially, this stage of the movement led to the recognition that reproductive rights and political rights were intertwined; birth control would give white women the freedom to pursue new opportunities made possible by the vote (Davis 1981). This freedom allowed white women to go to work while black women cared for their children and did their housework.

This second stage coincided with the eugenics movement, which advocated improvement of the human race through selective breeding. When the white birth rate began to decline, eugenists chastised middle-class white women for contributing to the suicide of the white race: "Continued limitation of offspring in the white race simply invites the black, brown, and yellow races to finish work already begun by birth control, and reduce the whites to a subject race preserved merely for the sake of its skill" (Popenoe 1926, p. 144).

Eugenists proposed a twofold approach for curbing "race suicide": imposing moral obligations on middle-class white women to have large families and on poor immigrant women and black women to restrict the size of theirs. For the second group, geneticists advocated birth control. The women's movement adopted the ideals of the eugenists regarding poor, immigrant, and minority women, and it even surpassed the rhetoric of the eugenists. Margaret Sanger described the relationship between the two groups: "The eugenists wanted to shift the birth-control emphasis from less children for the poor to more children for the rich. We went back of that [sic] and sought first to stop the multiplication of the unfit" (Sanger 1938). Thus, while black women have historically practiced birth control (Collins 1990; Rodrique 1990), they learned to distrust the birth control movement as espoused by white feminists—a distrust that continues to the present day (Collins 1990).

The third stage of the birth control movement began in 1942 with the establishment of the Planned Parenthood Federation of America. Although Planned Parenthood made valuable contributions to the independence, self-esteem, and aspirations of many women, it accepted existing power relations, continuing the eugenic tradition by defining undesirable "stock" by class or income level (Gordon 1990). Many blacks were suspicious of Planned Parenthood; men, particularly, viewed its policies as designed to weaken the black community politically or to wipe it out genetically (Littlewood 1977). From the beginning of this century, both public and private institutions attempted to control the breeding of those deemed "undesirable." The first sterilization law was passed in Indiana in 1907, setting the stage for not only eugenic, but also punitive sterilization of criminals, the feebleminded, rapists, robbers, chicken thieves, drunkards, and drug addicts. By 1931 thirty states had passed sterilization laws, allowing more than 12,145 sterilizations. By the end of 1958, the sterilization total had risen to 60,926. In the 1950s several states attempted to extend sterilization laws to include compulsory sterilization of mothers of "illegitimate" children (Morrison 1965). As of 1991, sterilization laws were still in force in twenty-two states (Reilly 1991). They are seldom enforced, and where they have been, their eugenic significance has been negligible (Collins 1990).

Numerous federal and state measures perpetuated a focus on poor women and women of color. Throughout the United States in the 1960s, the federal government began subsidizing family planning clinics designed to reduce the number of people on welfare by checking the transmission of poverty from generation to generation. The number of family planning clinics in a given geographical area was proportional to the number of black and Hispanic residents (Mass 1976). In Puerto Rico, a massive federal birth control campaign introduced in 1937 was so successful that by the 1950s, the demand for sterilization exceeded facilities (Presser 1973), and by 1965 one-third of the women in Puerto Rico had been sterilized (Gould 1984).

In 1972 Los Angeles County Hospital, a hospital catering to large numbers of women of color, reported a sevenfold rise in hysterectomies (Mass 1976). Between 1973 and 1976, almost 3,500 Native American women were sterilized at one Indian Health Service hospital in Oklahoma (Fried 1990). In 1973 two black sisters from Montgomery, Alabama, 12-year-old Mary Alice Relf and 14-year-old Minnie Lee Relf, were reported to have been surgically sterilized without their parents' consent (Aptheker 1974).[1] An investigation revealed that in the same town, eleven other young girls of about the same age as the Relf sisters had also been sterilized; ten of them were black. During the early 1970s in Aiken, South Carolina, of thirty-four Medicaid-funded deliveries, eighteen included sterilizations, and all eighteen involved young black women (Aptheker 1974). In 1972 Carl Schultz, director of the Department of Health, Education, and Welfare's Population Affairs Office, acknowledged that the government had funded between 100,000 and 200,000 sterilizations (Payne 1974). These policies aroused black suspicions that family planning efforts were inspired by racist and eugenist motives.

The first phase of the birth control movement, then, completely ignored black women's sexual subjugation to white masters. In the second phase, the movement adopted the racist policies of the eugenics movement. The third stage saw a number of government-supported coercive measures to contain the population of poor people and people of color. While blacks perceive birth control per se as beneficial, blacks have historically objected to birth control as a method of dealing with poverty. Rather, most blacks believe that poverty can be remedied only by creating meaningful jobs, raising the minimum wage so that a worker can support a family, providing health care to working and nonworking people through their jobs or through universal coverage, instituting a high-quality day care system for low- or no-income people, and improving educational opportunities (Edelman 1987).

INFORMED CONSENT

Informed consent is one of the key ethical issues in bioethics. In an unequal patient-provider relationship, informed consent may not be possible. The weaker partner may consent because he or she is powerless, poor, or does not understand the implications of consent. And when members of subordinate groups are not awarded full respect as persons, those in positions of power then consider it unnecessary to obtain consent. The infamous Tuskegee experiment is a classic example. Starting in 1932, over 400 poor and uneducated syphilitic black men in Alabama were unwitting subjects in a Public Health Service experiment, condoned by the surgeon general, to study the course of untreated syphilis. Physicians told the men that they were going to receive special treatment, concealing the fact that the medical procedures were diagnostic rather than therapeutic. Although the effects of untreated syphilis were already known by 1936, the experiment continued for forty years. In 1969 a committee appointed by the Public Health Service to review the Tuskegee study decided to continue it. The Tuskegee experiment did not come to widespread public attention until 1972, when the *Washington Star* documented this breach of medical ethics. As a result, the experiment was halted (Jones 1980). Unfortunately, however, the legacy of the experiment lingers on, as several chapters in this volume illustrate.

It may be tempting to assume that such medical abuses are part of the distant past. However, there is evidence that violations of informed consent persist. Of 52,000 Maryland women screened annually for sickle cell anemia between 1978 and 1980, 25 percent were screened without their consent, thus denying these women the benefit of prescreening education or followup counseling, or the opportunity to decline screening (Farfel and Holtzman 1984). A national survey conducted in 1986 found that 81 percent of women subjected to court-ordered obstetrical interventions (Caesarean section, hospital detention, or intrauterine transfusion) were black, Hispanic, or Asian; nearly half were unmarried; one-fourth did not speak English; and none were private patients (Kolder et al. 1987). When in 1981, a Texas legislator asked his constituency whether they favored sterilization of women on welfare, a majority of the respondents said that welfare benefits should be tied to sterilizations (Reilly 1991).

HOW A PROFESSIONAL PERSPECTIVE MAKES A DIFFERENCE

Thus far, I have shown some grounds for African-American perspectives on bioethics, based on black activist philosophy and the unequal health status of African Americans. I have also argued that a history of medical abuse and neglect toward people in an unequal power relationship commands our attention to African-American perspectives on bioethics issues. In this final section, I will argue that a professional perspective can voice the concerns of those not in the power circle. Two examples—black psychology and the white women's movement—illustrate that professional perspectives can make a difference in changing society's perceptions and, ultimately, policies regarding a particular population.

Black Psychology

Until recently, mainstream psychology judged blacks as genetically and mentally inferior, incapable of abstract reasoning, culturally deprived, passive, ugly, lazy, childishly happy, dishonest, and emotionally immature or disturbed. Mainstream psychology owned these definitions and viewed African Americans through a deficit-deficiency model—a model it had constructed to explain African-American behavior (Billingsley 1968; Dodson 1988; Edelman 1987; Jones 1980; Moynihan 1965). When blacks entered the profession of psychology, they challenged that deficit model by presenting an African-American perspective that addressed the dominant group's assessments and changed, to a certain extent, the way society views blacks. Real consequences of black psychologists' efforts to encourage self-definition, consciousness, and self-worth have been felt across many areas: professional training, intelligence and ability testing, criminal justice, and family counseling. Black psychologists have presented their findings before professional conferences, legislative hearings, and policy-making task forces. For example, black psychologists are responsible for the ban in California on using standardized intelligence tests as a criterion for placing black and other minority students in classes for the mentally retarded. The Association of Black Psychologists publishes the *Journal of Black Psychology*, and black psychologists contribute to a variety of other professional journals (White 1984). As a result of these and other efforts, most respected psychologists no longer advocate the deficit-deficiency model.

The Women's Movement

The women's movement is another example of a subordinated group defining its own perspectives. The perspectives of white women have historically been defined largely by white men; white women's voices, like black voices, have traditionally been ignored or trivialized. A mere twenty years ago, the question, "Should there be a woman's perspective on health?" was emotionally debated. Although the question is still asked, a respected discipline of women's studies has emerged, with several journals devoted to women's health. Women in increasing numbers have been drawn to the field of applied ethics, specifically to bioethics (Griffiths and Whitford 1988; Holmes 1989), and they debate issues such as maternal and child health, rights of women versus rights of the fetus, unnecessary hysterectomies and Caesareans, the doctor-patient relationship, and the absence of women in clinical trials of new drugs. Unfortunately, however, the mainstream women's movement is largely the domain of white women. This, of course, does not mean that black women have not been activists for women's rights; on the contrary, African-American women historically have been deeply involved in fighting both racism and sexism, believing that the two are inseparable. Many black women distrust the movement, criticizing it as racist and self-serving, concerned only with white middle-class women's issues (Collins 1990; Davis 1990; Giddings 1984). Black feminists working within the abortion rights movement and with the National Black Women's Health Project, an Atlanta-based self-help and health advocacy organization, are raising their voices to identify issues relevant to African-American women and men in general, and reproductive and health issues in particular (Fried 1990). Like black psychologists, these black feminists are articulating a perspective that is effectively promoting pluralism.

CONCLUSION

The disturbing health inequities between blacks and whites—differences in infant mortality, average life span, chronic illnesses, and aggressiveness of treatment—suggest that minority access to health care should be recognized and accepted as a *bona fide* concern of bioethics. Opening the debate can only enrich this new field, thereby avoiding the moral difficulties of exclusion. Surely the serious and underaddressed health concerns of a large and increasing segment of our society are an ethical issue that is at least as important as such esoteric, high-visibility issues as the morality of gestational surrogacy. The front page of the August 5, 1991, *New York Times* headlined an article, "When Grandmother Is Mother, Until Birth." Although interesting and worthy of ethical comment, such sensational headlines undermine the moral seriousness of a situation in which over 37 million poor people do not have access to health care.

There is a basis for developing African-American perspectives on bioethics, and I have presented examples of medical abuse and neglect that suggest particular issues for consideration. Valuable as our advocacy has been, our perspectives have not gained full prominence in bioethics debates. Thus, it is necessary to form a community of scholars to conduct research on the contributions as well as the limitations of perspectives of African-Americans and other poor and underserved peoples in this important field.

NOTES

A version of this chapter appeared in Annette Dula, "Toward an African-American Perspective on Bioethics," *Journal of Health Care for the Poor and Underserved* 2, no. 2 (1991):259–269.

1. More recently, Reilly has reported that, while the literature states that two sisters were sterilized, in fact only one of them, Minnie Relf, was. See P. R. Reilly, *The Surgical Solution* (Baltimore: Johns Hopkins University Press, 1991), p. 151.

Commentary by *J.L.A. Garcia*

Annette Dula urges that those working in medicine and in medical ethics attend to the neglected voices of people who approach issues in bioethics from what she calls "an African-American perspective." Such a perspective, she says, is based, first, on African-Americans' experiences with health and medicine, and second, on the "tradition of black activist philosophy." She illustrates what African Americans stand to lose when they are ignored, pointing to the infamous Tuskegee syphilis experiments and to the birth control movement's historic ties to the doctrines of eugenists. She points to psychology as a discipline where input from black professionals has helped reshape the dominant view and to the feminist movement to illustrate how ignored groups can influence the practice of professionals and force them to revise their preferred theories.

Dula's chapter raises some deep questions about the nature of morality and of our efforts to understand it which go to the heart of the ethical enterprise. What is an ethnic perspective on issues in biomedical ethics? Is it a matter of *what* a person thinks—the beliefs she holds, or of *how* she thinks—of the influences that help shape her reactions? How can there be such a thing? Is there just one perspective or more than one? How can we tell whether or not a particular person operates from such a perspective? Is being an African American sufficient? Is it necessary?

Ethnic perspectives in ethics seem to presuppose that certain intellectual positions can be identified with this or that ethnic group. Such an idea, however, is deeply problematic. I have argued elsewhere that it is better to conceive of an ethnic perspective less as a matter of what a person thinks than as a matter of how she thinks. Too often, efforts to identify such standpoints by their content seem to appeal to ethnic stereotypes, to vicious and antisocial behavior and attitudes, or to contrived and tendentious conceptions of racial or ethnic identity.[1] No mere listing of beliefs can plausibly identify one group, not only because some members of the group will not share the belief, but also because many outside the group may share it. Even if some beliefs were held by all and only African Americans, the interesting and important question will remain: how is holding the belief connected to being African American? Process, then, will matter more than results—more, that is, than content. If we are to talk meaningfully of ethnic perspectives on ethical or other issues, then we need to conceive of a person as speaking from such a perspective when the process by which she came to hold her beliefs is shaped in certain ways by experiences she has had, in part, because of her ethnicity, especially experiences common among members of her group. There will be as many perspectives as there are people, but only some of these will have been significantly influenced by the sorts of experiences that warrant identifying the viewpoint ethnically.

I say that for anyone's ethical standpoint properly to be called an "African-American" one, it would need to have been influenced by her ethnicity "in certain ways." This qualification is necessary, because there may be some ways in which a person's ethnic experience might affect her thought that are profoundly undesirable. Literary critic Shelby Steele adapts techniques that specialists use in interpreting the actions of literary characters to attempt to understand the behavior of some black Americans. Steele is especially concerned by black people he deems oversensitive on racial issues, and identifies a number of psychological mechanisms he thinks are at work in them. Thus, Steele finds black people who suffer from "integration shock"—"the shock of being accountable on strictly personal terms"; from "race-holding"—"using race to keep from looking at [one]self"; from "compensatory grandiosity"—"a form of dependency, a posture of personal or racial specialness that we rely on to keep the demons of doubt at bay"; and so on.[2] For a different group of black intellectuals, it is various people they deem insufficiently "conscious" of their blackness who get put on the theorist's couch. Thus, according to the press, one researcher has diagnosed a disorder, "Token Black Syndrome," whose victims (mainly first-generation status achievers) endorse negative stereotypes about most black people, and who are said to respond to this endorsement by endeavoring to minimize their similarities to other blacks. A second researcher is said to have discovered among some black people a "bleaching syndrome," whose "symptoms" include a total identification with white people and repudiation of other blacks.[3]

In my judgment, we should be suspicious of such claims, both from Steele and from his ideological opponents. They appear to be attempts to psychologize politics by identifying supposed mental disorders in people with whose politics the various authors disagree. This sort of ploy allows one to hold forth about the mechanisms that supposedly drive an intellectual opponent to think as she does, thus avoiding the hard work of rebutting what the opponent has said and of defending one's own ideas on their merits. Still, while we are right to be skeptical about such claims, there is always the possibility that some home truths lie behind all the quasimedical talk of "syndromes" and "shock." In any case, however infrequent such disorders may be, and whether or not they even exist, their possibility should serve to caution us that race and ethnicity can affect thought not only in positive ways but also in decidedly negative ones.

As Dula admirably shows, African Americans have had experiences of health and of medical institutions far different from those of most health care professionals; a perspective on issues in health care that is influenced by such experiences may differ dramatically from prevailing paradigms.

What will bioethicists learn when they begin to attend more carefully to the voices of underserved people? It is still too early to say in detail, of course, and I surely claim no privileged insights into this matter. A few tentative and speculative words may, nevertheless, be in order, if only to help stimulate further investigation.

First, from listening to those who live their lives as members of an oppressed minority, these professionals may learn to question the majoritarian presuppositions built into cost-benefit analysis. A policy that uses medical resources most "efficiently" by serving those likeliest to be restored to full health may also systematically work against those whose prospects have been reduced by lives of poverty.

Second, if health care professionals come to listen to people whose liberation from slavery and later discrimination was greatly advanced by legislation and formal enforcement mechanisms, they may learn to be less confident that doctors should proceed "unencumbered" by regulations from hospital administrators and government. These regulations, especially legislative ones, are more likely to have emerged from debates in which competing forces and interest groups were compelled to offer principled rationales and to defend them before people with diverse backgrounds, values, and constituencies. This procedure incorporates safeguards that are missing when a physician trusts only her own "professional judgment" and that of a few similar elites.

Third, medical professionals must give more thoughtful attention to the reflections of members of a community torn between a traditional affirmation of strong families and the grim social reality of families riven by abandonment and "illegitimate" birth. This might help them, as well as ethicists and public health officials, to place less emphasis on prevalent rhetoric about individual "choice" and to prefer policies that support family consultation and cohesion. At the same time, they must recognize that, for better or worse, in black neighborhoods especially, families are often configured in ways that are dramatically at variance with the "nuclear family" model familiar from the television situation comedies.

NOTES

1. See my remarks on the work of some social scientists in J. Garcia, "African-American Perspectives, Cultural Relativism, and Normative Issues," in *African-American Perspectives on Bioethics*, eds. Edmund Pellegrino and Harley Flack (Washington, D.C.: Georgetown University Press, 1992), pp. 11–66.

2. Shelby Steele, *The Content of Our Character* (New York: St. Martin's Press, 1990), esp. chaps. 2, 3, 4.

3. For the claims about recent research, I rely on Jack E. White, "The Pain of Being Black," *Time*, September 16, 1991, pp. 25–27.

3   Ethics, Ethnicity, and Health Care Reform

Jean J. Schensul and Barbara H. Guest

> The most disturbing finding is related to the signs of deterioration in access to medical care for the nation's poor minorities and the uninsured. In particular, the poor and African Americans have experienced a reversal of the gains in access to physician care made over the previous two decades, moving us further from securing more equitable access to care for all. (Freedman et al. 1987, p. 17)

INTRODUCTION

Events growing out of the civil rights movement of the 1960s redefined the relationship of ethnic minorities and poor peoples to the national health care system.[1] During the era of the Great Society programs, hunger, infant mortality, job training, community empowerment, and affordable housing were viewed as critical areas of human need to be addressed with innovative government funding and empowerment programs. As government agencies sought to address these problems, it became clear that good health was central to obtaining and maintaining employment, to increased self-esteem, and to the ability to care for family members and dependents. The nation was forced to address obvious health and socioeconomic inequities associated with race, class, and ethnic distinctions.

The national response was legislation that created community health centers, instituted health systems agencies, and funded federal block grants and innovative discretionary programs to improve access to health care to underserved communities. Financed by the federal government, community health centers were set up to correct inequities in the allocation of health services and to challenge the power relationships between the health establishment and the people being served. They were placed in medically underserved areas—in inner-city and rural areas where people could not afford adequate health care or where there were no practitioners—and hours were set up for the convenience of the community. People of the same culture and ethnicity were hired and received special training in order to work in these centers. Experimental organizational structures such as interdisciplinary health teams were employed, and family-oriented medical records were used to develop health histories for the entire family. Mental health services, nutritional counseling, substance abuse services, and dental care were all services offered by the neighborhood health center.

The health systems agencies (HSAs) were community health planning boards composed primarily of consumers. HSAs coordinated health planning, prevented duplication of high-cost technological and specialized services, and monitored hospital expansions. The federal block grants provided support for early and comprehensive access to perinatal care for poor and minority women. In addition, federal resources were made available for recruitment and retention of minorities in the health professions and for community-based health research and advocacy programs. By the end of the 1970s, the improvements in health status and access resulting from these measures were significant, although differences still remained in the health of lower income African-American, Latino, Indian, and poor white groups in relation to middle-class white populations.

These improvements came to an abrupt end in the early 1980s with a shift in federal policy away from community-based services. The change in political parties after the 1980 presidential election resulted in a fundamental philosophical shift in the national view of health care. Health care became a commodity, and marketplace competition was introduced into the health care delivery system. Benefits to poor people were rationed through such mechanisms as diagnostic related groups (DRGs). Not surprisingly, health status indicators began to show declines. Since that time, access to health care for the largest U.S. ethnic groups has steadily worsened.

Our discussion of the decline in health status and access to health services will be framed in the context of ethical arguments supporting greater equity in the distribution of health care. We will review current inequities in health status and barriers to access to health care of poor underserved groups, particularly African Americans and Latinos. Finally, we will suggest some directions for general reform within a proposal for nationalized health care and discuss our experience in developing and operating community-based treatment, prevention, and advocacy programs in Connecticut.

ETHICS OF ACCESS TO HEALTH CARE

With regard to equal access to health care, the U.S. Constitution is limited in two critical respects. First, it does not consider health or access to health care as a basic right (Mariner 1989). Second, it guarantees the rights of individuals, but not the rights of groups (Minow 1989). Ethicists concerned with access to health care have thus resorted to an argument based on individual needs, as exemplified by the following quote from Norman Daniels, a well-known medical ethicist writing in the 1980s: "All individuals should have equal opportunity to meet 'course of life' needs—needs common to all and incurred throughout a lifetime, including food, shelter, clothing, exercise, rest, [and even] companionship, and a mate" (Daniels 1983, p. 10). When these needs are not met, "normal functioning," which permits taking advantage of the "changing range of opportunities" that ensure equity, is impaired.

Health needs are not equally distributed in the population; they differ according to race, social history, class, and family background. Thus, to ensure fair equality of opportunity, special provision must be made to compensate for these varying health needs (Daniels 1983). Yet the cost of providing equal access to all types of treatment for health care is prohibitive. Consequently, universal access to "basic" health care has been proposed by policymakers and ethicists (Bayer et al. 1988; Enthoven 1993; Health Policy Advisory Center 1993). Arguing within the limits of the U.S. Constitution's guarantee of equal rights for the individual, Daniels suggests that in providing basic health care "it will be more important to prevent, cure, or compensate for those disease conditions that involve a greater curtailment of normal opportunity range" (Daniels 1983, p. 16).

A number of ethicists have opted for a multitiered system in which priority-setting by some socially and politically agreed upon decision-making process determines "basic," "less important," and "least important" needs. They argue that health is unequally distributed and health care is a societal rather than an individual product, society should be responsible for proactively establishing which health care needs should be met and in what order, and ways should be found for involving citizens in a priority-setting dialogue (Bayer et al. 1983).

It is also important to focus on equalizing access to care by improving the quality of existing care. Even if access to technology and special procedures remains inequitable, for example, because of geographic location, an ethical position requires quality basic care for all people, regardless of class, race, and ability to pay. Quality care must include not only sufficient basic services, but also respect for the patient's autonomy in decision making, as well as respect for the patient's cultural, racial, and sexual identity (see Ferguson, Chapter 11) (Dickman 1981; Friedman 1970).

In recent years, advances in medical technology have exacerbated the split in the U.S. health care system between traditional treatment services and a more comprehensive prevention-oriented public health approach to health care. There has been continuously increasing concern for accessing high-technology specialized services rather than for preventing disease and ensuring the general health of the community. This has meant an emphasis on specialization, higher costs, and the suburbanization of office outpatient care to meet the needs of middle and higher income patients (Dickman 1981). For the majority of low-income African Americans, Latinos, elderly people, and urban patients, care takes place in crowded hospitals or community clinics or emergency rooms with little followup or preventive care, rather than in the physician's private office. Whether the U.S. health care system and the Clinton administration can move once again, as in the 1960s and 1970s, toward responding comprehensively to issues of access, equity, and preventive services for poor and ethnic minority patients is the subject of continuing national debate.

HEALTH STATUS AND UNEQUAL USE OF HEALTH SERVICES

Disparities in Health Status

National sources from 1985 to the present time point to a continuing pattern of health differences and a worsening of health status among African Americans, Latinos, and other poor or ethnic minority groups (Council on Ethical and Judicial Affairs 1990). While it might be suggested that income level can account for these differences, data show that ethnicity alone is a good predictor of at-risk health status (Miller 1987). Inner-city African Americans and Latinos who rely heavily on public health institutions are at a greater risk for poor health status than whites in similar economic circumstances (Heckler 1985; Manton et al. 1987; Robinson 1987). Members of ethnic minority groups are more likely to be exposed to the hazards of inner-city and urban environments (including air and environmental pollution such as dust, roach and rat remains, poor housing, and traffic), occupational hazards (including pesticides, toxic substances, and accidents), and stress associated with poverty (including abuse and violence, homicides, and suicides). These circumstances are associated with higher rates of infectious diseases, chronic diseases, accidents, and premature deaths (Heckler 1985; Manton et al. 1987; Robinson 1987).

Adult African-American, Latino, and Native-American people are also at a higher risk for hypertension, cancer, diabetes, and heart disease than their white counterparts. The rates of breast cancer, for instance, are higher in black women than in white women (Baquet and Gibbs 1992). Five years after diagnosis of cancer, African Americans have cancer mortality rates 20 to 40 percent higher than the general population (Baquet and Gibbs 1992).

In addition to cancers and chronic diseases, stress, mental illness, substance abuse, and violence also directly affect morbidity and mortality. The rate of deaths due to homicide for males between 15 and 24 years of age is higher for African Americans than for either Latinos or whites; indeed, homicide is the leading cause of death for black males in this age group (President's Commission for the Study of Ethical Problems in Medicine and Biomedical and Behavioral Research 1983). Rates of mental illness are high, and indicators of positive mental health status are low for African Americans and Latinos living in the urban environment. An overwhelming majority of patients in the public mental hospitals are African Americans and Hispanics (Department of Health and Human Services 1986).

Reported high rates of substance abuse by both African-American and Latino urban males have also contributed to the steep rise in the incidence of HIV/AIDS in these populations. Much of HIV infection among African Americans can be attributed to intravenous drug use (IDU). For example, in Hartford, more than 65% of people with AIDS are African-American and Hispanic males who contract the disease through use of contaminated needles (Department of Health Services 1990; Singer et al. 1992a; Weeks 1991).

African-American, Native American, and Latino children are at very high risk for asthma, middle ear infection, allergies, upper respiratory infection, skin diseases, obesity, vision problems, learning disabilities, and misdiagnoses. While these problems appear in all ethnic groups, beliefs about etiology, patterns of use of health care facilities, home management of health problems, and interaction with the health care system are known to differ across ethnic groups. Furthermore, frequency and severity of infection, especially among Latino patients, is associated with limitations in access to health services, poor communication between providers and patients, inadequate referral and coordination of care, and poor followup (Allen 1988). These ethnic differences in access and quality of care must be addressed in order to ensure equity of information and quality of service delivery.

In 1982 no significant differences existed among ethnic groups for immunizations of all kinds (92% or more reported immunizations in all groups). In the last several years these percentages have changed dramatically for African-American and Latino inner-city communities, and for children in particular. Gaps in immunization among preschool children constitute a recently recognized public health problem. These gaps are occurring because health education and primary care for inner-city families are not promoted in a weakened and underfunded public health system that has reached the limits of its ability to serve. Prevention activities receive only 2.9% of health funding in the national budget. In response to the increased incidence of measles and tuberculosis outbreaks, prevention through immunization will be addressed by the Clinton administration's immunization plan.

Disparities in the Utilization of Health Services

Health care in the United States focuses on acute care needs and places limited value on prevention and on the maintenance of those suffering from chronic diseases. Yet for poor people there are difficulties in receiving care for both chronic and acute illnesses. Poor people treated for acute diseases often require more rehabilitation, medication, or continuous home care than they receive. Similarly, one of the primary characteristics of chronic health problems is the need for continuity of care. Stress, poor dietary habits, poverty, and environmental pollution have contributed to the large number of poor people who suffer from chronic diseases and to the severity of their suffering.

While people suffer from the same chronic diseases regardless of income, the poor are twice as likely to experience limitations of activity because of prevalence, severity, and persistence of these chronic diseases (Freedman et al. 1987). As stated in other chapters in this volume, their medical records may not be read or transferred from one hospital location to another. They may encounter linguistic, cultural, and racial prejudices in their interactions with the health care system. They rarely have the benefit of a regular physician, and thus they do not receive the continuous care they need to manage a chronic illness.

A number of recent articles point to significant differences among African-American, Hispanic, and white patients in the use of various types of health care. Again, these differences are tied to ethnicity rather than to income. Mark Schlesinger, for example, reported that African Americans in critical shortage areas make less use of health care than whites with comparable incomes (Schlesinger 1987). In 1982 significantly more whites than Hispanics, and more Hispanics than African Americans, stated that they had a regular attending physician (Ginzberg 1991). More African Americans than Hispanics and more Hispanics than whites used hospital outpatient or emergency rooms as primary sources of care (Anderson et al. 1986). Other reports have noted that Hispanic and African-American people without a regular source of care were least likely to visit the doctor (Aday et al. 1984; Trevino and Moss 1984). From 1980 to 1986 the gap in physician use between African Americans and whites grew by 25%. The percentage of African Americans without a regular source of care rose from 13 to 20 percent. Minority patients experience delays, diagnosis and treatment resulting in poor prognosis, and more frequent mortality (Mandelblatt et al. 1991). Physician shortages in low-income communities and physicians who refuse to accept Medicaid payment for services have forced minorities to use clinic and institutional forms of health care with their known limitations (Hanft and White 1987).

Financially motivated transfers of African Americans and Latinos from private to public hospitals increased dramatically from 1980 to 1986, raising the minority population of some public hospitals to more than 90% (Schlesinger 1987). Many more African Americans and Hispanics needed care in 1982 than in previous years, and more African Americans and whites reported trying to get help and failing than in previous years. These trends can only have worsened in the last decade (1982–92) with increasing regional unemployment, reductions in the insured population, increasing numbers of children and families living in poverty, reductions in support for public health services, and the reduction or elimination of prevention programs. In the following section we discuss barriers to care that account in part for reductions in health status and use of health services.

Barriers to Care

Barriers to care are often listed without further classification or interpretation (Flaskerud 1986). Here we will discuss several classes of barriers: structural, financial, cultural, and individual. Structural barriers are those inherent in the general economy as well as in the politics and economics of the health care system. Financial barriers are caused by individual economic problems. Cultural barriers are those referring to cultural differences between the target population and the professionals who operate the health care system. Individual barriers are defined as those lodged in the psychological construction, beliefs, and behaviors of the individual as distinct from his or her sociocultural and economic context.

Structural Barriers. Structural barriers to the health service delivery system for poor and low-income ethnic minority patients include inconvenient location, inadequate transportation systems, long waiting times, lack of physician coordination and follow through, reluctance of physicians (particularly specialists) to take Medicaid or uninsured patients, and lack of effective referral systems and case management (Melnyk 1988). Other structural characteristics of the health care system which create barriers especially for Hispanic, African-American, and other ethnic patients include the cost of health care (especially for the uninsured), policies concerning treatment of undocumented persons, and the limited number of ethnic minority health professionals.

Use of health care services would increase with the presence of ethnically and linguistically trained health staff in the community. Unfortunately, however, the number of African-American and Hispanic physicians has declined from the early 1970s. There are also fewer new minority medical students now than in the past. Lack of ongoing social supports, difficulties in meeting eligibility requirements, unresponsive medical school environments, the now-prohibitive cost of medical education, and the downsizing of the National Health Service Corps that supported medical student tuition in exchange for practice in a medically underserved area have all contributed to the decline (Hanft and White 1987). The need for African-American and Latino nurses, social workers, and case managers is also growing with proportionate increases in the number of patients from these ethnic groups. The lack of sufficient numbers of African-American, Native-American, Latino, and Asian professionals exacerbates the cultural discontinuities between these communities and the health care system (Anderson et al. 1986). Hanft and White noted in 1987 that if this trend continues, "we are in grave danger of slipping backward to the era before affirmative action, when there was an acute scarcity of minority health professionals and continuing disparities in health status between the majority population and minorities" (Hanft and White 1987, p. 266).

Financial Barriers. The health care system is a $700 billion enterprise, with inflation growing unchecked at around 15% each year. In 1992 health care costs accounted for 12.2% of the gross national product. Health care is becoming unaffordable, and the costs that are most heavily reimbursed by the insurance industry are hospital costs rather than physician visits or clinic care. Health insurance, which has traditionally been tied to employment, is no longer completely employer-supported. It is now common for employees to contribute to the cost of their health care plans. The deductible and co-insurance provisions of most health care plans cause individuals to pay more for their health care than they did before the enactment of Medicaid and Medicare; the elderly now pay more out-of-pocket costs with Medicare coverage than they did before enactment in 1965. This has forced more African-American, Latino, poor, elderly, and marginally employed people to do without coverage for health care. Twenty percent of African Americans, Cuban Americans, and Puerto Ricans and 30% of Mexican Americans are uninsured (Trevino and Moss 1984). In 1986 most of the 37 million people without health insurance were employed in part-time or low-paying jobs (McGinnis 1986).

The way the Medicare (Title XVIII) and Medicaid (Title XIX) programs were enacted as part of the Social Security Act in 1965 illustrates how the economics of health care creates barriers to care. Medicare provides reimbursement for health care and is available to everyone over the age of 62. It is administered at the state level by private insurance companies that reimburse services. Charges to Medicare are reimbursed in much the same way as health insurance, with annual deductibles and co-insurance payment on each visit.

Eligibility for Medicaid, on the other hand, is linked to income rather than to age. It covers the cost of health care for individuals with limited incomes and is administered at the state level by social service agencies. Eligibility is determined by a means test, and frequent recertifications are required in order to maintain eligibility. Medicaid may serve as a disincentive to self-sufficiency and employment, particularly for women who are heads of households with children who need health care. Low-paying employment may remove a person from eligibility range, without providing adequate health care benefits.

Medicaid has formalized and institutionalized an already existing inequity in the health care system. Since most physicians will not accept Medicaid's low level of reimbursement, those eligible for Medicaid are forced to use public clinics and emergency rooms. Services in these institutions are not completely covered by Medicaid, causing them to operate at serious financial risk. In addition, the number of people who are both poor and elderly is increasing, along with the cost of health care. Over 60 percent of Medicaid reimbursements are now directed toward paying the nursing home costs of the elderly.

Cultural Barriers. Cultural barriers to health care access are differences in beliefs, behaviors, expectations, explanations for wellness, disease and disease management, and language between the patient/community culture and that of the service provider/institution. Such differences impede communication between the two and result in perceptions of "inadequate treatment" on the one hand and "poor compliance" on the other. Communication problems spring from negative or incorrect perceptions of the provider about patient differences in lifestyle, economic status, responsibility, and health beliefs. For example, providers may discount the use of herbs, rubs, teas, and other home remedies as well as spiritual and folk healers (Schensul and Schensul 1982). They may also make judgments about patients' appearances, emotional reactions, and ability to understand the problem and follow directions in treatment (Singer 1987; Singer et al. 1988). Many patients feel that the physician belittles their perception of the problem, thereby underscoring the power differentials between patient and provider. These inequalities exist not only between patient and provider, but also between the medical establishment and the community as a whole.

Individual Barriers. Individual beliefs and preferences may play a role in creating barriers to the use of health care services. While we acknowledge that individuals do make choices based on their beliefs and experiences, and that these choices are important to understand, too often individual barriers are used to blame poor people for their poor health. In fact, poor people are caught in a web of structural, financial, and cultural obstacles over which they have little control. Thus, while individual barriers must be addressed, a public health or social science perspective that examines group patterns rather than individual cases is necessary to identify and confront the broader societal barriers that prevent classes of people from equal access to quality care.

APPROACHES TO HEALTH CARE SYSTEM REFORM

Since the enactment of Social Security legislation in the 1930s, experts in health care reform concerned with issues of accessibility have emphasized public health care financing over quality of care in the public and private service sectors. All the reforms that resulted from the enactment of Social Security legislation in the 1930s through to the enactment of Medicare and Medicaid legislation in the 1960s were concerned with the financial aspects of the health care system, but left untouched both fee-for-service physicians' practice and the insurance-based reimbursement system. Indeed, even the current managed care competition proposals put forward by the Clinton administration may not dismantle the foundations of the insurance-based system, because they rely on programs "run by large insurance companies that can intrude in the patient-health care provider relationship through surveillance, financial incentives, and other controls" (Health Policy Advisory Center 1993, p. 22). Only the community health center concept introduced in the 1960s has offered a structurally distinct and innovative approach to changing the way health care is delivered.

CHCs as a Model for Reform: Meeting the Needs of Poor and Culturally Diverse People

The community health center (CHC) is a successful approach for the community-based coordination of primary health care and prevention for all patients and in particular those residents who do not have coordinated and continuous access to quality health care in other settings. The CHCs of the 1970s were critical in promoting the development of ethnic health personnel. Furthermore, they were central to the development of an informed, organized, economically more stable group of citizen advocates who were prepared to participate on decision-making boards and committees. The CHC environment supported improvements in health status, in prevention of health problems, and in promotion of an integrated model of community health and development. They increased advocacy on behalf of the health service needs of poor and ethnic patients formerly locked out of the decision-making process. These early steps should influence more recent thinking in health policy reform.

Health system reform must start by recognizing, as CHCs did, that medical care is only one aspect of health care and health maintenance. An improved, federally funded, coordinated system of medical care will reverse some of the current inequities in access to care and quality treatment. Since many of the health problems faced by poor people in the United States are the result of inadequate financial resources, poor nutrition, poor and congested housing conditions, and toxic urban environments, a national commitment to full employment, affordable housing, and adequate education is necessary to improve the overall health status of poor, African-American, Latino, and other ethnic minority and low-income peoples in the United States. Some recent community-based health care programs have been successful in serving the community needs (see Hertz and Williamson, Chapters 18 and 8, in this volume). In their attempt to reform health care, policymakers must not discard successful programs, but rather ought to use them as a model.

A national health care plan will organize universal coverage. To ensure universal coverage, however, it must also include structural reform designed to benefit lower income and ethnic and culturally diverse peoples who represent an increasingly large proportion of the overall population. While several proposals for health care reform have been discussed and one will be implemented under the Clinton administration (Health Policy Advisory

Center 1993), CHCs and HSAs of the 1960s and 1970s should serve as the model for community health care. In a community-based model, administration would fall to state and local health departments. Placing the medical care system in the health department integrates its functioning with public health and environmental efforts. The system would not be a unified federal system but would function in relation to health care needs assessed in each locality. Federal responsibilities would include the establishment of uniform standards for quality assurance, and quantity and accessibility of health services. Financing these structural changes would be accomplished through progressive taxation on income and corporations, as well as excise taxes on tobacco, alcohol, and toxic and hazardous industrial waste materials.

Any health care reform package must ensure equitable access, quality service, and prevention programs for poor and ethnic communities. It must address the need for additional minority health care personnel, affirmative action in training, and recruitment of health care workers. A just reform package must specify how the CHC will guarantee culturally appropriate services and how it will convince private physicians to incorporate poor people into their practices. The emphasis in medical training must be on community-based primary health care and related public health options. Furthermore, resting the financing for an equitable, rationed health care delivery system on taxation of tobacco, alcohol, and toxic substances—critical elements that contribute significantly to the burden of chronic disease in ethnic minority communities—is at least ethically, if not practically, questionable (Nichter and Cartwright 1991).

In addition to acknowledging the role of public health departments in prevention and health promotion, a national health policy must also spell out how to integrate medical care and public health systems. This is important since many chronic and acute problems of low-income communities can be prevented through public health education and specifically targeted non-medical interventions. This integration has been the goal of our efforts in Connecticut.

Integration of Public Health and the Community: Hartford Examples

In our opinion, a just health care system must include community involvement and public health education for prevention. It is essential to create programs to strengthen the training of ethnic personnel—programs that provide culturally specific curricular materials and emphasize community-based primary health care and related public health options. In addition, the full potential of communities of color should be utilized in the development, implementation, and evaluation of the community health center. A just system should include professional training and mobility for all candidates for community-managed boards. The system must ensure informed citizen participation in defining the boundaries of treatment, and the relationship between treatment, prevention, and community development. To serve all people equitably regardless of ethnicity, class, culture, gender, age, or other factors, we must also provide coordinated treatment and prevention-oriented services in a cohesive network of institutions. This must begin with a broad-based dialogue that includes public health advocates (including professional social scientists, humanists, policymakers, and politicians) and that emphasizes action.

In Hartford, Connecticut, we have applied this ethnically responsive approach to the development of community health research, training, and intervention programs. We offer our experiences as a model for action. In our multidisciplinary approach, anthropologists and other public health advocates have been involved in the creation of new community health and mental health services, centers, and programs. We have been active in community health research and advocacy organizations such as the Hispanic Health Council and the Institute for Community Research. We have also been involved in community action and service in the areas of pediatric impairments, AIDS and IV drug use, pregnancy, addiction, genetic screening and counseling, and neonatal intensive care followup (Schensul and Schensul 1992).

We have developed culturally and community-appropriate approaches that are to be incorporated in both new and existing service centers. These have been tested in the areas of maternal and child health (Schensul et al. 1987), AIDS prevention (Singer et al. 1992b), substance abuse prevention (city and state), otitis media (Allen 1988), pediatric impairments (Schensul and Allen 1985), Alzheimer's disease (Schensul et al. 1992; Wetle et al. 1989), and other areas. We have collaborated with the community on policy formulation on hunger, pediatric care, developmental assessment methods, abuse of women, and health care for the uninsured. Vehicles for collaboration include basic research, intervention projects, demographic surveys, advocacy training programs, curriculum development, and community health education efforts.

We have also worked to ensure that health training programs recruit and retain ethnically diverse students and trainees, and that their educational programs are culturally appropriate as part of the retention process. Perhaps the most notable example of such programming in Connecticut is the Hartford Area Health Education Center which was designed to change university curricula, build alternative community-oriented service models, recruit high school students, and engage in community health education. The Hispanic Nurses preaccreditation training program funded by a local community foundation in 1990–91 for the University of Connecticut School of Nursing helps nurses from Puerto Rico prepare for their accreditation examination, an examination that is culturally discriminating and that they must take in

English. In one year, this program successfully assisted over fourteen recently arrived Puerto Rican nurses in passing the state examination.

Social scientists and public health advocates can also play important roles in promoting a more comprehensive vision of prevention, which encompasses both a public health and community development perspective. Incorporating this perspective into public arenas can educate audiences and move them beyond issues of "compliance" and into questions concerning structural barriers to health and health care utilization. We have used public panels, forums, presentations at public hearings, and press conferences to educate and empower the community. Other public discussions focus on such controversial topics as needle exchange programs, rationing of health care, infant mortality, the effects of hospital amalgamations on primary health care for urban children, and school-based health programs.

CONCLUSION

We have reviewed some issues in the creation of an equitable health care system. It is clear that the 1980 change in government policy toward health care resulted in poorer health status and limitations in access to health care for African Americans, Latinos, and other historically marginated groups in the United States.

We argued that applied social scientists, health personnel, community health advocates, and policymakers should work to create new, community-based and culturally appropriate controlled health care options. As we continue to move toward restructuring the currently inadequate health care system, health social scientists must remember that the strength of the discipline lies in understanding communities in national systems, and that our repertoire of applied methods favors strategies for collaborating with communities to assist institutions and policy-making bodies to meet their needs.

To conclude, we strongly argue in favor of a broad-based public dialogue concerning the future of health care, health care funding, and the framing of prevention programs in the United States. This view has been eloquently noted in an excellent article on citizen involvement in health reform and the allocation of health care resources: "Citizens need to clarify their health care rights and establish a just system to ensure those rights. . . . We must come to a consensus on the meaning of health care before we discuss or legislate levels of access. Only through dialogue can we fairly consider distributive justice" (Cassidy 1988, p. 299).

We believe that health social scientists, ethicists, public health administrators, and other policy-oriented health advocates working in community settings in the United States and elsewhere have a significant role to play in facilitating this dialogue.

NOTE

1. By ethnic minority, we refer to the categories used in the United States Census: black (including African Americans and people of the African Caribbean), Hispanic (Mexican, Cuban, Puerto Rican, and people of the countries of Central and South America), Asian/Pacific (Hawaiian and people of the countries of Southeast Asia), and Native American (differentiated by tribe). In addition to the distinctions implied by country or tribal origin, there may in each instance be numerous intragroup differences with regard to place of birth, migration patterns, education level, degree of acculturation, gender, and age. Furthermore, when comparing the health status of members of ethnic minority groups to that of people of European origin, it is critical to disaggregate by class.

Commentary by Stephen Toulmin

In this chapter, Jean Schensul and Barbara Guest advocate working "to create new, community-based and culturally appropriate controlled health care options," and they argue in favor of "a broad-based public dialogue concerning the future of health care, health care funding, and the framing of prevention programs in the United States." The core of the chapter consists of two richly illustrated central sections, on "Health Status and Unequal Use of Health Services" and "Approaches to Health Care System Reform," respectively—for which one may alternatively read "What is wrong" and "What needs doing." They also include a preliminary section called "Ethics of Access to Health Care" to which I will return shortly.

The two central sections pursue some important themes in the political history of the American health care debate in the 1980s. I will not take issue with the material they present here—I myself can add no independent evidence to their documentation. Nor do I believe that, in 1993, many people would question their general thesis: that is, that at a time when publicly supported medical care fails to meet the needs of at least 37 million Americans, from all sorts of ethnic communities, poor blacks and Latinos systematically came off worst. On the contrary, although they sometimes present their material more rhetorically than coolly, the general thrust of their empirical arguments is difficult to ignore or deny. The Reagan/Bush era of politically rewarded greed was an especially hard time in which to be black and poor and sick. The institutional changes that marked that period, for example, the introduction of a system of funding hospital costs by "diagnostically related groups" of illnesses, bore down hardest on those who were most dependent on public aid for their medical services.

There is only one more moral question in these sections that calls for special comment. It is helpful to the reader that the authors underline the gross disparities in access to medical care available to different ethnic communities; but they do not sufficiently distinguish between two central moral issues that their inquiries bring to light. On the one hand, it is morally deplorable that *anyone* should be as deprived of proper access to medical care as so many people have been. On the other hand, it is deeply unsettling—and politically obnoxious—that this should happen *disproportionately* to individuals from the so-called minority communities. Yet it is distracting to run these two issues together, as though they were two parts of a single question. To the contrary, the full force of the authors' argument will be clear only if we step back and consider the two issues separately.

First, let us look at their section, "Ethics of Access to Health Care," in which they begin by looking to the U.S. Constitution as an exhaustive compendium of American political ethics and note with regret that "With regard to equal access to health care, [this document] is limited in two critical respects." They go on to quote Norm Daniels' views about priorities in the definition of the "basic" components in health care, implying that Daniels argues "within the limits of the U.S. Constitution's guarantee of equal rights for the individual."

Treating the Constitution as a moral compendium has unfortunate results: in particular, it blurs the distinction between legal, political, and moral questions, and so it leads to a fogging of the very issues about which one most needs to achieve clarity and illumination. Testifying before the Judiciary Committee of the Senate as a nominee to the Supreme Court, Robert Bork insisted on limiting the scope of the law to the manifest content of the text of the Constitution and Statutes—what philosophers call "positive law." He objected to judicial reinterpretation of that text—even more to references to any "natural law" capable of supplementing or overriding the plain sense of that text—as importing into judicial decisions a reliance on "personal preferences and satisfactions" irrelevant to any determinate judgment of the Court. In his view no personal *ethical* commitments can have any *legal* force.

The present authors take the opposite tack. They imply that everything of moral significance ought to be represented, either explicitly or implicitly, in the Constitution; nowhere do they address the true basis of their central moral argument, which lies less in constitutional law than in the consensus of many older moral traditions—going back on the one hand to Aristotle, and on the other hand to the Talmud, Jesus, and earlier moral teachers. As to that, we can read Norm Daniels as looking back quite as much through Rawls to Kant and earlier philosophers, as to a supposed "guarantee of equal rights for the individual" in the U.S. Constitution. Fortunately, perhaps, the shared thrust of our moral traditions antedates the work of the Founding Fathers.

The moral confusion in the present chapter most needing to be sorted out is one that it shares with too many popular American discussions of ethical and political questions. The authors slide between the terms *equity*, *equitable*, or *inequities* in some places, and questions of proportionality and appropriateness to special needs and situations on the one hand, and on the other hand the wish for an exact numerical division of resources. By the end of their argument, we are relieved to find that the balance of their concerns does really lie with equity rather than equality, although it would have been helpful to have the idea of "culturally" appropriate health care options spelled out more clearly. Do they just mean hiring Spanish-speaking nurses for clinics serving Latino patients? Or do they imply that ethnic diseases call for appropriately ethnic doctors? (What if the world expert on Tay-Sachs turned out to be a Gentile?)

Another pair of contrasted themes in their argument is "dialogue" versus "control." Many of us would agree with the thrust of the final section, in which the authors move in the direction of greater participation by patients in discussions of their own needs and care. Yet this argument needs to be carried through to a clear conclusion. We should not just think about drawing individual patients into their own clinical diagnosis and treatment: the deeper need is for community representatives or subscribing patients to have a role in the management of their families' health maintenance organizations (HMOs) or the like, which is *at least* equal to the role of PTA groups in the management of neighborhood public schools. The practice of drawing subscribing patients into the management of HMOs or other group practices is not unknown in places like Palo Alto, where there is already a community of background or experience among the physicians and patients in question. What I *hope* the present authors are dreaming of is a situation in which this practice is extended to community health centers serving poorer and less educated constituencies. It is unsettling to find them arguing the case for "community-based and culturally appropriate *controlled* health care options." What is meant in this context by "controlled"? Who is doing this "controlling"? Are we in danger of falling back into a patronizing model, in which a public dialogue is effectively open only to well-meaning, user friendly health care professionals, not to the patients and their families themselves? (Who knows where a shoe pinches better than the person who wears it?)

In conclusion, to return to a topic touched on earlier: the need to distinguish *moral* questions about the wrong that is done to *all* those human beings who are denied access to health care—regardless of ethnicity—and *political* questions about what we can do to prevent this wrong being done disproportionately, for reasons of institutional structure or reimbursement procedures, to people who are poor, sick, and from ethnic groups that are already exposed to systematic neglect. Certainly, the sense of moral outrage that is proper in response to *medical deprivation*, whoever the victim, can carry over and inform our concern for political campaigns to rectify the *disproportionate* loss or suffering of those most adversely affected by the deprivation. While all that the moral outrage requires of us is a principled stand against the current wrong, the political solution demands a more energetic commitment to advocating, and voting for, new policies and procedures that can alone remedy the injustices from which victims of ethnic discrimination especially suffer.

4   Surrogates and Outcast Mothers: Racism and Reproductive Politics

Angela Y. Davis

INTRODUCTION: THE CULT OF MOTHERHOOD

New developments in reproductive technology have encouraged the contemporary emergence of popular attitudes, at least among the middle classes, that bear a remarkable resemblance to the nineteenth-century cult of motherhood. This cult of motherhood "attempts to press women in the direction of child-bearing and . . . in this sense women's motivations [for motherhood] are socially shaped" (Stanworth 1987, p. 17). Women who don't comply with this ideology are considered disturbed or abnormal. In the late nineteenth century, white and middle-class women were imprisoned within a privatized home sphere by this ideology, as the rise of industrial capitalism led to the historical obsolescence of the domestic economy. Despite small advances, their imprisonment continued until the advent of the modern women's movement. Middle-class white women then moved from the home to the workplace, challenging the cult of motherhood ideology.

Now, late-twentieth-century technologies that allow the possibility of transcending biological reproductive incapacity are resuscitating the old motherhood ideology in bizarre and contradictory ways. Infertile women who can afford to take advantage of these new technologies—often career women for whom motherhood is no longer a primary or exclusive vocation—now feel it necessary to initiate a motherhood quest that is even more compulsive and oppressive than the ideological imprisonment of the nineteenth century. These women are compelled by the "mystification of motherhood," the socially created desire for children which is central to conservative politics today (Overall 1987). Consider, for example, the anti-abortion campaign, which has made efforts to deny all women the legal rights that would help shift the politics of reproduction toward a recognition of women's autonomy with respect to the biological functions of their bodies.

In this chapter, I will show how the reproductive role of women has been historically and socially constructed and is largely synonymous with the failure to acknowledge women's reproductive self-determination. This role has been informed by a peculiar constellation of racist, classist, and misogynist assumptions. I will discuss the role of these assumptions in the ideology of motherhood, showing how they have led to exploitation of women and fragmentation of motherhood, especially in African-American women, in both historical and contemporary contexts. Furthermore, I will provide examples of current inconsistencies in the ideology of motherhood that have resulted in the vilification of young, working-class, single mothers, especially in African-American communities. Using surrogacy as an example, I will show how new reproductive technologies maintain or deepen misogynist, anti-working-class, and racist marginalization. Finally, I will suggest a reconceptualization of reproductive issues that does not exploit women, especially poor women and women of color.

In the United States, the nineteenth-century cult of motherhood was complicated by class- and race-based contradictions. Poor immigrant and slave women were not allowed to participate in the cult of motherhood. For example, poor women who had recently immigrated from Europe were cast, like their male counterparts, into the industrial proletariat and, therefore, were forced to play roles as workers, contradicting the increasing representation of women as wives and mothers. Racial contradictions, on the other hand, resulted from conflating slave motherhood and the reproduction of the slave labor force; the moribund slave economy effectively denied motherhood to vast numbers of African women. Thus, slave women, like white women, were imprisoned within their reproductive role. The same sociohistorical reasons—racist/classist/misogynist assumptions as well as the industrial revolution—that forced white women to stay at home and raise children while their husbands went out to work caused slave women to be valued in accordance with their role as breeders. Of course, both motherhood, as it was ideologically constructed, and breederhood, as it historically unfolded, were contingent on the biological birth process. However, motherhood presumed to capture the moral essence of womanness, while breederhood, on the basis of racist presumptions and economic necessity, denied the very possibility of participation in this motherhood cult.

During the first half of the nineteenth century, when the industrial demand for cotton led to the obsessive expansion of slavery at a time when the importation of Africans was no longer legal, the slavocracy demanded of African women that they bear as many children as they were biologically capable of bearing. Thus, many women had as many as twenty children.[1] At the same time that nineteenth-century white women were being ideologically incarcerated within their biological reproductive role—essentialized as mothers—African women were being forced to bear children, not as evidence of their role as mothers, but for the purpose of expanding the human property held by slave owners. The breeder role imposed on African slave women bore no relationship to their own definition of motherhood. As Toni

Morrison's novel *Beloved* (Morrison 1987) points out, some slave mothers even committed infanticide as a means of resisting the enslavement of their progeny.

SLAVE WOMEN AND SURROGACY:
THE FRAGMENTATION OF MOTHERHOOD

Slave women were "birth mothers" or "genetic mothers" (to employ terms rendered possible by the new reproductive technologies), but they possessed no legal rights as mothers. Considering the commodification of their children, and indeed, of their own persons, their status was similar to that of the contemporary "surrogate mother" (who carries a fetus to term for another woman for economic and sometimes altruistic reasons). The term *surrogate mother* might be invoked as a retroactive description of the status of slave women because the economic appropriation of their reproductive capacity reflected the inability of the slave economy to produce and reproduce its own laborers.

The children of slave mothers could be sold by their owners for business reasons or as a result of a strategy of repression. Slave women could also be forced to give birth to children fathered by their masters. They knew fully well that the white fathers would never recognize their black children as offspring. As a consequence of the socially constructed invisibility of the white father—a pretended invisibility strangely respected by the white and black community alike—black children would grow up in an intimate relation to their white half-brothers and -sisters, except that the biological kinship, often revealed by a visible physical resemblance, would remain shrouded in silence. Slave women who had been compelled, or had agreed, for their own reasons, to engage in sexual intercourse with their masters would be committing the equivalent of a crime if they publicly revealed the fathers of their children (Jacobs 1987). These women knew that it was quite likely that their children might also be sold, brutalized, or beaten (or all three) by their own fathers, brothers, uncles, or nephews.

If I have lingered over what I see as some of the salient reproductive issues in African-American women's history, it is because they seem to shed light on the ideological context of contemporary technological intervention in the realm of reproduction. Historical and contemporary reproductive interventions have caused serious fragmentation of motherhood in slave times, and of maternity in modern times. Within the contemporary feminist discourse about the new reproductive technologies (such as in vitro fertilization, surrogacy, and embryo transfer), concern has been expressed about what is sometimes described as the "deconstruction of motherhood" in which motherhood is no longer a unified biological process. "In place of 'mother', there will be ovarian mothers who supply eggs, uterine mothers who give birth to children, and . . . social mothers who raise them" (Stanworth 1987, p. 16).

While the new technological developments have rendered the fragmentation of maternity, the economic system of slavery fundamentally relied on alienated and fragmented motherhood, as women were forced to bear children whom masters claimed as potentially profitable labor machines. Birth mothers, therefore, could not expect to be mothers in the legal sense. Legally, these children were chattel and thus motherless. Slave states passed laws to the effect that children of slave women no more belonged to their biological mothers than the young of animals belonged to the females that birthed them (Scarborough 1963).

At the same time, slave women, particularly those who were house slaves, were expected to nurture, rear, and mother the children of their owners. It was not uncommon for white children of the slave-owning class to have far more emotionally intense relationships with the slave women, who were their "mammies," than with their own white biological mothers. Thus, the slave economy called into question the conception of motherhood—although white women gave birth, black women were the nurturers of these white babies, and indeed were frequently "wet nurses" as well. They nourished the babies in their care with the milk produced by their own hormones. Black women, therefore, were not only treated as surrogate wombs with respect to the reproduction of slave labor, but they also served as surrogate mothers for the white children of the slave owners.

Versions of a well-known lullaby, which probably originated during slavery, powerfully portray the surrogacy role of black slave women who were forced to neglect their own children while lavishing their affection on the children of their masters. The following version appears to have been directed to the white babies:

> Hushaby,
> Don't you cry
> Go to sleep, little baby.
> And when you wake,
> You shall have a cake
> And all the pretty little ponies. (Scarborough 1963)

In all likelihood, this alternative version was sung to slave babies:

> Go to sleep, little baby,
> When you wake
> You shall have
> All the mulies in the stable.
> Buzzards and flies
> Picking out its eyes,
> Poor little baby crying,
> Mamma, mamma! (Scarborough 1963)

As these lullabies suggest, slave mothers (as surrogates) were forced not only to give up their own children for the economic benefit of their owners, but also to be more attentive to the white babies than to their own. In this way, slave mothers were both exploited as breeders and prevented from nurturing their own children.

SURROGACY AND EXPLOITATION OF POOR WOMEN

The economic history of Mexican, Irish, West Indian, and Chinese women, as well as other immigrant women—like the economic history of African-American women—reveals a persisting pattern of employment as household servants for the wealthy. They have cleaned the houses, they have nurtured and reared their employers' babies, and they have functioned as surrogate mothers. Considering this history, is it not possible to imagine that poor women—especially poor women of color—might be transformed into a special caste of hired pregnancy-carriers? Certainly, such fears are not simply the product of an itinerant imagination. In any event, whether or not such a caste of women baby-bearers eventually makes its way into existence, sociohistorical experiences constitute a backdrop for the present debate regarding the new reproductive technologies.

The discussion of surrogacy inevitably leads to a debate on surrogacy for profit, by virtue of corporate involvement and intervention in the new technologies. Thus, it becomes necessary to acknowledge the historical economic precedents for surrogate motherhood. Those economic patterns that led to surrogacy in the first place are likely to persist under the impact of the technology in its market context.

Those who opt to employ a surrogate mother will participate in the economic as well as ideological exploitation of her services. The commodification of reproductive technologies in general, and the labor services of pregnant surrogate mothers in particular, means that someone is being exploited. The woman who becomes a surrogate mother earns relatively low wages. A few years ago, the going rate was $22,000–$25,000 (Overall 1987). Considering the fact that pregnancy is a twenty-four hour a day job, what might seem like a substantial sum of money is actually not even a minimum wage. This commodification of motherhood is quite frightening because it allows women and their partners to participate in a program that seems only to generate life, but in reality generates and even celebrates sexism and profits as well.

The economic model evoked by the relationship between the surrogate mother and the woman, or man, who makes use of her services is that of a feudalistic bond between servant and employer. In the United States domestic work has been performed primarily by women of color as well as by poor immigrant women of European descent. Racism and class bias reflected in the historical structure of domestic work are also likely to be reflected in the politics of surrogate motherhood. Currently, there is an absence of large numbers of surrogate mothers of color. Based on historical features of racism and sexism, however, it seems likely that in the future, poor women of color will be exploited as baby-bearers for the wealthy.

AN AFRICAN-AMERICAN APPROACH
TO INFERTILITY

Once upon a time (and this is still the case outside the technologically advanced capitalist societies), a woman who discovered that she was infertile had to reconcile herself to the impossibility of giving birth to her own biological offspring. She would, therefore, either try to create a life for herself that did not absolutely require the presence of children, or choose to enter into a mothering relationship in other ways. There was the possibility of foster motherhood, adoptive motherhood, or play motherhood.[2] This last possibility is deeply rooted in the black community's tradition of extended families and relationships based both on biological kinship, though not necessarily biological motherhood, and on fictive kinship, which is rooted in personal history and is often as binding as biological kinship. Even within the biological network itself, however, relationships between, for example, an aunt and a niece or nephew might be as strong as or stronger than those between a mother and daughter or son (McAdoo 1980).

One example of a fictive kinship comes from my own family. My mother grew up in a family of foster parents with no siblings. Her best friend had no sisters and brothers either, so they invented a sister relation between them. Although many years passed before I became aware that they were not "really" sisters, this knowledge had no significant impact on me: I considered my Aunt Elizabeth no less my aunt later than during the earlier years of my childhood. Because she herself had no children, her relation to me, my sister, and two brothers was one of a second mother. If she were alive and in her child-bearing years today, I wonder whether she would bemoan the fact that she lacked the financial resources to employ all the various technological means available to women who wish to reverse their infertility. I wonder if she would feel a greater compulsion to fulfill a female vocation of motherhood.

The new reproductive medicine sends out a message to those who are economically capable of receiving it: motherhood lies just beyond the next technology. While working-class women are not often in the position to explore the new technology, infertile women of the upper classes, or the wives or partners of infertile men who are financially able to do so, are increasingly expected to try everything, from embryo transplants to in vitro fertilization to surrogacy. The consequence is an ideological compulsion toward a palpable goal: a child one creates either via one's own reproductive activity or via someone else's.

CONTRADICTIONS IN THE IDEOLOGY
OF MOTHERHOOD

The ideology of motherhood sends out contradictory messages to women, based on their class or race. In this section I will present three inconsistencies regarding the value of motherhood: (1) criticism of young black mothers, (2) sterilization based on race and class, and (3) separation of incarcerated mothers from their children.

While infertile affluent white women are often pushed into a motherhood quest because of the availability and accessibility of the new technologies to them, teenagers of color are severely criticized for participating in the cult of motherhood. If the emerging debate regarding the new reproductive technologies is presently anchored to the socioeconomic conditions of relatively affluent families, the reproductive issue most frequently associated with the poor and working-class women of color is the apparent proliferation of young single parents, especially in the African-American community. For the last decade or so, teenage pregnancy has been represented ideologically as one of the greatest obstacles to social progress in the most impoverished sectors of the black community (Moynihan 1967). In actuality, the rate of teenage pregnancy in the black community, like that among white teenagers, has been declining for quite a number of years. According to a National Research Council study, fertility rates in 1960 were 156 births per thousand black women aged 15–19 (Jaynes and Williams 1989). This figure dropped in 1988 to 94 per thousand (Henshaw 1993).

What distinguishes teenage pregnancy in the black community today from its historical counterpart is the decreasing likelihood of teenage marriage. There is a constellation of reasons for the failure of young teenagers to consolidate into two-parent families. The most obvious one is that it rarely makes economic sense for an unemployed young woman to marry an unemployed young man. The deindustrialization of the national economy, with the resulting shop closures in industries previously accessible to young black male workers, has dramatically decreased the number of young men capable of contributing to the support of their children (Malveaux 1988). For a young woman whose pregnancy results from a relationship with an unemployed youth, it makes little sense to enter into a marriage that will probably bring in an extra adult, as well as a child, to be supported by her own mother/father/grandmother, and so on.

It angers me that such a simplistic interpretation of the material and spiritual impoverishment of the African-American community as being largely rooted in teenage pregnancy is so widely accepted. This is not to imply that teenage pregnancy is unproblematic; it is extremely problematic. I cannot assent, however, to the representation of teenage pregnancy as "the problem." There are reasons why young black women become pregnant or desire pregnancy. I do not think I am far off-target when I point out that few young women who choose pregnancy are offered an alternative range of opportunities for self-expression and development. Are those black teenage girls with the potential for higher education offered scholarships permitting them to study at colleges and universities? Were teenagers who chose pregnancy ever offered even a vision of well-paying and creative jobs?

Is it really so hard to grasp why so many young women would choose motherhood? Isn't this path toward adulthood still thrust on them by the old and persisting ideological constructions of femaleness and the cult of motherhood? Doesn't motherhood still equal adult womanhood in the popular imagination? Don't the new reproductive technologies further develop this equation of womanhood and motherhood? I would say perhaps that many young women make conscious decisions to bear children in order to convince themselves that they are alive and creative human beings. As a consequence of this decision, they are characterized as immoral for not marrying the fathers of their children.

I have chosen to evoke the reproductive issue of single motherhood among teenagers in order to highlight the absurdity of locating motherhood in a transcendent space where motherhood is deified for affluent white women and yet vilified for poor black teenagers—both of whom voluntarily seek motherhood. In this context, there is a glaring inconsistency: motherhood among black and Latina teens is constructed as a moral and social evil, yet they are denied accessible and affordable abortions. Moreover, teen mothers are ideologically assaulted because of their premature and impoverished entrance into the realm of motherhood, while older, whiter, and wealthier women are coaxed to buy the technology to assist them in achieving an utterly commodified motherhood.

A second contradiction in the contemporary social compulsion toward motherhood can be found in the persisting problem of sterilization abuse. While poor women in many states have effectively lost access to abortion, they may be sterilized with the full financial support of the government. While the "right" to opt for surgical sterilization is an important feature of women's control over the reproductive functions of their bodies, the imbalance between the difficulty of access to abortions and the ease of access to sterilization reveals the continued and tenacious insinuation of racism into the politics of reproduction. The astoundingly high, and continually mounting, statistics regarding the sterilization of Puerto Rican women expose one of the most dramatic ways in which women's bodies bear the evidence of colonization (Salvo et al. 1992). Similarly, the bodies of vast numbers of sterilized indigenous women within the presumed borders of the U.S. bear the traces of a 500-year-old tradition of genocide (Dillingham 1977). There is documented evidence that the federal government promoted and funded sterilization operations for young black girls during the 1960s and 1970s (see Dula, Chapter 1, in this volume). However, as yet there is no evidence of large-scale sterilization of African-American and Latina teenage girls. The forces that led to sterilization abuse, including racism, classism, and sexism, are the same forces that would permit the exploitation of healthy, young, poor women—a disproportionate number of whom would probably be black, Latina, Native American, Asian, or from the Pacific Islands—as pregnancy carriers for women who can afford to purchase their services.

A third contradiction in the ideology of motherhood is the separation of incarcerated mothers from their children. The majority of all women in jails and prisons are mothers, and 7 to 10% of incarcerated women are pregnant (Barry 1989). Women's correctional institutions still incorporate and dramatically reveal their ideological links to the cult of motherhood. Even today, imprisoned women are labeled "deviant" not so much because of the crimes they may have committed, but rather because their attitudes and their behavior are seen as blatant contradictions of prevailing expectations—especially in the judicial and law enforcement systems—of women's place. They are mothers who have failed to find themselves in motherhood.

The strategic role of domesticity in the structure and correctional goals of women's prisons revolves around the notion that to rehabilitate women, you must teach them how to be good wives and good mothers. Federal prisons such as Alderson Federal Reformatory for women in West Virginia, and state institutions like the California Institute for Women and Bedford Hills in the state of New York attempt to evoke family life architecturally, albeit mechanistically. Instead of cells there are cottages, where women "learn" how to keep house, wash and iron clothes, do the dishes, and so on. What bearing does this have on the politics of reproduction? There is a flagrant contradiction in a prison system that emphasizes training for motherhood and at the same time refuses to allow incarcerated women to pursue any meaningful relationship with their children.

In the San Francisco Bay Area, there are only three alternative institutions where women serving jail sentences may live with their children—the Elizabeth Fry Center, Mandela House, and Keller House. In all three places combined, there is space for about twenty to twenty-five women and their children. In the meantime, thousands of women in the area suffer the threat—or reality—of having their children taken away from them and made wards of the court. Imprisoned women who admit that they have drug problems and seek to rehabilitate themselves often discover that their admissions are used as evidence of their incapacity to be good mothers.

In the jails and prisons where they are incarcerated, they are presumably being taught to be good mothers, even as they are powerless to prevent the state from seizing their own children. Except for a small minority of alternative "correctional" institutions, where social stereotypes are being questioned (although in most instances, the structure of incarceration itself is left unchallenged), the underlying agenda of this motherhood training is to turn aggressive women into submissive and dependent prison "mothers," whose children are destined to remain motherless.

The incarcerated young mothers are not the only ones who are criminalized. A significant portion of the population of young black, Latina, Native American, Asian, Pacific, and poor European immigrant mothers are criminalized simply because they don't adhere to the ideological representation of motherhood. For example, a poor teenage black or Latina girl, who is a single mother, is regarded as criminal just because she is poor and has had a child "out of wedlock."

The process of criminalization affects young men in a different way—not as fathers, but rather by virtue of a more all-embracing racialization. Any young black man can be potentially labeled criminal: a shabby appearance is equated with drug addiction; an elegant and expensive self-presentation is interpreted as drug dealing.

While this process of criminalization is apparently unrelated to the construction of the politics of reproduction, it has contributed to the increase in single motherhood in black and Latino communities. For example, the 25% of African-American young men in jails and prisons (Mauer 1990) cannot engage in any significant parenting projects.

RECONCEPTUALIZING REPRODUCTIVE ISSUES

In pursuing the degree to which racism and class bias inform the contemporary politics of reproduction, I am suggesting that we need to reconceptualize reproductive issues. It is not enough to assume that women—whose bodies are distinguished by vaginas, ovarian tubes, and uteri—should be able to claim "rights" to exercise control over the processes of these organs, such as the right to abortion. Certainly, women should have controlling rights on their bodies, but they should not be exploited because of their race, ethnicity, and class backgrounds. A woman may sign a surrogacy contract, but inequities in education, power, and economic status may mean that she has not been truly informed of the consequences of signing the contract. Social/economic/political circumstances that oppress and marginalize poor women cannot be ignored without affirming the same structures of domination that have led to such different but related politics of reproduction in the first place.

Several strategic constellations should be taken into consideration in reconceiving an agenda of reproductive rights. I do not present the following points as an exhaustive list of such goals, but rather I am trying to allude to a few of the contemporary issues requiring further theoretical examination and practical/political action. The multiple arenas in which women's legal abortion rights are presently being assaulted and eroded account for the struggle for reproductive rights, from birth control and abortion to the new technologies. Yet the failure to regard the economic accessibility of birth control and abortion as equally important as the right to them results in the inevitable marginalization of poor women's reproductive rights. With respect to a related issue, the "right" and access to sterilization is important, but again, it is equally important to look at those economic and ideological conditions that track some women toward sterilization, thus denying them the possibility of bearing and rearing children in numbers they themselves choose.

Although the new reproductive technologies cannot be construed as inherently affirmative or violative of women's reproductive rights, anchoring the technologies to the profit schemes of their producers and distributors results in a commodification of motherhood that complicates and deepens power relationships based on class and race. Beneath this marriage of technology, profit, and the assertion of a historically obsolete bourgeois individualism lies the critical issue of the right to determine the character of one's family. The assault on this "right"—a term I have used throughout this chapter, which is not, however, unproblematic—is implicated in the ideological offensive against single motherhood. It is also reflected in the homophobic refusal to recognize lesbian and gay family configurations, especially in the persisting denial of custody (even though some changes have occurred) to lesbians with children from previous heterosexual marriages. This is one of the many ways in which the present-day ideological compulsion toward motherhood further resonates inconsistency. Moreover, this ideology of motherhood is wedded to a stubborn denial of the very social services women require in order to make meaningful choices to bear or not to bear children. Such services include health care, child care, housing, education, jobs, and all the basic services human beings require to lead decent lives. The privatization of family responsibilities resulting from lack of access to these services takes on increasingly reactionary implications, particularly during an era when so many new family configurations are being invented that the definition of family stretches well beyond traditional borders. This is why there must be a reconceptualization of family and of reproductive rights that moves from the private to the public, from the individual to the social.

NOTES

*This chapter is an edited version of a keynote address for a Women's History Month conference on "Re-conceiving Reproduction" at Le Moyne College, Syracuse, N.Y., March 8, 1991.

1. My own grandmother, whose parents were enslaved Africans, was one of thirteen children.

2. The tradition of black women acting as "play mothers" is still a vital means of inventing kinship relations unrelated to biological origin.

Commentary by Anita L. Allen-Castellito

Angela Davis maintains that women in the United States—especially low-income and working-class women of color—are poorly served by the nation's reproductive policies, practices, and politics. A "peculiar constellation of racist, classist, and misogynist assumptions" structure how and why women procreate. As a consequence, meaningful "reproductive self-determination" is illusive. Self-determination is beyond our reach. In the United States women live under the spell of an ideology of mandatory maternalism.

Akin to the nineteenth-century "cult of true womanhood" (Welter 1966), the prevailing ideology prescribes maternal roles for all women. The particular maternal role assigned an individual by the ideology of mandatory maternalism depends on her economic class and race. Once, affluent white women bred heirs while enslaved black women bred slaves; today, many upper income professionals are working mothers, dependent on low-income women of color to rear their children. To be sure, constitutional protection for access to contraception and abortion won in the 1960s and 1970s facilitates procreative self-determination. Yet, Davis contends, the ideology that mandates motherhood also "mystifies" it, constructing motherhood as the ostensibly free choice of housewives, wage earners, and professional women alike.

Constitutional scholar Laurence H. Tribe argues that reproductive technology promises women greater autonomy (Tribe 1990). Davis advances just the opposite perspective. According to Davis, U.S. citizens are using new technology to perpetuate the status quo. Technological innovation promises to make every woman a mother. Indeed, in the 1990s even a woman without a uterus can mother a child genetically related to her husband, and even to herself if she has ovaries.

First, a sterile wife can purchase a surrogate who will have her husband's child and then surrender the child for adoption. The attempt to buy one's way into a maternal role through surrogacy sometimes fails, however. Dr. Elizabeth Stern's effort stands out as a notorious failure. The famous *Baby M* case was Mary Beth Whitehead's ultimately successful battle against the Sterns in the New Jersey Supreme Court to retain maternal rights she once contracted away.[1] Second, a woman without a uterus can purchase the right to have her physician harvest an egg from her ovaries, fertilize it *in vitro*, and then implant the resulting embryo into another woman's body for gestation and delivery. Mark and Crispina Calvert underwent these procedures with the help of an African-American surrogate gestator who gave birth to their European and Asian ancestry child. In a widely publicized California case, *Johnson v. Calvert*, gestator Anna Johnson went to court seeking parental rights.[2] Analogizing the black surrogate gestator to a wet nurse, the judge in Anna Johnson's case denied that she had any parental rights whatsoever over the child that she had carried and delivered.

Viewed from Professor Davis's perspective, Elizabeth Stern, Mary Beth Whitehead, Crispina Calvert, and Anna Johnson are all high-tech victims of the ideology of mandatory maternalism. Dr. Stern and nurse Calvert are also victims, driven to pursue the most expensive and emotionally risky paths to motherhood. Overvaluing a certain kind of genetic affiliation, women and their partners often eschew the low-tech motherhood options that Professor Davis endorses. These include acceptance of infertility, creating lives that do not require children, and entering mothering relationships through foster care, adoption, or friendship. Paid surrogates Mary Beth Whitehead and Anna Johnson are victims of the maternalism ideology because they willingly viewed their own bodies as market commodities. Historically, lower income and black women have been conditioned to make themselves available to the affluent. The ideology that makes women with money believe they must buy motherhood leads women without money to believe they must sell it.

Employing black women like Anna Johnson as gestational surrogates for men and women of other races is especially reminiscent of the era of U.S. slavery when many whites and a few blacks literally owned black women's wombs. Anna Johnson can be compared to Polly, a black woman unlawfully sold into slavery as a child who went to court claiming that she, not a white man, owned her daughter.[3] While contemporary surrogacy is not slavery, the morally problematic character of womb-renting and baby-buying in a context of overall social inequality is well brought out by analogies to slavery.

Davis raises an exceedingly complex and important ethical challenge: how, in the age of miraculous technology and pervasive racism, to supplant the ideology of mandatory maternalism with an ideology of reproductive self-determination. The ethical argument for a new, postmaternalist conception of womanhood could be expressed as a case for gender equality. Reproductive self-determination surely advances the cause of gender equality, for women freed from caretaking roles are at liberty to compete with men on an equal basis.

But there is an argument for reproductive self-determination independent of the liberal ideal of gender equality. Reproductive self-determination helps to make women more fit for all their public and private roles. Control over when and if we reproduce is imperative if we are to exploit our many talents and meet our many responsibilities. In my view, a world in which the female half of the population contributes to the full extent of its full human potential is better than a world in which women are cloistered in the private sphere as caretakers. A morality that makes developing, rather than wasting, adult female potential an imperative is also a morality that demands procreational autonomy.

Idealizing where we would like to be as a society is one thing, but getting there is another. Davis maintains that our society is under the grip of an ideology mandating maternity. An ideology is a cast of mind, a way of life. How can so fundamental a transformation in our society occur? There is cause for optimism, I believe, since, despite the ideology of mandatory maternalism, many women already enjoy a great deal of genuine reproductive autonomy. On the other hand, at the federal level, some of this autonomy is threatened. *Roe v. Wade*, the 1973 Supreme Court decision that established abortion as among women's constitutional privacy rights, is vulnerable (*Roe v. Wade* 1973). The Supreme Court has taken a decidedly conservative turn (*Webster v. Reproductive Health Service* 1989; *Planned Parenthood v. Casey* 1992).

In addition, under current law the distribution of reproductive autonomy is arguably unjust. Low-income women have a lower degree of meaningful reproductive autonomy than middle- and upper income women. The legal right to use birth control or obtain an abortion is meaningless for a woman who cannot afford either. The Supreme Court continually upholds interpretations of access to reproductive services that permit state and federal government to assist the poor pregnant woman who wishes to deliver, but turn away the poor pregnant woman who wishes to abort.[4] The Supreme Court has even held that poor women may be denied the right to talk about abortion with a physician employed by a federally funded health care facility (*Rust v. Sullivan* 1991). This "gag rule" has been revoked by the Clinton administration, which is also considering a health care plan that funds abortion, although it faces stiff opposition in Congress (Rubin 1993).

Public policy regarding the maternal fitness of poor women is a mass of contradictions. Black women who, despite poverty, youth, disease, and dysfunction, aspire to have children of their own find only qualified support in law and society. Stereotyped on the one hand as unfit and irresponsible, black women are valued as minimum wage nannies and may be exploited as surrogate gestators. Adult women of color are often dismissed as oversexed welfare queens, but, it is in fact women of color who have raised a significant portion of white America's most successful children. Pregnant teens and their families are condemned, and yet, as Davis points out, many who condemn pregnant teens subscribe to an ideology of mandatory maternalism that actually encourages young women to turn to maternity as a source of self-esteem. More concretely, they oppose sex education and contraception in the schools.

Concern about the death of the urban black family reached a peak in the 1980s, but little was done to aid its survival.[5] The poverty and educational deficits that lead to criminality and self-destructive drug dependence remain. Our society seems more prepared to finance jails than jobs. Specifically, we now seem more prepared to jail pregnant drug users and female child abusers than to finance education, housing, social services, and police protection that could reduce the need for criminal prosecution. Limited resources and well-meaning conservative economics explain some of the reluctance among policymakers to dedicate public funds to solving problems of poverty. But Angela Davis is surely correct that racism and misogyny have a role in the current paralysis. Poor women need family planning, contraception, abortion, prenatal care, genetic screening, and pediatric advice. If poor women of color are to have meaningful access to reproductive health care services, ideologies of race and class must be displaced along with the ideology of mandatory maternalism. This tripartite displacement is the complete ethical challenge.

NOTES

1. In *Re Baby M*, 109 N.J. 396, 537 A.2d 1227 (1988). See also Anita L. Allen, "Privacy, Surrogacy, and the Baby M Case," *Georgetown Law Journal* 76, 1759 (1988).

2. Reporter's Transcript, *Johnson v. Calvert* (No. X 63 31 90 consolidated with AD57638) (Cal., Super. Ct., October 22, 1990). This verdict was upheld by the California Supreme Court in May 1993. The ruling will surely be appealed. See also Anita L. Allen, "The Black Surrogate Mother," *Harvard Blackletter Journal* 8, 17 (1991).

3. See Lucy Delaney, "From the Darkness Cometh the Light, or Struggles for Freedom," in *Six Women's Slave Narratives* (New York: Oxford University Press, 1988; originally published St. Louis, MO: J. T. Smith, 1891). See Anita L. Allen, "Surrogacy, Slavery, and the Ownership of Life," *Harvard Journal of Law and Public Policy* 13, 139 (1990), for a discussion of Polly's story and the moral analogy between surrogacy and slavery.

4. After *Roe v. Wade*, 410 U.S. 113 (1973), the Supreme Court in *Maher v. Roe*, 432 U.S. 464 (1977), *Poelker v. Doe*, 432 U.S. 519 (1977), and *Harris v. McRae* 448 U.S. 297 (1980) held that state and federal governments may refuse to pay for the elective abortions of poor women. The Court upheld denial of Medicaid funding for abortions, other than abortions elected by victims of rape or incest or those whose lives were at risk, even though the federal government routinely paid for poor women's prenatal care. In *Webster v. Reproductive Health Service*, 492 U.S. 490 (1989), the Court relied on the earlier three abortion funding cases to uphold the constitutionality of Missouri legislation prohibiting abortion by state employees and facilities.

5. Forty-three percent of all black women with children under the age of 18 lived in poverty in 1989. An increase in the economic gap between black and white women is predicted, if current trends continue. See David Swinton, "The Economic Status of African Americans: 'Permanent' Poverty and Inequality," 53, 63 in *The State of Black America 1991*, ed. J. Dewart, New York: National Urban League, 1991.

5 Lack of a Moral Consensus on Health Care: Focus on Minority Elderly

Marian Gray Secundy

INTRODUCTION

The last decade has seen a significant encroachment on the ideology of equality in access to health care. Retrenchment and restrictions are reflected in increasing cost containment strategies, stricter quality control attempts, and efforts to rely less on federal programs than on private sector initiatives. Entitlement programs that some had come to view as a permanent part of the landscape have been trimmed back. The notion of automatic support for health care for the elderly and the disadvantaged, which had almost become an ideological given, has recently been challenged openly. We have been urged to reassess directions, to restructure current systems, and to acknowledge that we cannot and ought not try to serve everyone's health needs equally. The extent to which the federal government has responsibility for service delivery and benefits is being reexamined. We have come to accept the limitations on access and quality, without ever having an open dialogue about the reality of these limitations. In the face of the gross disparities in health status between ethnic minorities and whites, we can legitimately ask if the notion of health care based on free market capitalism can really work in an even minimally acceptable way.

In this chapter, I will discuss the disturbing and worsening health status of the African-American elderly population as a means of questioning this country's commitment to the provision of adequate health care for all. I will comment on the lack of moral consensus among the general population and discuss what we should do to ensure health care access, noting that even policymakers and health care providers tend to pay mere lip service to this ideal; they seldom back their words up with positive efforts to eliminate the disparities in health status. Finally, I will suggest that as long as we insist on viewing health care as a commodity within a free market capitalist system, gaining equity in health care may be impossible.

HEALTH STATUS OF THE
AFRICAN-AMERICAN ELDERLY

Minority elders in the United States, particularly those of limited income, are the most vulnerable to the vicissitudes of current health care policy. Their quality of care and access to care are severely compromised. To a large extent, the problems they face are cyclical and feed on one another. For instance, substandard housing and poor nutrition associated with lower economic status contribute to the poor health status. Morbidity and mortality rates remain high for elderly minorities (Jackson 1990). They make less use of health care, their chronic diseases are greater, payment mechanisms fewer, availability of high-level acute care and long-term care facilities more limited, and lifestyles more problematic.

To a large extent, the poor health status of minority elders is due to their overrepresentation in lower socioeconomic groups. For older black women, the poverty rate is close to 55%; for the population at large, it is 12% (Cutler 1991). Census figures recorded in 1989 indicated that for the age group 65 and older, 30% of blacks were in poverty, 20% of Hispanics, and 14.5% of Pacific Islanders (Kamikawa 1991). Analysts note, however, that minority elders (including blacks, Hispanics, and Pacific Asians) are represented in less than 3% of all elderly poverty programs, compared to 10% of elder whites, who consume 97% of those benefit outlays (Kamikawa 1991). Clearly, ethnic minorities are receiving lower benefits.

No matter what the economic strata, minorities receive less insurance coverage for health costs, experience less continuity of coverage, and confront psychological, social, and structural barriers, both perceived and actual. For many poor people, hospitals have replaced the general practitioner's private office as the main locus of care, and hospital and medication costs have soared to prohibitive levels. One elderly lady with an annual income of only $6,000 recently reported bills of $200 per month for medications. There are also racial disparities in service utilization under Medicare (Krause and Wray 1991). Entitlements change weekly as do eligibility requirements. One cannot depend on any particular stability on this front. Currently, co-payments and deductibles are rising and are increasing out-of-pocket costs so that in 1991, Medicare paid less than half of the health expenditures of the elderly in the United States. If the other half was not available, care was not provided. Furthermore, in 1991, 70% of Medicare expenditures covered hospital costs, but only 3% of those expenditures paid for home health care and less than 1% for nursing homes (Estes 1988). These disparities in health care access and health lead to disparities in work disability as well. More elderly minorities are forced to miss work than whites owing to more untreated chronic conditions and greater bed disability. Clearly, health status influences economic status in a cyclical and downward-spiraling fashion.

Any attempt to analyze the moral context that has led to such problems involving access to health care for minority elders must acknowledge certain historical realities and identify common assumptions that have driven past health care policy. In the next section, I will identify some of these assumptions and note that until they are substantially altered, the grim realities for minority elders will not change and may in fact worsen.

U.S. COMMITMENT TO EQUITY IN HEALTH CARE: FACT OR FICTION?

This country has only given lip service to notions of equality and equity in health care. Our commitment to capitalism and private enterprise makes efforts to provide meaningful access and quality care extraordinarily difficult, if not impossible. Furthermore, liberal assumptions that minority elders and the poor ought to have a special right to health care are not necessarily shared by a majority of the U.S. population. They may voice support for this as an ideal, but only when it requires no personal cost or inconvenience. While the public is aware of the vulnerability of the elderly and recognizes that some state financing is necessary to maintain a minimal level of health care, no moral consensus has been reached regarding how much is appropriate. Indeed, there is much dissension between the halls of academia, where philosophers and theologians argue about theories of social justice, and the wider social arena, where politicians and policymakers play out their own notions of fairness and justice. Politicians are responding to their constituents, to their economic and policy advisers, and to their own senses of morality; their priorities are set by virtue of what is most valued in their particular constituencies, and these values are bound to vary widely. Without a moral consensus on the issue, is it even realistic to consider the possibility of approximating equity in access and care?

The United States has a history of limited federal initiatives, minimal financial support, and narrow objectives regarding health care. As far back as 1797, Thomas Paine's proposal for national pensions for the indigent elderly was turned down (Achenbaum 1988). The early 1900s brought veterans' benefits and the civil service retirement system, but the focus for health care was on family and individual responsibility, supplemented by the involvement of voluntary organizations and religious groups. In 1935 the federal purview and services to the U.S. elderly were expanded with the enactment of the Social Security Act, but while Social Security has become the largest domestic program and contributed largely to the needs of our aging population, equity in access and quality of health care has remained elusive. The last decade in particular has seen greater imbalances in access to health care than any decade prior to the enactment of Social Security. Indeed, the climate of the 1980s, which placed high priority on cost containment and valued market forces through the private sector, dramatically highlighted this country's limited commitment to the needs of the less advantaged. The changing demographics of the twenty-first century may, however, provide a significant challenge to this trend.

A variety of proposals for improving the state of health care for the elderly and for the nation in general are currently before this country's legislative bodies. Unfortunately, these proposals have minimal chance of success, given this country's emphasis on capitalism and free market trade. Although the Clinton administration is giving greater attention to the real health needs of the people, there is as yet no moral consensus about the critical nature of prevention, lifestyles, and reductions in environmental and occupational risks—changes the United States must make to improve health in the long term. Continued prioritization of cost containment as the first order of the day also seriously restricts meaningful advances. To date, many legislative initiatives focus on shoring up acute care medicine and other short-term, high-tech, costly "solutions." They are sustaining the current system which, as Carroll Estes (aging and long-term care expert) points out, has "an acute care bias: in which one is paid better to be sick than to stay well." Estes goes on to observe that "there is a failure/refusal to acknowledge the inherent link between inadequate health care when one is young with health status in old age." She notes that existing policies have facilitated economic growth and expansion of the medical technology industry, the medical profession, and biomedical research, ensuring that existing disparities remain intact. Finally, Estes observes that today's philosophy is one of "marketing health and other social services as if they were commodities with a belief that costs will be kept down and that profit incentives will increase competition" (Estes 1988, p. 44). Essentially, in her view, those previously (albeit briefly) espoused goods of equity, access, and public accountability have been abandoned. The goals of cost control efficiency and access will be difficult, if not impossible, to meet by selling health for a profit. Estes predicts a continuing stratification and a system characterized by increasing inequalities in access and quality of care.

We can only hope that her predictions are wrong and that the work of Hillary Rodham Clinton's Health Care Task Force will result in a reversal in "business as usual" and give attention to prevention, access, chronic and long-term care, and qualitative services that are responsive to the needs of all our aging citizens.

CONCLUSIONS

Clearly, the United States has demonstrated limited commitment to equity in health care. Although philosophers and policymakers have discussed the ideal of the right to health care, generally they have merely paid it lip service. The social programs that were instituted to promote greater social equity have recently been reexamined and trimmed back. The United States is in the midst of a health care crisis. Limited federal initiatives, significant but insufficient federal funding, and misdirected or poorly directed funding sources are problematic and contribute to the health status of minority elders. That status is a clear example of the severe limitations of the current system.

As a nation, we are being forced to look for more appropriate and just alternatives. Enhancements might require "diversity assessments" of existing and proposed policies to identify barriers and to evaluate programs in terms of their impact on ethnic minorities (Capitman 1991). The feasibility of using functional measures rather than chronological age as a measure of eligibility for health and social benefits appears to be promising. In addition, continued attention to increasing incentives to provide culturally and linguistically sensitive health promotion, prevention, and chronic care services will be essential.

For now, it is important not to turn our heads from the critical gaps in health care coverage for our minority and disadvantaged elderly. They continue to be unempowered, confronting greater morbidity and mortality, having less access to quality care, and utilizing fewer appropriate resources. While the role of government is not clear to most of us, it is clear that we are all in some very visible and real way morally responsible for solving this problem, or at least for explaining the impossibility of that task. If we continue to operate as if medical care is only an economic good and not a fundamental human good, our problems in these areas will persist. Can we continue to turn our heads, harden our hearts, and go about our tasks when faced daily with tragic, frightened, angry voices, and disturbing headlines and stories such as the following?

—Millions of elders are being dumped out of hospitals "sicker and quicker."

—Patients are dumped daily for lack of insurance. Three die in transit to city hospitals per day.

—"My mother could not get her prescription filled for her diabetic medication. She has now had a leg amputation at a cost of $25,000. The medicine costs $40 a month. Medicare would only pay for the surgery."

—Americans spend more on cosmetics and potato chips than they spend on health care.

—Paying patients have their cancers diagnosed in earlier stages and have better survival rates than do indigent patients.

—More black elderly in poverty receive care in urban emergency rooms than in physician offices.

—The poor and the old are in the greatest need of new medical technology. Yet, the hospitals in which they receive care are less likely to be eligible for this technology under federal reimbursement systems.

Commentary by Howard Brody

Secundy cites data to illustrate how our present health care system is not meeting the needs of minority elderly. She also contends that as long as we rely on market forces to allocate health care resources, the system will continue to respond very poorly to these needs. I agree that the present U.S. health care system lends little support to those who would argue that reliance on market forces will solve our current problems. Fortunately, we appear to be entering an era when defenders of market approaches are increasingly being placed on the defensive. Still, a great many questions must be answered before we can be sure that any new scheme proposed to meet the needs of minority elderly and others in our society is ethically sound.

Are specific proposals for health care allocation fair to minority elderly? While at first it might appear enticing to select some abstract ethical theory and then try to derive from it an ideally just proposal for health care for the elderly, I believe it is much more realistic to look at various practical proposals and assess them from an ethical standpoint, even though all such proposals fall short of an idealized standard of justice. One could, for example, consider the plan for Medicaid rationing that has been developed in the state of Oregon and that was approved for implementation in early 1993. Oregon proposes to extend Medicaid coverage to all of its poor citizens, whereas only about half of them are now covered. To fund this proposal, however, the state wants to cut back on some expensive and presumably less beneficial health services for all Medicaid recipients. A number of advocates for the elderly have charged that this plan is unjust. However, the plan has been attacked more vigorously by advocates for children, who argue that many of the Medicaid dollars currently go for long-term care for the elderly, making relatively less available for infants and the young.

Is it ethically appropriate to divide society into competing interest groups when arguing for the ethical justification of plans of health care distribution? Are the elderly better served if we limit the use of expensive life-extending resources for them, assuming the tradeoff will vastly increase the number of elderly who gain basic coverage? Does such a rationing scheme have particular and disproportionate negative impact on minority citizens, compared to the rest of society?

Is "minority elderly" a status of special entitlement? Is being a member of a minority group, or being elderly, by itself an indicator of a special moral status that deserves disproportionate allocation of health resources? Plausible arguments could support either of these contentions. Some evidence suggests that even after correcting for the effects of poverty, minority elderly still have disproportionate health needs. We could justify additional services based on these increased needs. Alternatively, we could point to historical

METHODIST COLLEGE LIBRARY
Fayetteville, N.C.

abuses and discriminatory practices, and argue for enhanced health care for minority citizens as a form of retributive justice. We could argue for special health programs for the elderly on the basis of increased need for health care in that age group; furthermore, in allocating health care resources to the elderly, it could be argued that all of us are allocating resources for ourselves, in the form of a sort of savings account, since all of us hope some day to be among the elderly. The important thing to notice here is that the moral values appealed to cannot be those of pure equity. Secundy appeals primarily to equity when she argues for a change in the present health care system and a rejection of marketplace-based proposals. We may need a longer list of the important moral values that a just health care system would embrace.

Should we allocate funds for health care or for relief of poverty? After what has just been said, it may seem strange to suggest that at some point, it becomes unethical to allocate additional money for health care for the minority elderly. However, this point follows from observations about the role of poverty in worsening one's health status. Poverty is not the only factor contributing to the health needs of the minority elderly, but it is an important factor.

Any just approach to health care distribution must answer to what extent one makes the poor healthier by buying them more health care access, as compared to making them healthier by improving their overall standard of living. This question can be answered only by empirical evidence and not by ethical reflection. When resources are limited, it is unethical to spend our limited dollars inefficiently. Purchasing additional access to health care for some poor citizens may constitute an inefficient use of resources, when compared to other programs that address the core problems of poverty.

What philosophical view of aging and death ought to inform health resource allocation? When we talk about allocating health resources to the elderly, regardless of racial or ethnic group, we make assumptions about what it means to grow old and to die, and about the proper role of health care in dealing with those natural processes. It has been widely noted that modern U.S. society is afflicted with some value assumptions that, at first glance, at least appear to be quite irrational. These include a marked unwillingness to spend considerable sums of money to stave off death even for short periods of time; and a radically individualist notion of rights, which appears to give short shrift to any deep conception of community and culture.

While the minority elderly may have additional health care needs compared to the rest of society, when it comes to philosophical conceptions of aging and death, they may indeed have special resources. It may well be that within the cultural practices and beliefs of some of these minority citizens, our society could find a more positive model of the graceful acceptance of aging, an appreciation of what the elderly contribute to the community, and an acceptance of the inevitability of death. These conceptions in turn could guide resource allocation in more rational directions—for example, tilting spending for the elderly toward humane long-term care and toward medical interventions that enhance function in daily living, rather than life extension in intensive care units for patients who have no hope of regaining independent function.

Of course, there is a considerable danger here as well. If a particular group within society has been accustomed over the years to getting much less than its fair share, it would not be surprising if cultural beliefs arose within that community that emphasized how to make do with the limited share that one received. It would hardly be just for the society to use the existence of those cultural beliefs to justify the perpetuation of the unfair system of distribution in the future. Nonetheless, at least some evidence suggests that some of the expensive, life-prolonging medical care administered in our hospitals today is in fact care that the majority elderly really don't want. A more rational conception of the role of medical care in treating the elderly patient might lead to considerable savings in that sector. Those savings might be reinvested in programs that would more directly meet the needs of the minority elderly.

PART 2

DISPARITIES IN ACCESS AND HEALTH STATUS: AN ETHICAL ISSUE

6 Race, Prenatal Care, and Infant Mortality

John D. Lantos

INTRODUCTION

Infant mortality in the United States is nearly twice as high for African-American babies as it is for white babies and has been getting relatively worse for them than for white babies. In 1947 the ratio of black/white infant mortality was 1.6/1; by 1989 it was 2.3/1 (Wegman 1992). This worsening black/white infant mortality ratio has occurred while overall infant mortality rates for both groups have steadily fallen (Jaynes and Williams 1989, p. 398). Many researchers maintain that the disproportionately higher rate of infant mortality among African Americans is a result of racial and class discrimination in the delivery of health care. Others have contested this viewpoint, and claim that higher infant mortality rates among African Americans reflect genetic factors rather than soluble social, medical, and political problems in health care delivery. This chapter provides a general overview of some factors that affect infant mortality, briefly examines studies that seem to support the genetic position, and discusses the political implications of adhering to the genetic explanation of racial differences in infant mortality.

MEASURING INFANT MORTALITY

Infant mortality is defined as death before one year of age and has been divided into two components: neonatal mortality and postneonatal mortality. Neonatal mortality is death before 28 days of age, and postneonatal mortality is death between 28 days of age and a baby's first birthday. In the fifteen years between 1950 and 1965, the overall infant mortality rate remained relatively constant in the United States. During that time, the neonatal mortality rate was approximately 20 per 1,000 live births, while the postneonatal mortality rate was about 7 per 1,000 children. In the next fifteen years, dramatic decreases in both mortality rates occurred, leading to an overall infant mortality rate of 10.1 per 1,000 live births by 1987. Provisional data for 1991 indicate that the infant mortality rate in the United States dropped to 8.9 per 1,000 (Wegman 1992). This decline in infant mortality rates can be attributed to advances in high technology, hospital-based management, and regional neonatal intensive care units.

Infant mortality rates are often used as a yardstick of social welfare; comparisons between countries or ethnic groups provide an indication of the adequacy of a number of social services as well as the general health of the population. Infant mortality is a health index that can reflect the results of a number of very different and not easily distinguishable health interventions. Because it is not always clear which particular interventions lead to improvements in infant mortality, high rates have been used to justify interventions as varied as universal access to prenatal care (Committee to Study the Prevention of Low Birthweight 1985; Joyce and Grossman 1988); widespread use of neonatal intensive care (Lee et al. 1980); increased funding for Headstart programs (Emanuel 1986); national programs to provide nutritional supplements to women, infants, and children (Stockbauer 1987; Kotelchuck et al. 1984); family planning programs (Grossman and Jacobowitz 1981); legalized abortion (Glass et al. 1974; Lanman et al. 1974); and decreased military expenditures (Woolhandler and Himmelstein 1985). To understand the factors associated with infant mortality rates, it is necessary to examine neonatal mortality and postneonatal mortality separately. Different interventions can selectively influence each of these components.

Factors That Affect Neonatal Mortality

The factor that is most strongly associated with neonatal mortality is low birthweight, and the most important determinant of birthweight is maternal health status. Mothers with poor nutritional status generally have infants of lower birthweight. Programs that improve maternal nutrition have been shown to increase birthweight (Kotelchuck et al. 1984; Maso et al. 1988; Rush et al. 1988). According to the General Accounting Office, the nutritional improvements that resulted from participation in the Women, Infants and Children (WIC) supplemental food program led to a 16 to 20% decrease in the proportion of low-birthweight babies (General Accounting Office 1984).

Access to prenatal care and other health care services leads to improvements in birthweight, even in high-risk populations (Geronimus 1986). Studies that carefully control for socioeconomic status and access to medical care have found that differences in the use of prenatal care accounted for 10 to 15% of the difference in the incidence of low birthweight (Starfield 1985). That means that if everybody obtained early prenatal care, the rates of low birthweight (LBW) would be expected to fall by 10 to 15%. While improved nutrition and prenatal care certainly do increase birthweight, it is clear that they alone do not account for the total differences in infant mortality between blacks and whites in the United States.

Prenatal care can lead to increases in birthweight. Once a baby is born, however, neonatal intensive care is the only intervention that can lower mortality rates. Accordingly, the advent of neonatal intensive care led to a drop in birthweight-specific neonatal mortality: for babies weighing 500 to 700 grams at birth, neonatal mortality rates dropped from 850 per 1,000 in 1978 to 800 per 1,000 in 1983. For newborns weighing 900 to 1,000 grams, neonatal mortality rates dropped from 525 per 1,000 in 1978 to 300 per 1,000 in 1983 (Goldenberg et al. 1985).

The availability of family planning services and abortion has also been shown to be associated with decreases in neonatal mortality (Starfield 1985). For example, the estimated effect of a reduction in the number of abortions in this country to the 1969 level of 4 per 1,000 pregnancies would be to increase neonatal mortality rates by 25% for whites and by 6% for blacks (Hadley 1982). The beneficial effects of family planning and abortion availability may occur primarily because they allow women to decide when and how often to become pregnant. Such freedom may lead to improved maternal health and nutritional status, which in turn lead to higher birthweights.

While the above factors affect neonatal mortality rates for both black and white infants, there may also be racial differences in birthweight-specific mortality. For example, low-birthweight black babies generally have slightly higher survival rates for a given birthweight than low-birthweight white babies. This survival advantage reverses for babies or normal birthweight (Alexander et al. 1985). The explanation for racial differences in birthweight-specific neonatal mortality is unknown.

Factors That Affect Postneonatal Mortality

Postneonatal infant mortality is influenced by birthweight and prenatal care, but it is largely accounted for by a few diseases. The most prevalent are congenital anomalies and Sudden Infant Death Syndrome (SIDS). Most congenital anomalies strike infants of different races equally and are not considered preventable. Deaths due to SIDS, by contrast, are more frequent in children of lower socioeconomic classes, children of young mothers, low-birthweight babies, siblings of children who have died, and African Americans (Kraus et al. 1989). All of these factors suggest that SIDS deaths may be avoidable. To date, however, no reliable method of preventing SIDS has proven efficacious. Postneonatal mortality rates have been steadily falling throughout the century. In this country, they declined from over 60 per 1,000 live births at the turn of the century to below 4 per 1,000 in 1987 (Kleinman and Kiely 1990). Postneonatal mortality rates for African Americans have been roughly double the white rate for the last twenty years (La Veist 1990). However, in most studies, socioeconomic class is the variable most strongly associated with high postneonatal mortality, so it is difficult to determine what percentage of excess postneonatal mortality among blacks can be attributed to socioeconomic status.

RACE, CLASS, AND INFANT MORTALITY

The associations between race, class, and infant mortality appear to be straightforward. Blacks in the United States have infants of lower birthweight as well as higher infant mortality rates as compared to whites. Furthermore, infants born to women of lower socioeconomic class have higher mortality rates than children of more economically advantaged women.

While no studies have successfully teased apart the interplay of race and class, a number of them have attempted to sort out the relative contribution of each of these factors. These studies either compare blacks in the lowest risk groups with similarly situated whites or blacks in the highest risk groups with other high-risk ethnic groups. For example, one study of birthweight rates in Chicago found that even when matched for income, maternal education, and maternal age, low-risk whites had half the occurrence of low birthweight babies as low-risk blacks. Even within groups that controlled for income, maternal education, and maternal age, blacks were two or three times more likely to have low-birthweight babies than whites (Collins and David 1990). Similar results were obtained from a study in Los Angeles (Gould and LeRoy 1988). In both studies, the authors caution against overinterpretation of their results and suggest that crude measures of socioeconomic status might overlook important but difficult-to-measure differences. J.W. Collins and R.J. David write, "even with household income data for each birth we could not have 'controlled' for Black-White economic differences since income cannot be equated with purchasing power." They speculate that unmeasurable effects that result from "generations of poverty" may explain their results and that "it may require more than one generation of non-poverty and adequate services to see an impact on infant birthweight" (p. 679).

Yet, when the highest risk blacks are compared with high-risk mothers from other racial groups—notably Hispanics and Southeast Asian immigrants—being black is still more strongly associated with low birthweight, despite controlling for a variety of pregnancy and health-related factors, including psychosocial, socioeconomic, and health services delivery (Leven et al. 1989). In spite of similar levels of poverty and other traditional risk factors for high infant mortality, Hispanics and Southeast Asians have lower infant mortality rates than blacks.

On the face of it, these studies suggest that a genetic or racial factor is involved in infant mortality. Writers like Collins and David bend over backwards to suggest that there may be nongenetic risk factors that we do not yet understand and cannot measure, but are unable to suggest specifically what these might be. For the remainder of this chapter, I will discuss the political implications of arguments that affirm or deny the possibility that differences in infant mortality might reflect biologically based racial differences, rather than simply disparities in socioeconomic status.

THE POLITICAL IMPLICATIONS OF RACIAL DIFFERENCES

Hiding behind the abstract and supposedly value-free statistical arguments in infant mortality studies are some disturbing political implications. If racial differences in birthweight or infant mortality can be attributed to poverty or inadequate medical care, then social, medical, and political changes could close the present gap between white and black infant mortality rates. These changes might include access to family planning services (including abortion), prenatal care, neonatal intensive care, and better nutrition.

On the other hand, the suggestion that racial disparities in infant mortality stem from genetic rather than medical or social causes has serious political implications. If higher black infant mortality is a function of racial or genetic factors, rather than a result of poverty or lack of access to care, then public policymakers could argue that intervention would be futile, ineffective, and financially wasteful; political changes cannot alter genetics. This theory supports and justifies a defeatist, laissez-faire attitude toward reducing infant mortality among blacks.

In the political rhetoric of infant mortality, it might seem important to specify what proportion of excess infant mortality among black Americans, if any, should be "written off" as unavoidable. But even if a certain amount of infant mortality is unavoidable because of genetic or racial factors, at present it is irrelevant whether such differences can be entirely eliminated because we do not have technology that can make use of the knowledge. However, it is clear that we do have the ability to greatly reduce the racial differences in infant mortality rates through social, medical, and political changes.

The Children's Defense Fund (CDF), a Washington-based advocacy group for children, proposes that by the year 2000, the national infant mortality rate should be no more than 7 deaths per 1,000 live births and that no county or racial or ethnic group should have more than 11 deaths per 1,000 live births. While acknowledging that it may be impossible to completely eliminate racial differences in infant mortality, CDF insists that the differences between the most advantaged and the least advantaged members of society must be narrowed, rather than widened (Children's Defense Fund 1991). Even if equality is not a possible endpoint, we must make progress toward it.

In the 1980s steadily falling infant mortality rates were largely accounted for by improvements in neonatal intensive care and in birthweight-specific mortality rates. These improvements are unlikely to continue because neo-natal intensive care appears to be reaching its full potential. Thus, the limit of viability has remained roughly 500 grams for the last decade. There have been few recent improvements in survival rates for the lowest birthweight babies, despite more aggressive treatment (Hack and Fanaroff 1989). Attempts to achieve the CDF goals for the year 2000 will necessitate wide-spread implementation of programs to increase birthweight among black babies. These will require improved access to family planning (including abortion), adequate nutrition, and prenatal care. There will also need to be more general structural changes in the health care delivery system as well as improved educational and employment opportunities (see Ferguson, Young, and Woods, in Chapters 11, 22, and 10, respectively, of this volume).

Most other industrialized countries have implemented programs to assure that all women of child-bearing age have access to most of these services. As a result, these countries have achieved lower infant mortality rates than the United States. There is nothing mysterious about infant mortality. We know what needs to be done to save babies' lives, the only question is whether we have the political will do it.

Commentary by Kathryn Moseley

John Lantos cites a well-known yet alarming statistic: African-American infants die at twice the rate of white infants. The gap is widening at a time when overall infant mortality has improved. Because it is in large part pre-ventable, infant mortality is a reflection of the adequacy of social services. This is why it is used to compare international public services.

Three elements influence infant mortality, and all three can be modified by social policy. Birthweight is inversely correlated with infant mortality and is directly influenced by improved maternal nutrition and overall health. Neonatal mortality (death before the twenty-eighth day of life) is decreased by services like family planning and abortion that allow women to space their pregnancies more appropriately. Postneonatal mortality is improved by attention to disease prevention.

Infant mortality is also tied to socioeconomic status (SES), a measure of education and income. Not surprisingly, a higher proportion of infants born to poor women die than those born to middle-class women. There are also apparent racial or genetic factors. Black infants have a higher mortality re-gardless of their mother's SES. Studies that compare SES-matched whites and blacks reveal that blacks still have two to three times as many low-birthweight infants as whites. When compared with other ethnic minorities, high-risk (low SES, poor prenatal care) black women still deliver more low-birthweight infants than other ethnic minority women with similar risk factors. Lantos states that we can interpret this difference in two ways: that racial discrimination in accessing medical care and employment has led to this difference or that racial or genetic differences cause the variation. These two views have very different policy implications. Lantos states it simply. "If higher black infant mortality is a function of racial or genetic factors, rather than a result of poverty or lack of access to care, then public policymakers could argue that intervention would be futile, ineffective, and financially wasteful." There are important ethical issues here. First and foremost, is society's obligation to provide treatment for disease mitigated by the presence of a racial or genetic propensity to disease, especially when the racial or genetic factors cannot be cleanly separated from social and environmental factors? As Lantos observes, the economic opportunities and lifestyle available to an African-American woman with a high school education are not those of her white counterpart.

Society has an obligation to provide for the health of its members. Health is not a commodity, but is part of the community welfare and should be paid for by the community, much as education and law enforcement are taxed. Social programs such as Medicare and Medicaid acknowledge this obligation, but the extent of that obligation is a subject of ongoing debate. Nevertheless, society's response to other diseases with genetic and racial components has been positive. Deaths due to genetically linked disease such as muscular dystrophy and hemophilia are not accepted as inevitable. Rather, research is ongoing to improve treatment and seek a cure. The Human Genome Project promises many answers to the causes and eventual cure of many genetic diseases. There are also diseases for which environmental and genetic factors are tightly linked, for example, diabetes and coronary artery disease. Again, research continues on both fronts. While infant mortality is not a disease per se, it has much in common with diseases that have a complex etiology. To write off a segment of the population because of an inherited tendency toward certain diseases would mark a drastic change in policy.

A second issue is one of resource allocation and justice. Medical research is funded in large part by the tax dollars of U.S. citizens, including African Americans. Research on genetic diseases such as cystic fibrosis is paid for out of these tax dollars. Cystic fibrosis affects one in 2,500 white infants, but only 1 in 17,000 black infants, or one-tenth the number of affected white infants. There is treatment, but no cure or preventive strategy is available other than abortion. Low birthweight affects much larger numbers of both black and white infants. Effective preventive strategies are known, yet may not be widely implemented because of a genetic or racial component. Little research (if any) has been done to uncover this racial factor. This is not to suggest that funding for research in other genetic diseases should diminish or cease, but that a major cause of mortality in black infants is being singled out for a form of not-so-benign neglect. In other areas of medical research, the discovery of a genetic component to a disease would be the impetus to further research, a new challenge to overcome. Here, it is suggested that we shrug our shoulders, and not only accept the status quo, but also withhold strategies known to improve the nongenetic elements.

If health care *is* a community good, paid for out of community resources, then it should benefit *all* of society's members. To quote Lantos, "it is clear that we do have the ability to greatly reduce the racial differences in infant mortality rates through social, medical, and political changes. . . . (I)t is irrelevant whether such differences can be entirely eliminated." Blaming the excess black infant mortality on racial factors and doing little to ameliorate the social conditions associated with it reveals a deeply rooted racism. That attitude must not be tolerated.

7 The AIDS Epidemic and the African-American Community: Toward an Ethical Framework for Service Delivery

Stephen B. Thomas and Sandra Crouse Quinn

INTRODUCTION

On June 5, 1991, the world marked the second decade of the Acquired Immunodeficiency Syndrome (AIDS) epidemic (CDC 1991b). According to Dr. Jonathan Mann, founder of the World Health Organization's (WHO) Global AIDS Programme, "AIDS has involved not one but three successive global epidemics" (Panos 1990, p. i). These three phases may be characterized as the first epidemic of hidden infection with Human Immunodeficiency Virus (HIV); the second epidemic of AIDS illness and death (the fatal end stage); and the third epidemic of social and political repercussions.

This third epidemic is a direct challenge to our compassion, judgment, and humanity. It has evoked serious moral and ethical dilemmas at every level of our society, from the drug injection dens of New York City to the boardrooms of major corporations. Should insurance companies be allowed to deny medical coverage to people infected with HIV? Should physicians be tested for HIV? Should children with AIDS be allowed to attend school? Should HIV testing include name reporting and contact tracing? Should condoms be distributed in public schools? Should pregnant women infected with HIV be counseled to have abortions? Should people who knowingly transmit HIV be subject to criminal charges? These and many more questions have no easy solutions.

In our attempt to find answers, we simultaneously expose the degree of our humanity and inhumanity. Sometimes our search for answers demands a forced choice between protection of individual rights and protection of the social welfare. Our human need for answers encounters a mountain of intolerance, a canyon of racism, and a river of indifference. It is within this context that we must come to understand the wisdom in Dr. Mann's statement:

Protecting the human rights and dignity of HIV-infected people, including people with AIDS . . . is not a luxury—it is a necessity. It is not a question of the rights of the many versus the rights of the few; the protection of the uninfected majority depends upon and is inextricably bound up with the rights and dignity of the infected persons. (Panos 1990, p. iii)

World history offers several parallels to what happens when an unfamiliar infection attacks a population for the first time. The plague of the fourteenth century is a spectacular example of how disease can change social systems. When bubonic plague swept through Europe, there was a first epidemic of infection, a second epidemic of sickness and death, and a third epidemic of fear and persecution, as thousands of Jews were massacred as the supposed cause of the Black Death. Yet unlike the plague bacillus, which has an incubation period of days, the latent period of HIV is measured in years, and the long time lag between the first two epidemics has intensified the impact of the third (Panos 1990). The third epidemic has exposed the impoverished blackface of AIDS on a stage set for a historical test of individual freedom and social justice, two basic values that serve as the foundation of our democratic society.

The first decade of AIDS was characterized by an almost singleminded focus on interrupting the cycle of HIV transmission. Our approach to AIDS prevention reflected an illusion that everyone in our society is an educated individual eager to do the right thing if only given all the appropriate information. The spread of HIV has highlighted the complex relationship of social class, gender, and race in a society where health care facilities are impoverished, access to care is inadequate, and prevention technology is devalued. In the second decade of AIDS, we must use the knowledge that existing public health efforts have failed to stop the disproportionate spread of HIV infection among black Americans.

This chapter presents the cold epidemiological facts that lay bare a moral tragedy—black Americans are being killed by a disease that is almost totally preventable. We believe that, by presenting the facts on AIDS within the context of public health as social justice, we move closer to finding ethical solutions that utilize the power of tolerance, understanding, and information. These are the weapons needed to combat the third epidemic of the social and political repercussions of AIDS.

EPIDEMIOLOGY OF HIV INFECTION AMONG BLACKS

Since AIDS was first recognized and reported in 1981, more than 242,000 persons with the disease have been reported to the Centers for Disease Control. Of these, more than 66% have died. HIV infection has emerged as a leading cause of death among men and women under 45 years of age and children 1 to 5 years of age. Although whites still constitute a majority of the AIDS cases, blacks are contracting AIDS in numbers far greater than their relative percentage in the population: blacks constitute 12% of the U.S. population, yet represent approximately 29% of reported AIDS cases. In addition, 52% of all children (under age 13 at time of diagnosis) with AIDS are black. Among cases in women, approximately 52% are black (CDC 1992b).

With the disproportionate impact of AIDS among blacks, special emphasis must be placed on reaching this population with effective HIV education and AIDS risk-reduction programs. In order to understand the ethical issues that may pose barriers to HIV education and AIDS risk reduction, it is crucial to have a better understanding of the behavioral risk factors and attitudes within the black community.

BEHAVIORAL RISK FACTORS FOR HIV-INFECTED POPULATIONS

Black Youth

The problem of HIV infection and AIDS among adolescents is much greater than the official count would suggest. Evidence shows that, given the long HIV latency period (8 to 10 years), a majority of the 35,635 individuals who had AIDS and were in their twenties in 1991 most likely were infected with HIV when they were teenagers (CDC 1991b; Miller et al. 1990). The impact of HIV infection among adolescents is magnified by the potential for these sexually active young people to become parents themselves, transmitting the virus to yet another generation. The 1980 Census Bureau statistics indicate that young people currently (1991) between 11 and 24 years of age represent an unusually small segment of the population. Consequently, AIDS could cause sufficient premature illness and death in this group to seriously threaten the nation's economy (Department of Health and Human Services 1987).

Statistics for adolescents ages 13 to 19 years have only recently been reported separately from adults. The actual number of teenagers diagnosed with AIDS as of September 1992 was relatively small (912), less than 1% of the total AIDS population. The majority of them fall into the exposure categories of hemophilia/coagulation disorders (30%), male homosexual/bisexual contact (24%), heterosexual contact (15%), or injection drug use (13%) (CDC 1992b). A disproportionate share of the adolescent AIDS burden is carried by minority youth. Approximately 38% of teen AIDS cases are among blacks, who make up only 15% of the teen population (CDC 1992b; Miller et al. 1990). Certain subgroups of adolescents may form bridges from currently infected adults to a larger group of adolescents, particularly in light of the teenage tendency to participate in risk-related behaviors. As one commentator put it: "As the virus spreads from individuals initially infected (adult homosexual men, blood product recipients, and injection drug users) to their partners and beyond, the risk-related behaviors of adolescents put some teenagers directly in the path of the epidemic" (Hein 1989, p. 144).

Adolescents sexually involved with older partners, who often have had numerous sexual partners, provide a perfect bridge for the transmission of HIV. Black adolescents are the AIDS epidemic's next high-risk population.

Black Men

There is one major difference in the distribution of HIV infection by transmission category between white and black men who contract AIDS. Whereas 7% of white men with AIDS are injection drug users (IDUs) or had sex partners who were IDUs, fully 36% of black men with AIDS fall in that category. Most black men (43%) with AIDS acquired HIV infection through homosexual/bisexual contact (CDC 1992b). This fact has been obscured by a culturally based reluctance in the black community to accept the idea that black men have sex with other men. In addition, 8% of black men contracted AIDS through a combination of homosexual or bisexual contact and injection drug use (CDC 1991b).

There has been considerable behavioral change among some white gay men, who have altered risky behaviors. This change was largely reflected in decreased frequency of unprotected anal intercourse and fewer sex partners. (Unfortunately, there are signs that gay men are returning to risky behaviors [National Commission on AIDS 1991a]). However, progress made in AIDS risk reduction within the mainstream gay community may not have efficiently reached black men who have sex with other men (Thomas and Hodges 1991).

Black Women

AIDS is the leading cause of death for black women in New York and New Jersey (Chu et al. 1990). In 1988 black women died from HIV infection at a rate nine times higher than that of white women (CDC 1990b). AIDS has become the nation's fifth leading cause of death in the United States for women 15 to 44 years of age (American Public Health Association 1991; CDC 1991a).

Approximately 55% of black women with AIDS are classified as IDUs. Thirty-four percent of cases among black women are the result of heterosexual transmission. According to the CDC, approximately 59% of heterosexually transmitted cases among black women are the result of being the sex partner of an IDU (CDC 1992b). The cumulative incidence of AIDS cases acquired through heterosexual contact is more than eleven times higher for black women than for white women (Holmes et al. 1990).

The association between injection drug use and HIV infection is well established. However, for female IDUs, risk of HIV infection comes from multiple factors. Researchers have found that female IDUs, in addition to sharing contaminated needles, are likely to be multiple drug abusers and that their use of crack cocaine, in particular, increases their participation in unprotected sexual activity (Miller et al. 1990). These researchers report that female IDUs are also likely to participate in risky behaviors such as multiple sex partners and sex for drugs. Women who use intravenous drugs are more likely to have a primary relationship with a male IDU than with a nondrug user (Karan 1989). Female IDUs are also susceptible to physical abuse and rape that may place them at risk for infection.

Female sex partners of male IDUs are often unaware of their partner's mode of injection of drugs, and consequently are not aware of their own risk for HIV infection (DesJarlais et al. 1984; Miller et al. 1990). In addition, although they may not use drugs intravenously, sex partners of IDUs use alcohol and drugs that may have an impact on their participation in high-risk sexual behavior (Kane 1990). Because sex partners of IDUs are somewhat invisible, they have not been readily available to AIDS treatment and HIV prevention programs (Miller et al. 1990).

Mounting evidence exists for an association between high-risk sexual behaviors and the use of other (non-IV) drugs, including alcohol, cocaine, and crack cocaine (Miller et al. 1990). Others report an association between cocaine use and syphilis that serves both as a cofactor itself for HIV infection and a proxy measure of unprotected sexual behavior (Rolfs et al. 1990). In 1988 the incidence of gonorrhea was approximately twenty-one times higher for black women than for white women. In 1987 the incidence of syphilis was approximately thirty-one times higher for black women than for white women (Holmes et al. 1990).

BARRIERS TO HIV EDUCATION AND AIDS RISK REDUCTION

Homophobia

To date, there is no full picture of the character and consequences of black homophobia. Homophobia appears to be greater within minority subcultures than in mainstream American culture (Freudenberg 1989). While observers do not have the quantitative evidence to confirm this belief, to support their claim they point to the disinclination of some black mainstream organizations to associate themselves with what is still perceived as a gay disease, and to the tendency of some black families to disown gay children who come out of the closet. This is unfortunate because, as previously stated, most black men (43%) with AIDS acquired HIV infection by having sex with other men (CDC 1992b). Cultural barriers prevent open discussion of homosexual behavior, and black men who have sex with other men may not self-identify as gay or bisexual. If instead they identify by their ethnicity, they may be hidden within the social, economic, and community-based activities of the broader, predominantly heterosexual, black community (Mays 1990). In addition, black men who may participate in sex with other men during periods of incarceration or extended military duty return to female sex partners once they go back to their community.

The Problem of Drugs

Public health research and practice operate in an environment of societal values and political ideology. For example, needle distribution programs for IDUs are a frequent source of political debate. Efforts to develop needle distribution programs have been stymied by political controversy, moral questions, and outraged cries of genocide from blacks. In many black communities where drug abuse is epidemic, needle distribution programs are perceived as contributing to the drug problem, particularly when such programs are promulgated in the absence of access to adequate drug treatment services. The image of black IDUs reaching out for drug treatment only to receive clean needles from public health authorities provides additional grist for the genocide mill (Thomas and Quinn 1993).

Lack of access to adequate health care, including drug treatment services, is a critical issue for black women. The lack of health care insurance, the presence of overburdened public clinics, and the lack of transportation or child care interfere with ready access to general health care and prenatal care (Quinn 1993). Carol Levine and Nancy Dubler describe access to care for poor, black women as "extremely limited to nonexistent" (Levine and Dubler 1990). Access to drug treatment for substance-abusing women is influenced by factors beyond their control: high cost, lack of insurance, inadequate transportation, and poor accessibility. Treatment programs also frequently refuse admission to pregnant women, do not offer or coordinate prenatal care, fail to provide child care, and do not offer the range of support services needed by drug-dependent women. In addition, poverty and poor education are commonplace. HIV-infected women describe themselves as dependent on men for self-esteem. In areas where drug use is epidemic, the economic rewards of selling drugs, coupled with inadequate education, contribute to the lack of consideration of alternative futures (Karan 1989; Levine and Dubler 1990).

Women's Rights

The reproductive rights of HIV-infected women cannot be separated from societal values, political ideology, moral issues, and concern over access to primary health care. The CDC and state health departments advocate HIV testing programs and counsel HIV-infected women to avoid pregnancy in an effort to prevent perinatal transmission. Yet Levine and Dubler (1990) specifically describe abortion as problematic because federal funds—and in many states, local public funds—cannot be used to obtain abortion services. However, implementation of these public health methods in the black community is potentially volatile and disastrous. The promotion of condoms as a means to prevent HIV infection is viewed with suspicion by blacks. Levine and Dubler state that "many African-Americans view any attempt to interfere with or discourage reproduction as part of a plan for genocide" (Levine and Dubler 1990, p. 333). Without a sensitivity to these views, strong advocacy of testing, avoiding pregnancy, or abortion—in the face of limited access to health care—will reinforce fears of genocide and alienate blacks from health care providers.

HIV TESTING POLICY AND POTENTIAL DISCRIMINATION

Early in the 1980s the nation's blood supply was in danger of being contaminated with HIV, leading many to fear infection of the general population. The perception that AIDS was certain death stimulated panic and a backlash against those persons thought to be potential HIV "carriers." In the early years of the epidemic, there was no way to determine whether one had been infected with HIV (Institute of Medicine 1988).

The need to protect the nation's blood supply stimulated a search for an effective HIV test. In 1985 the Elisa and Western Blot test for HIV antibodies became available, and for the first time, those wishing to determine their HIV status could do so. With testing available, issues regarding confidentiality of test results became paramount. Currently, state legislative requirements surrounding HIV testing range from (1) providing anonymous, voluntary testing; (2) offering confidential testing; (3) reporting names of HIV-positive individuals to the state public health authority; and (4) requiring mandatory testing for certain populations (Quinn 1992).

It is assumed that the foremost purpose of testing is to promote the adoption of risk-reduction behaviors. However, knowledge of HIV status may be insufficient to stimulate behavior change; many other factors contribute to decisions about risk-reduction behaviors (Coates et al. 1988). Frank Rhame and Dennis Maki move beyond advocacy for testing solely as a means of risk reduction for HIV infection and suggest several significant public health benefits to HIV testing. For one thing, broader testing might lead to general acceptance of testing, which would reduce the reluctance of those at risk to pursue it. Furthermore, widespread testing might help to undermine the we/ they mentality and the stigma associated with HIV/AIDS. Rhame and Maki suggest that testing itself would serve as a motivator for risk-reduction behaviors and could serve as a basis for partner notification programs and identification of candidates for clinical research trials (Rhame and Maki 1989).

The benefits of HIV testing appear clear; nevertheless, broader testing may drive those at highest risk underground. In addition, public health professionals should be sensitive to the concern that the benefits of testing may be outweighed by the potential for discrimination. Because of the stigma associated with AIDS and the fear of discrimination, many individuals at high risk for HIV infection may avoid testing when, despite confidential testing, state requirements demand the reporting of names of persons who test seropositive. At the end of 1992, "26 states had imposed some form of HIV name reporting; the names of people with AIDS are reportable in all states" (Cooper 1992, p. 12). Name reporting of HIV-positive persons provides public health officials with the opportunity to encourage followup care, estimate future health planning needs, and better utilize partner notification programs (Demkovich 1989). Name reporting of those testing HIV-positive may, however, result in reduced demand for testing. Research in New York City indicates that mandatory name reporting would inhibit urban blacks and Hispanics from seeking testing (Fordyce et al. 1989). When South Carolina adopted the mandatory reporting of names of HIV-positive persons to public health officials, the number of homosexual men seeking testing decreased by approximately 50% (Lamboi and Sy 1989). Furthermore, health professionals should recognize that name reporting, particularly in low-incidence states, may pose a significant risk of discrimination for the individual (Quinn 1992). Partner notification or contact tracing is standard public health practice in sexually transmitted disease control. However, it has not been adopted quickly and universally in AIDS cases owing to the stigma attached to homosexuals and injection drug abusers and the potential for discrimination resulting from repressive attitudes (Potterat et al. 1989).

The emphasis on HIV testing and counseling without adequate access to clinical trials and appropriate treatment for AIDS evokes memories of the deliberate withholding of treatment by the researchers in the Tuskegee Study, which is discussed later in this chapter. Public health professionals must ensure that HIV testing and counseling are accompanied by specific informed consent, full discussion of treatment options, and appropriate referrals for primary care and clinical trials.

AIDS: IS IT GENOCIDE?

It is crucial to understand how attitudes and beliefs influence the black response to HIV education programs. Several reports in the popular black media suggest that blacks mistrust government reports on AIDS, believe that AIDS is a man-made virus, respond negatively to people who say AIDS came to America from Africa, and believe AIDS is a form of genocide. Public health and HIV education programs must compete with these beliefs that are already established in the community.

The Nation of Islam has disseminated literature in the black community that describes AIDS as a form of genocide, an attempt by white society to eliminate the Negro race (Smith 1988). "Tony Brown's Journal," a popular public television talk show, focused a series of programs specifically on the issue of AIDS as a form of genocide. The *Los Angeles Sentinel,* the largest black newspaper on the West Coast, ran a series of stories that suggested that blacks had been intentionally infected with HIV. *Essence Magazine* also ran a story titled "AIDS: Is It Genocide?" in which Barbara J. Justice, a New York City physician, asserted that "there is a possibility that the virus was produced to limit the number of African people and people of color in the world who are no longer needed" (Bates 1990, p. 78). Fears about genocide have also been reported by public health professionals and community-based organization staff who work in black communities. Yet there has been little systematic examination of these attitudinal barriers within the context of HIV education.

The Tuskegee Syphilis Study, wherein hundreds of rural illiterate black syphilitic men were deceptively told that they were receiving treatment for the disease, is the longest nontherapeutic experiment on human beings in medical history (Jones 1981). The legacy of this experiment, with its failure to educate the study participants and treat them adequately, laid the foundation for today's pervasive sense of black distrust of public health authorities (Thomas and Quinn 1991). The study was intended to last six to nine months. However, the drive to satisfy scientific curiosity resulted in a forty-year experiment that followed these men to "End Point" (autopsy).

The ultimate reason why the Tuskegee Syphilis Study continued for forty years was a minimal sense of personal responsibility and ethical concern among a small group of U.S. Public Health Service (PHS) officials who controlled the study. This attitude was reflected in a 1976 interview with Dr. John Heller, director of Venereal Diseases at the PHS from 1943 to 1948, who stated, "the men's status did not warrant ethical debate. They were subjects, not patients; clinical material, not sick people" (Jones 1981, p. 179).

Black fears and attitudes arising from the Tuskegee Syphilis Study and other abuses must be assessed in order to develop effective AIDS education programs for the black community. The Southern Christian Leadership Conference (SCLC) conducted a survey in 1990 to determine HIV education needs among 1,056 black church members in five cities. Thirty-five percent of respondents believed that AIDS was a form of genocide, and another 30% were unsure. In addition, 44% believed that the government was not telling the truth about AIDS and 35% were unsure. Furthermore, 34% believed that HIV is a man-made virus, while an additional 44% were unsure (Thomas and Quinn 1991).

Public health professionals must recognize that the belief in AIDS as a form of genocide is a legitimate attitudinal barrier rooted in the history of the Tuskegee Syphilis Study. Many public health authorities who work with black communities are uncomfortable responding to the issue of genocide and the Tuskegee Study because they do not know the facts. The common response is to ignore these issues. This approach may result in a loss of credibility and further alienation. One culturally sensitive response would be for public health professionals to discuss the fear of genocide evoked by the AIDS epidemic. They must be willing to listen respectfully to community fears, know and share the facts of the Tuskegee Study when it arises as a justification of those fears, and admit to the limitations of science when they do not have all the answers. This approach may assist public health authorities to regain the necessary credibility and trust needed to successfully implement HIV risk-reduction strategies in the black community.

Community-Based HIV Education

The impact of HIV infection and AIDS in black communities is exacerbated by other sources of poor health status and social inequities. Therefore, AIDS risk-reduction programs must be built on solid assessments of community perceptions and needs, and must include ongoing involvement of community members in program planning and evaluation.

Public health professionals must know how to develop and implement effective community-based HIV education programs that are ethnically acceptable and culturally sensitive. Strategies such as the use of program staff indigenous to the community, the use of incentives, and the delivery of health services within the target community were used to successfully recruit participants in the Tuskegee Syphilis Study. These public health techniques are used by AIDS risk-reduction programs today, and the value of these community-based strategies should not be diminished by their association with the Tuskegee Study.

Successful HIV education and AIDS risk reduction will require a long-term commitment and collaboration among federal agencies, state and local health departments, community-based organizations, private industry, philanthropies, and institutions of higher learning. Such collaboration must be based on trust among the agencies and the black community. Given the legacy of Tuskegee, the credibility of public health service providers from outside the black community is severely limited.

The CDC's program to provide direct funding of African-American community-based organizations (CBOs) in order to deliver HIV education represents a significant development. However, while CBOs may have ready access to a community and have established credibility with the target population, they often lack the infrastructure necessary for long-term success (Thomas 1991; Thomas and Morgan 1991). Consequently, CBOs will require consistent technical assistance and long-range funding from government and private agencies. To ensure that the specter of Tuskegee will not impede progress, decision-making power must be so distributed that collaborating agencies allow CBOs to maintain control over program integrity.

RESTORATION OF TRUST: ROLES FOR PUBLIC HEALTH PROFESSIONALS

Black Americans' trust in the public health system can be regained through a variety of measures. We have an ethical responsibility to combat discrimination against HIV-infected individuals and persons with AIDS. As researchers, we can conduct knowledge and attitude surveys to monitor public attitudes toward HIV-infected individuals and persons with AIDS. Based on our research, educational interventions can be designed and implemented that address issues of stigma, fear about AIDS, and discriminatory attitudes specific to a given community. Public health professionals must advocate for black Americans to have increased access to clinical trials, so that information about AIDS can be expanded and the benefits of potential treatments can be realized. The successful inclusion of blacks in clinical trials, however, will require the willingness of researchers to conduct their investigations in convenient settings trusted by the black community. In addition, investigators must recognize that mere compliance with protection of human subjects procedures is insufficient. Since researchers who conducted the Tuskegee Study made a conscious decision to withhold information about syphilis from participants, blacks today may not fully trust that they are being told the whole truth about HIV. In order to successfully overcome distrust, community members must be fully informed about research procedures, costs, and benefits, and they must be represented on research advisory committees. Researchers should conduct their work with respect to the humanity of study participants regardless of the social and cultural gulf that may divide investigator and subject. Ultimately, cultural sensitivity can best be manifested through the professional obligation to advocate for AIDS policies that provide for the protection of civil rights and access to health care services (Quinn 1992).

Public health professionals bear a responsibility to exceed their traditional service delivery roles and to use public health as a means of facilitating social change (Thomas 1990). We have a major role to play as advocates for HIV-infected individuals, persons with AIDS, and those groups at greatest risk for infection. These groups have limited advocacy organizations and resources to protect their rights. We have a responsibility to communicate the needs of these constituencies to policymakers and to monitor legislation on HIV/AIDS that could potentially affect their civil rights (Quinn 1992).

In addition, AIDS in the black community must be understood within the context of other leading causes of preventable death that may result in decreased population growth and decreased life span. It is necessary to deal with the AIDS epidemic in the context of a comprehensive national plan to improve the health status of black Americans in order to assuage fears that AIDS will be used to stigmatize the black community and deny social justice. Public health must be used as a means of achieving social justice.

PUBLIC HEALTH AS SOCIAL JUSTICE: AN ETHICAL FRAMEWORK

AIDS policy decisions in the first decade of this epidemic were greatly influenced by strong gay advocacy groups that sought adequate protection for those seeking HIV testing services. As the public health system sought to implement traditional public health measures such as partner notification and confidential testing, gay advocacy groups lobbied for the adoption of favorable laws. As the focus of public health concern continues to shift away from white homosexual men to poor black drug users and their sexual partners, the influence of those who have spoken on behalf of the gay community has begun to wane (Kirp and Bayer 1992).

AIDS risk-reduction policy is based on the assumption that we as individuals can control our health destinies in significant ways. The emphasis on changing personal behavior assumes equality of access to health care, education, income, and quality of life. It assumes that all individuals have comparable control of their lives, and therefore fails to recognize the structural and social factors that minimize that control for some minority groups. On the one hand, risk factors such as unprotected sex and sharing of drug injection needles appear to be supported by this assumption of individual control over lifestyle. On the other hand, it is unrealistic to expect an individual to overcome the forces that prevent access to drug treatment on demand combined with failure to distribute clean needles to IDUs. In addition, it is unreasonable to expect an individual to overcome economic barriers to preventive, primary, and hospital care. To expect individual blacks to overcome the multiple barriers that contribute to their persistent health disadvantage is to ensure that a large segment of the black community will not benefit from advances in AIDS treatment and prevention research.

History reminds us that science is subject to racism, classism, and sexism; we must be cognizant of those influences on research, policy, and prevention. We must also be mindful that race is not an independent risk factor. In other words, compared to whites, blacks do not have higher morbidity and mortality rates simply because they are black. The relationship between poor health and socioeconomic status has been well documented (Jaynes and Williams 1989). People with the least education, people who live in the least desirable neighborhoods, and people who work at the least prestigious jobs are all more likely to die earlier than people on the other end of these scales. Within this context, disease prevention policies that place responsibility solely on individual black men and women are simply unjust.

Poor black drug users have not influenced public policy in the same way that white homosexual men have done. In addition, those who speak on behalf of drug users often lack the commitment to privacy and informed consent that characterizes the position of gay organizations. Public policy directed toward the poor is often authoritarian, and it is precisely such authoritarianism that evokes the worst traditions of public health, as the Tuskegee Study shows. The time has come for increased support for traditional public health approaches to screening, reporting, and partner notification. It is crucial that policy decisions incorporate strong protections for those who already suffer from discrimination. Without adequate protection, such as anonymous testing, case reporting without name identifiers, voluntary partner notification, and strong confidentiality regulations, high-risk individuals who already distrust the public health system may not seek HIV testing or AIDS prevention services. Consequently, we might expect rapid growth in the numbers of unknowingly infected individuals, higher mortality rates than among those whose infection is detected early, tremendous budgetary strains on the public health system, and increasing numbers of HIV-infected babies. This could spark public support for repressive policies against those suspected to be infected with HIV (Quinn 1992).

As U.S. citizens become increasingly aware of AIDS as a significant health problem in the black community, there will be both opportunity and danger. The opportunity is to deal comprehensively with the problem as a whole, to see it as a social catastrophe brought on by years of economic deprivation and benign neglect, and to meet it as other disasters are met, with adequate resources. The danger is that AIDS will be attributed to some innate weakness of black people and used to justify further neglect, and to rationalize continued deprivation. The AIDS epidemic has exposed the harsh reality of diminished economic resources, limits of medical technology, and confusion over how best to attribute responsibility for prevention of HIV infection.

As knowledge about HIV infection and AIDS continues to grow, and this disease affects our social, medical, and legal fabric, existing exceptions to traditional public health policy will be reconsidered and more traditional policies are likely to be adopted. However, the underpinnings of antidiscrimination legislation and regulations must be maintained. Based on those protections, HIV education and AIDS risk-reduction program efforts can maximize success.

The promise of public health for black Americans must be directed toward societal goals that maximize human potential and minimize risk factors limiting that potential. The mission of public health involves fulfilling society's interest in assuring conditions in which people can be healthy; the substance of public health is characterized by organized community efforts to prevent disease and promote health. From this perspective, community activism, community development, and social action are legitimate tools needed to attack complex health issues such as infant mortality, violence, drug abuse, and AIDS. Public health professionals must forge a direct link between the

AIDS-related health care needs of black Americans and the efforts to design and implement national health care reform. The approach must employ the same vision, commitment, and vigilance that transformed the civil rights movement into a source of empowerment for disadvantaged people. From this vantage point, our country's response to AIDS could truly be a measure of our nation's greatness.

Commentary by William M. King

There is much food for thought in this chapter, in particular the discussion of the Tuskegee Syphilis Study and how it has laid a foundation for African-Americans' pervasive sense of distrust of public health authorities whose research and practices are constrained by the values and political ideologies of the environments in which they operate.

The thrust of Thomas and Quinn's argument is directed at what they call the third epidemic of social and political repercussions of disease presence. What they seek is a reconceptualization of traditional public health approaches as a form of social justice, employing the powers of tolerance, understanding, and information to rectify the moral tragedy that black people "are being killed by a disease that is almost totally preventable."

Yet, I am troubled by some of the assertions they make, weaving back and forth from a general population to a more specific population, namely, African Americans, whose history and experiences in the United States have remanded them to the periphery of the society, leaving them to fend for themselves the best way they can. Too, the character of their presentation raises a number of questions that even they concede will be difficult to answer, if only because they are beyond the scope of any one discipline to answer. For those answers will contain policy-setting precedents that have real time consequences for the self-interests of those being called on to respond.

Because disease germs are the most democratic creatures on the planet—having the potential to strike anyone regardless of social class, race, gender, nativity, sexual orientation, whatever—it is clear that we will need to rethink, as they suggest, our approaches to treatment and prevention, if only because germs have a way of mutating faster than the protective screens we erect to contain them can change themselves.

Historically, they imply, our past treatment policies and practices appear to have much in common with the notion of triage—we treat the ones we believe have the greatest potential for survival and contribution to the society. Clearly, this is a value-laden decision based on our perception and interpretation of the evidence placed before us in accord with certain carefully crafted criteria of evaluation.

Because current "AIDS risk reduction policy is based on the assumption that we as individuals can control our health destinies in significant ways," because of the turf protection mentality that is the essence of the operational reality of bureaucracy, and because of the disingenuous treatment of black people in a white society, I question whether what they propose is achievable in the near term. I am further discouraged inasmuch as the principal instrument of health care delivery in the United States is a fee for service model that fits in rather nicely with the economic rationales of the society. This, in and of itself, speaks volumes, as they observe, about limited access to health care among the poor and dispossessed of the society. The underserved are then further stigmatized if they are homosexual or intravenous drug users, because it can then be contended that they are making no effort to normalize themselves. Thus, they can be perceived as getting exactly what they deserve.

Unfortunately, these same persons live with and among us, interact with us, and therefore have the potential to act as transmitters of inflictions that we would rather sweep under the carpet in our quest to preserve certain myths about ourselves. Thus, I would go further than Thomas and Quinn in their call for redefinition. I would argue that, in addition to facing up to the barriers imposed on us by the false morality we so readily embrace, we also need to accept the reality that opportunity itself is differentially distributed in the United States along race, class, and gender lines. The fact that this is a society predicated on the principles of exclusion and exploitation, our so-called democratic political rhetoric notwithstanding, is easily evident in the most cursory examination of our history. And until such time as we look at ourselves more clearly, no public policy will do more than preserve the status quo.

8   Women and Children Living with HIV: Impact of Racism and Poverty

Mildred Williamson

INTRODUCTION

AIDS (Acquired Immunodeficiency Syndrome) is an infectious disease caused by the Human Immunodeficiency Virus (HIV) that results in the failure of the immune system, leaving the body unable to fight infections. Infection with HIV can occur through unprotected sex with infected persons, injection with infected blood, or perinatally from an infected mother to her fetus. HIV-infected persons have been known to live free of symptoms for ten or more years (Lemp et al. 1990).

Among documented AIDS cases in the United States, 46% are among people of color and 30% involve African Americans. Although African-American and Latina women represent 19% of the nation's female population, they account for 78% of AIDS cases among women (CDC 1992b). AIDS has become the nation's fifth largest killer of women of child-bearing age, and in New York and New Jersey it has been the leading cause of death for women between the ages of 15 and 44 since 1988 (CDC 1992b). The number of HIV-infected women and children of color is growing dramatically. Most are low-income people and rely on Medicaid and public health facilities for their primary health care.

The majority of pediatric AIDS cases are perinatally acquired, meaning that the child was born to an HIV-infected mother. About 20% of all U.S. AIDS cases involve children under the age of 18, and the number of HIV-positive children is estimated at two to ten times the number of reported cases of children with AIDS. HIV infection in adults is determined by a simple blood test for antibodies to the virus. With infants, however, this diagnosis is more difficult: HIV antibody tests taken before the fifteenth month of age do not provide accurate information (Simonds and Rogers 1992). Different types of tests exist but are not widely available. Virtually all infants born to HIV-positive women test positive for the antibody, but only about 25% are actually infected. The others carry the mother's antibodies, which disappear over time. In addition, more than 80% of all youth whose mothers have died or will die of HIV/AIDS (an estimated 36,560 youth) are offspring of African-American and Latina women (Michaels and Levine 1992).

In the general population, contact with homosexual or bisexual men is the main identified risk factor for the majority of reported AIDS cases, followed by intravenous drug use (Department of Health and Human Services 1990). However, among women the opposite is true. The leading risk factor for women has been their own IV drug use, accounting for more than half the cases. The next leading risk factor for women, which accounts for over one-third of the cases, is heterosexual contact, either with an HIV-infected intravenous drug user (IVDU) or with an HIV-infected bisexual man (National Commission on AIDS 1991a).

This chapter looks at the particular social circumstances of women and children of color living with HIV infection. Their complex and difficult situation must be understood if they are to be provided with adequate social services. I will outline some basic requirements for social service delivery for this population, and as an example I will briefly describe the Women and Children HIV Program at Cook County Hospital.

CAUGHT IN A WEB OF CO-RELATED RISKS

Black and Latina women living with—or at risk for—HIV infection are likely to be caught in a web of co-related risk factors, including substance abuse, other sexually transmitted diseases, tuberculosis, and incarceration. In addition, they are trapped by a desperate inner-city environment where violence, joblessness, substandard housing, and lack of access to health care reinforce their dire social situation. Substance abuse may lead to risky sex practices and exposure to sexually transmitted disease; legitimate distrust of the medical establishment may cause pregnant substance abusers to avoid prenatal care; and prisons and homeless shelters expose women (who may be immuno-compromised) to tuberculosis (TB) and other diseases.

HIV infection is the most deadly component of a larger epidemic of sexually transmitted diseases (STDs), including syphilis and herpes, which threatens the well-being of African-American and Latina women and children (Perrow and Guillen 1990). Although declining in the majority population, the incidence of STDs is increasing rapidly in communities of color.[1] The STD epidemic can in part be traced to crack, a cheap, smokable form of cocaine that has saturated poor communities of color across the nation (Wilkin et al. 1991). Crack cocaine produces a quick addiction and results in behaviors driven by the need to obtain more of the drug. Selling sex for drugs is common among crack users. The influence of crack may make an addict unconcerned about condom use, even if the individual knows about safer sex practices. Sex partners of crack users are likely to include IV drug users, some of whom are infected with HIV or other sexually transmitted diseases.[2]

It is well known that drug and alcohol use by pregnant women has adverse effects on birth outcomes and that the number of babies born to (mostly cocaine) addicted mothers is rising. What is new is the escalating number of babies born with congenital syphilis, and, for the first time in decades, there are reports of syphilitic stillborns (Chicago Department of Health 1991). Because syphilis is completely preventable and treatable, the poor outcomes of these reported pregnancies indicate that the mothers were untouched by any health care system, delivering their babies with very late or no prenatal care.

Some states actually discourage African-American and Latina women substance abusers from seeking prenatal health care, because they criminalize chemically dependent pregnancy. For example, in a Pinellas County, Florida, study, Dr. Ira Chasnoff, a national expert in the clinical management of chemically dependent pregnant women, compared toxicology screens among 200 black and 500 white women. Sixty-three percent of the black women were at or below the poverty level; 65% of the white women were middle class. He found that, despite this difference in socioeconomic class, their drug use was almost the same, approximately 14 and 15.4%, respectively. More black women tested positive for cocaine, and more white women for marijuana. Cocaine use during pregnancy is more dangerous than marijuana use, which may account for the disproportionate reporting.

Chasnoff also looked at births in the county over a six-month period: 4,300 white babies and 793 black babies were born. The mothers of 133 of these newborns—48 white and 85 black—were reported for child abuse after positive toxicology screens. That is, 10% of all the black mothers were reported to the child protection system, while only 1% of the white mothers were reported, although toxicology screening indicated almost equal drug use among black and white women. Chasnoff contends that physicians are more likely to take the drug histories of black women, more eager to perform urine tests on this group, and more inclined to report black women who test positive to child welfare authorities. He concludes that unfortunately this criminalization results in driving black women out of prenatal care (Chasnoff 1990).

An increasing number of women are becoming involved with the criminal justice system. Although there are relatively few incarcerated women as compared to men, still, the population of women prisoners has skyrocketed over the past decade. In 1980 approximately 13,000 women were in federal and state prisons. By the end of 1989, the number had more than tripled, to almost 41,000. In 1989 alone, the female prison population grew by 25%, compared with a 13% growth in the male prison population (National Commission on AIDS 1991a). The General Accounting Office estimates that between 60 and 80% of female prisoners have alcohol and drug dependency problems, and among prison entrants, HIV infection is more prevalent for women than for men (National Commission on AIDS 1991b). With an increasing number of black and Latina women in prison and in homeless shelters, TB is becoming recognized as a significant health threat to this population. Tuberculosis, which has historically afflicted poor people, is one of the opportunistic infections associated with HIV disease. With the rise in multidrug-resistant strains of tuberculosis, the compromised immune systems of HIV-infected women, and the prison system's inability to isolate infected individuals and provide adequate health care, incarceration will prove deadly for an increasing number of women.

TB has been on the rise in the United States since 1985, with over 20,000 cases reported, mostly among blacks and Latinos. Not surprisingly, TB outbreaks have been reported among persons congregated in enclosed spaces such as nursing homes, shelters for the homeless, hospitals, schools, and prisons (Benenson 1990).

Drugs—and the violence and property loss associated with them—are literally destroying many black and Latino neighborhoods. The quality of the living conditions—material, social, and spiritual—serves as a backdrop for initial drug use and inevitable relapse. The testimony of Robert Fullilove, MD, before the National Commission on AIDS provided this insight: "We think relapse is related to environmental factors, the degree to which people live in neighborhoods where the neighborhood itself is a toxic agent that promotes addiction" (Fullilove 1991, p. 14).

THE WOMEN AND CHILDREN WITH HIV PROGRAM: COOK COUNTY HOSPITAL

Cook County Hospital is the only public hospital in Chicago and Cook County, Illinois, and it is the last resort for the area's medically underserved minority communities. The Women and Children HIV Program (WCHP) started with a weekly afternoon clinic session in 1988 and expanded in 1989 to include additional psychosocial services, including chemical dependency counseling and extensive health education. WCHP began a second weekly clinic session in 1991, adding the services of a nutritionist and extensive clinical trial availability. Eleven women physicians—internists, infectious disease specialists, pediatricians, family practitioners, and an obstetrician/gynecologist—serve in the clinic along with other health and social service professionals, making up a multiracial and bilingual (English- and Spanish-speaking) team.

Staff have gained expertise in conducting health education with women of color at risk; providing medical and psychosocial services to HIV-infected women, their partners, and children; and attracting and working with community-based organizations. The demographics of the client population mirror the national statistics. More than 830 women, their partners, and children have been served by the program. The majority (550) have been women. Most (68%) of the women are African Americans; the remainder are white (17%), Latina (14%), and Haitian or Native American (1%). Most women are either IV drug users (60%) or had unprotected sex with an HIV-positive man (25%). Another 10% report both IV drug use and unprotected sex with an HIV positive man.

According to the Illinois Department of Public Health, the Women and Children HIV Program cares for 80% of the state's known HIV-infected women and 35% of the state's known HIV-positive child population. It was the first medical program in the Chicago area to provide services for the whole family at a single site, and as of this writing, it remains the only such program. Some of the families served have prior or current involvement with the state's child welfare agency. A few of the patients have been jailed; between 10 and 15% do not have telephones; and it is estimated that 10% are homeless or have been homeless in the past.

CONSIDERATIONS FOR CARE PROVIDERS AND ACTIVISTS

Because the primary mode of transmission for heterosexuals with AIDS has been IV drug use and sharing needles with infected persons, efforts have been made to establish free needle exchange programs, with the goal of saving the lives of addicts who are unwilling or unable to discontinue their use of drugs. National Institute on Drug Abuse (NIDA)-sponsored programs have found that, as cooperating addicts exchange dirty needles for clean ones, they often respond favorably to obtaining drug treatment and report decreasing IV drug use. Similarly, high proportions of addicts also report decreases in sharing injection equipment. Unfortunately, however, the same respondents less frequently report reductions in sexual risk behaviors than they do drug-associated risk behaviors (Hatziandreu et al. 1990).

Many people in the black community fear that needle exchange programs encourage drug use. The concern stems from the observation that health officials are eager to invest in free needles for widespread distribution, but not in expanding effective free or low-cost substance abuse treatment programs. Many African Americans are also suspicious about law enforcement authorities who cannot seem to round up known drug dealers whom streetwise children can often easily identify. Yet these same authorities use excessive force with would-be suspects.

Long-term residential drug treatment is the chronic drug user's best hope for recovery. Unfortunately, there are far too few slots in treatment programs. In Illinois alone, the Department on Alcohol and Substance Abuse estimates that there are approximately 80,000 addicts, but only about 9,000 treatment slots (American Public Health Association 1990). Less than 1% of federal antidrug monies are targeted for drug treatment for women, and the fraction is even lower for pregnant and parenting women (Bowsher 1990).

Chemically dependent women often have other problems along with their addiction. They are more likely to have been victims of abuse, to have unstable living arrangements, and to have limited family support and poor self-esteem. They may suffer additional health problems associated with poverty and lack of health care. These women often lack work experience, and they may be unemployed. They may have several children, and yet lack adequate parenting skills. Few treatment programs accommodate persons with little or no money, persons with children, or persons with concurrent mental illnesses. Programs that are woman-centered and culturally sensitive are rare. While state drug agency directors report that more clients than ever before are female multiple drug users, most treatment centers serve predominantly young men (Hatziandreu et al. 1990).

Health care providers must be prepared to encounter values, attitudes, and priorities in their patients that are radically different from their own and that on the surface may appear irrational and counterintuitive. For example, HIV may not be the patient's first priority; the majority of these families battle to survive economically and emotionally under difficult conditions. Adequate housing, paying the electric bill, and food are their main priorities, along with their struggles to overcome chemical dependency. This is especially true for asymptomatic HIV-positive individuals, who commonly deny their HIV status. Therefore, the concrete needs of patients must first be met if they are to comply with clinic appointments and treatment regimens, or to participate in clinical studies.

Nor can the health care provider assume that an HIV-positive woman would want to avoid pregnancy or, if she becomes pregnant, would want to terminate the pregnancy. Childbearing can be a source of strength, even power, for a woman, especially if she has previously lost custody of a child through the child protection agencies. Therefore, counseling becomes important, and to be effective it should result in a personalized plan for risk reduction (CDC 1993b). Counseling should thoroughly explain the risks of unprotected sex and the possible consequences of terminating or completing a pregnancy. A woman's decision must be informed and her own; the provider should then be guided by her decision. Women need to know that they will be treated with dignity, without racism or sexism, and that their concerns will be taken into consideration. This approach to service delivery implies that the client-patient is worthy of respect and is capable of making her own decisions.

In addition to acknowledging differences in values and priorities, health care workers must anticipate and address expectations of racial prejudice (DesJarlais et al. 1991). Black America's complex attitudes toward white America—and vice versa—cannot be treated as bothersome background noise. Only if we acknowledge these disconcerting realities have we a chance to escape their constraining force (Dalton 1989). The National Commission on AIDS discusses inequality and concludes:

The HIV epidemic did not leave 37 million or more Americans without health care—but it did dramatize their plight. . . . HIV did not cause the problem of homelessness—but it has expanded it and made it more visible. . . . HIV did not cause the collapse of the health care system—but it has accelerated the disintegration of our public hospitals and intensified their financing problems. . . . HIV did not directly augment problems of substance use—but it has made the need for drug treatment for all who request it a matter of urgent national priority. (National Commission on AIDS 1991a, p. 4)

These are the points of advocacy that must be addressed if we are to make a dent in this epidemic, and if desperately needed improvements in the quality of life are to be made for people of color and all people in the United States. We need to honestly confront poverty and inequality (including sexism and homophobia), and resolve to eliminate them. This is the key to responding to AIDS as the frightening human emergency that it is.

NOTES

1. Sexually transmitted diseases are most frequently reported by public medical facilities, which are disproportionately used by poor people of color. White middle-class persons may more likely be served by private physicians who may not regularly report STD incidence. This, in part, may account for the statistical decline in the majority population.

2. The pattern is different among sex-industry workers (prostitutes). HIV infection rates among sex-industry workers are relatively low; these workers are far more likely than crack users to insist that their partners use condoms (Perrow and Guillen 1990).

Commentary by Ruth Purtilo

Mildred Williamson correctly places the problem of the majority of women and children living with HIV in the context of poverty and racism. While not all such persons are poor and of color, the majority are, and the character of their suffering is not incidental to that fact. The reader will not be surprised by her observations showing the higher incidence of HIV positivity among poor people and especially among poor African-American women and children. Nor will her emphasis on major conditions causing the disproportionate suffering in these groups come as news. Among the conditions she emphasizes are the lack of access to health care and (when it is available) its emphasis on treatment at the exclusion of prevention and education; the concurrent debilitating effects of other conditions such as TB, STD, and substance abuse; the poor person's feelings of low self-esteem imposed by not being able to measure up to societal ideals; and the responses to their overall situation (e.g., substance abuse, depression, violence). All of this is exacerbated by the society's seeming inability or unwillingness to treat such persons with the respect they deserve and to provide effective measures to decrease that suffering. The author sketches the contours of a model program fashioned to meet the real needs of persons in these untenable situations. The program is characterized by counseling in a nonjudgmental way, recognition of what can and cannot be changed in the client's existing life and relationships, and intensive education geared to enabling informed decision making by the clients themselves. All of this is offered over and above appropriate medical care.

Two themes from Williamson's sensitively drawn profile of HIV-infected women and children bear further reflection. The first is that the author correctly targets the problem of a health care system that is "out of sync" with the needs of such persons. As I read her chapter, I recalled a motto in a Chicago Loop "El" station in the late 1960s, which I have thought about many times hence. It said, "A racist is someone who thinks black people are just as good as white people." Since then, I have learned more fully what it means to work within a health care system in which the "gold standard" is middle-class whiteness. Almost all health care professionals, administrators, bureaucrats, and policymakers are white, are in the middle class or above, and come from cultural and socioeconomic heritages that may deem poverty and people of color as necessary evils to be tolerated (or worse).

In a world where becoming "as good as a white person" is the gold standard, few poor people and no people of color will be able to measure up. Our health care system, "the best in the world" for its acute care, has been promulgated and sustained by persons defining the gold standard. It has long focused on disease rather than on prevention, has increasingly shown its preferential option for the well off, and springs from an ethos of individual self-sufficiency. Given the white and middle-classness of the canvas, it should come as little surprise that the current HIV epidemic is painted in life-and-death decisions, conceived as an illness/condition to be abhorred because it affects the autonomy of individuals, and carries the assumption that treatment should be paid for by those individuals (or their "surrogates"—the third-party payers).

While it comes as no surprise, even the anticipated can be morally wrong, and the singlemindedness of our approach is. At the time of this writing, several health care reform plans are before us, signaling that not everyone is in agreement with our present focus and biases. No one proposal completely accommodates those whose lives do not fit the gold standard of white middle-class values, though several elements of a number of the proposals do bear attention: the approaches that provide for universal access, separate the receipt of high-quality care from ability to pay and from employment, allow only a just remuneration for professional services, include cost containment measures driven by cost effectiveness and *have a preferential option for the poor*, and create a context into which some of the narrowness of our present approaches would be challenged.

The second theme is that Williamson correctly moves the source for relief of the suffering out of the medical care arena and into the larger life situation of the women and children who are the subjects of her comments. In her scheme, the disproportionate spread of HIV in her population becomes another manifestation of more fundamental quality-of-life dilemmas. Giving attention to one's (or the child's) HIV infection competes with attaining other basic goods. Should I buy a taxi ride to the clinic or buy coal? Dare I lose the solace of a crack high, knowing there is no way to buy it but with my own body? Does the coughing of pneumonia create any more discomfort than the cramp of hunger?

These dilemmas are completely foreign to most health care professionals, government or private policymakers, and administrators. Williamson suggests, though not directly, that a great barrier to moving the focus of attention from treatment to more essential prevention and education is disbelief by those in power that such dilemmas actually exist. In a highly individualistic and, many say, narcissistic middle class, HIV is imagined to be the most terrible blow possible. It is feasible that the relatively better off will further marginalize those who are poor, of color, and concerned with problems other than their HIV infection as simply not caring about themselves, especially if those who are suffering do not see medical care as the sole (and appropriate) means of seeking relief from such suffering.

In conclusion, Williamson's observations provide an opportunity for us to reflect on the nature and scope of a form of suffering in our society that has been largely ignored. As I am an ethicist working in a health care setting, Williamson creates an opportunity for me to carry her insights to health care educators, policymakers, and practitioners. Although the issues are societywide, health professionals are well situated to lead in the types of reforms needed to address these travesties. To fail to do so not only runs counter to the age-old medical ethics adage directing the professional to "cure when possible, comfort always" but ignores the professionals' larger social responsibility to use their skills and insights to create a community of mutual respect for all. To fail to do so when the stakes are so high becomes complicity.

9

Health Care and the Rural Poor: Focus on Appalachia

Bruce David White

I am a physician practicing in my native beautiful and mountainous Appalachia. While the focus of this volume is on African Americans, I want to insert a reminder that there are other poor populations who suffer just as acutely as African Americans and other ethnic groups. In particular, the health and social needs of Appalachians and other rural peoples have been grossly ignored and neglected. Recent government statistics describing the health care plight of the rural poor in the United States are astounding. Consider these facts from a 1991 Department of Health and Human Services Center on Budget and Policy Priorities report (Department of Health and Human Services 1991):

- The rural poverty rate is higher than the national average for the first time in history, and it is expected to continue to climb.
- There are only 97 physicians for every 100,000 rural residents in this country, while there are 225 physicians per 100,000 U.S. urbanites.
- There are 111 rural counties in the United States with no physician at all; another two-thirds of these counties have neither an obstetrician nor a pediatrician.
- Nearly 17% of rural residents under age 65 have no health insurance coverage, compared with 15.4% in urban areas. About 40% of U.S. agricultural workers and their families have no health insurance at all.
- Among small businesses in 1989, 72% in urban areas provide health insurance to employees, compared with 54% in rural areas.
- For the period 1981–88, 216 rural hospitals closed while 64 urban hospitals closed.

These impersonal health care statistics do not tell the full story about one particularly poor region: Appalachia. The geographical term itself is synonymous with "poor" and "backward." The *Random House Dictionary of the English Language* contains the following definition for Appalachia: "a region in the Eastern United States, in the area of the Southern Appalachian Mountains, marked by *poor economic conditions*" (emphasis added). This scenically beautiful, mountainous region has long been characterized with phrases usually reserved for particularly devastated areas. Appalachia's underdeveloped economy has little commercial potential; its industry depends heavily on diminishing natural resources. Government subsidies for agriculture do not protect farmers from devastating declines in world cash crop markets. Unemployment is high in the available workforce. Moreover, there are significant numbers of high school dropouts and teenage pregnancies, and little public interest has been shown in providing quality educational opportunities.

During the Great Society years of the Johnson administration, Appalachia and its people were a special target for reform. At that time, the U.S. government thought that it could really improve the living conditions of citizens in poorer regions of the country through massive aid programs. The government would prove this ability by helping to transform Appalachia. Innovative and novel approaches were instituted to make as great an impact as quickly as possible. Many of the country's Volunteers in Service to America (VISTA) workers went to Appalachia in the 1960s and 1970s to help residents there, just as Peace Corps volunteers had traveled overseas to help the natives of impoverished, Third World countries. In many ways, Appalachia resembles an underdeveloped nation with its abject poverty, high infant mortality rates, and shorter life expectancies. The Appalachian Regional Commission was established to coordinate economic advancement programs and to consolidate federal funding efforts to improve the area citizens' opportunities for a better quality of life. Physicians with a commitment to the National Health Service Corps were recruited for Appalachia, just as they were for the Indian reservations and urban ghettos. At least three new medical schools were established in Appalachia: East Tennessee State University in Johnson City, Tennessee (1975); Marshall University in Huntington, West Virginia (1974); and the West Virginia School of Osteopathic Medicine in White Sulphur Springs, West Virginia (1977). These schools were established both to increase training opportunities locally for medical students, residents, and physicians and to improve patients' access to tertiary care medical centers.

Unfortunately, these and subsequent programs have not sustained significant improvements in the general living conditions or health care services for Appalachian residents. According to the government report cited at the beginning of this chapter, rural residents—a quarter of the nation's population, of whom Appalachian citizens are a significant part—are in poorer health and more likely than their urban counterparts to have a more difficult time finding and paying for health care.

The culture of Appalachia is just as unique as African-American, Latino, Southeast Asian, Indian, or Native-American cultures. The people who live in my region of Appalachia are peculiarly proud of their heritage. They are the descendants of defiant and courageous settlers who disobeyed the orders of British King George III to cross the mountains and live in Indian territories in order to build a better life for their families in freedom. They are descended from the self-sufficient colonists who drafted the first instrument of self-government west of the Alleghenies. They are the descendants of proud Revolutionary patriots who gathered at the Sycamore Shoals of the Watauga and then marched to victory at the battle of Kings Mountain. Their ancestors were the same pioneers who were Daniel Boone's, Davy Crockett's, Georgie Russell's, Andrew Jackson's, and Isaac Lincoln's friends and neighbors. They are the great-great-grandchildren of citizens who raised several Union regiments to fight in the Civil War.

The Appalachian character cannot be described with adjectives and symbolic historic phrases alone. It is better conveyed through a personal illustration. The first story occurred twenty years ago. I took my future wife, Sarah, "home to meet the family" in 1974. We drove over 525 miles from Memphis to spend the weekend at my parents' home in Upper East Tennessee. To show Sarah where my mother grew up, we traveled from Elizabethton to Mountain City thirty miles away. Mountain City is the county seat of Johnson County, Tennessee, with a population then of about 4,000. We first visited my Aunt Beulah who lived on the outskirts of town. We saw that she was busy in her backyard when we drove up her graveled driveway. She was stirring something in her big, black kettle over an open flame. She was carefully skimming off the floating, yellowish, semisolid mixture from the top of the boiling liquid which she then spooned into a quart-size, glass canning jar. We had arrived near the end of her project. She had spent most of the morning making lye soap, which she planned to take as a "housewarming present" to the new family that had moved in across the road.

This gesture of hospitality was typical of my Aunt Beulah. She not only made her own soap, but she also grew her own vegetables and fruits in her garden, canned goods for the cellar and put up goods in the freezer, raised her own hens for eggs and poultry, and raised her own cattle and pigs for meat. Just before our visit she had assembled her quilting rack in the parlor for the winter. She was expecting my grandmother and Aunt Marie over that afternoon to help begin quilting Christmas presents. She offered to serve us fresh meat for lunch—she had slaughtered one of her hogs earlier in the week and was baking hog's head. She planned to make mince meat with the leftovers for Sunday's "Dinner-on-the-Ground" after morning worship service.

Aunt Beulah lived with my Uncle Frank. They were both widowed, met at church, and married about ten years later. Uncle Frank had retired with disability after his first heart attack. He had trouble with his blood pressure, and almost every time he went to the doctor some change in medication was required. The doctor lived thirty miles away in Boone, North Carolina.

Because of this distance they relied very heavily, and still do, on the local pharmacist for over-the-counter remedies, and they avoid going to the doctor except perhaps as a last resort. Other than a few added conveniences— primarily electric power, with attendant appliances, made available through Roosevelt's New Deal Tennessee Valley Authority—my Aunt Beulah and Uncle Frank lived much the same way that my grandparents had lived. She grew or raised her own food. Her family's health care was still dependent on one doctor some way off.

Some attempts have been made to change this health care barrier of distance in the last twenty years. Notably, the county built a hospital and tried to help several family doctors establish their practices. After a few years, however, the hospital closed because the county could not continue subsidizing their losses, and most of the physicians moved—many to Boone, North Carolina. The hospital facility is now a nursing home. East Tennessee State University is about forty miles away; its medical school and its three family practice residency programs have a number of specialists and subspecialists.

The second story occurred recently here in Nashville. I was working as a consultant to a large referral hospital with several specialized units. In this capacity, I had the opportunity to speak with many physicians who care for patients from all over Middle Tennessee. On this particular occasion, I learned about an elderly farmer who had lived all his life on the family farm where he and his wife had reared their six children, much like my Aunt Beulah. This man had just had coronary artery bypass surgery. He was doing well, better than was thought possible, and expected to go home within a few days. The farmer and his wife were already planning to sell the farm to pay his hospital and medical expenses. They did not know of any other way to pay their hospital bills. They were quite concerned and felt very uncomfortable owing any debts. However, after some financial counseling about their Medicare benefits, they were relieved to learn that they would not have to sell their farm. When the farmer left the hospital, he thanked his surgeon and gave him a sack of fresh vegetables from the farm.

Similar stories of rural patients could be recounted by other people all across this nation. I feel sure that my experiences of caring for rural patients are typical. Efforts to solve the problems of health care for rural residents must address not only the difficulty of distance but also the unique features of rural culture. Rural citizens differ from their urban cousins in many ways. Their needs are different—in some ways greater. The primary cultural differences are ingrained in character. Rural Appalachians speak slower with a distinctive mountain drawl; they are wary of strangers, fiercely loyal, proud, independent, strong-willed, responsible, self-reliant, and highly self-sufficient in ways that contrast with urban residents. These qualities can create special challenges and opportunities for health care providers. It can be just as difficult to recruit physicians to rural areas as to other economically depressed localities. The doctor may be the only one for miles, on call all the time. There are few specialty consultants nearby; very few resources and limited technological assistance are available. There are no cultural frills such as restaurants, theaters, orchestras, libraries, social amenities, or even friends with similar backgrounds. Even with these hardships, the opportunity to meet the social service needs, especially the health care needs, of rural residents is just as critical and can be just as rewarding as meeting the needs of those who live in urban ghettos and on the Indian reservations. There is an immediate need to address the health care problems of rural residents. People in the rural heartland are hurting. The rural health care problems of this country are unique—because of cultural differences and great distances between population centers. But these problems are deserving of sensible answers that are rooted and grounded in an understanding of and respect for rural life. The health problems of rural communities are no less demanding of remedy than those of African Americans, American Indians, Pacific Islanders, or Latinos.

Commentary by Kate Brown

Bruce White has reminded us that the needs of poor people in Appalachia are every bit as compelling as those of Hispanics and Asian-, African-, and Native-Americans. He presents a fascinating tapestry of facts and personal experiences depicting several important ethical dimensions of the current crisis of rural health care delivery and policy. White situates his analysis in his own experience as a native of Appalachia. He juxtaposes a description of the magnificent beauty and proud culture of the area with a picture of a population's health status that, in his own words, is comparable to that of an underdeveloped nation. White's plea is for this impoverished, but deserving, area of the country to be given assistance that is meaningful within the context of the cultural and geographic realities of Appalachia. He illustrates some of these realities in the story of his Aunt Beulah stirring her wood-fueled soap kettle where she is making a gift for a new neighbor and in the report of an elderly farmer in Nashville who, after learning that he will not have to sell his farm to pay for his bypass surgery, leaves a bundle of fresh vegetables with his surgeon.

One obvious ethical concern raised by White is the lack of adequate health care services for the people of rural Appalachia. There, as elsewhere in our country, people deserve adequate, affordable, and timely health care. This claim can be defended both through the language of individual rights and through a communitarian sense of common, empathetic need. Two special twists to this claim, however, are relevant to the rural context.

First, there is the question of what kinds of health care are universally deserved. I share the widespread worry that financial, or "bottom line," reasoning will dictate an intolerably low standard of care for rural residents. People need to know that they can receive competent, respectful care for their preventive and primary health care needs at a local level—whether in the city or country. We also need to recognize that there are good reasons for making different kinds of health care available in different settings. Rather than working toward the goal of a CAT scan in every rural hospital, we need first to ensure that a strong local base of primary and preventive services is available. We must also ensure the financial means, transportation, and support services that would give rural residents access to more populated centers where such technologies are more appropriately located.

This vision of triage requires comprehensive planning and coordination, two principles that are sorely lacking in the competitive model of commercialized health care delivery currently supported by government and provider policies. Furthermore, it requires a reframing of the desired standard of care. To the extent that we demand a model of health care characterized by specialists and sophisticated technologies, we risk devaluing the essential quality of "relationship," a quality that remains a rich endowment of rural life.

This aspect of life in Appalachia is skillfully illustrated in the brief vignettes shared by White. In each case, the reciprocal themes of self-sufficiency and interdependence are interwoven in stories of mutual connection. Although the need for health care services in Appalachia is profound, we are reminded by these stories that assistance must be given in ways that support a rural version of justice. Respect between rural people is often based on one's ability to reciprocate in mutually sustaining ways. As White writes, these are proud, loyal, strong-willed, responsible people who would be degraded by a handout. Although the farmer who gave his surgeon a gift of vegetables may not have had the financial means to pay for his surgery, he still gave back. Instead of money as the currency of exchange, he gave, symbolically, the gift of his life, of his livelihood. Rural health care can only flourish in an environment that fosters economic opportunities and community enrichment of the kind that enables such reciprocal relations.

10 Homelessness: A Risk Factor for Poor Health

Kristy Woods

> So that to *all*, *everywhere*, skilled succor may come in the hour of need.
> —Sir William Osler

INTRODUCTION

This chapter documents my personal experience as a physician at a free general medicine clinic from 1984 to 1987. The clinic, located in an underserved area of Chicago, was housed in a Salvation Army residence facility for recovering alcoholics and participants of a work-release state prison program. Medical care was provided to the facility's tenants and to uninsured and underinsured community residents, which included a large number of homeless men and women referred from city shelters and drop-in centers. The medical staff included two full-time physicians (in internal medicine), four part-time physicians (a psychiatrist and three general practitioners), a dentist, and a dedicated nursing staff and social service team. The clinic had approximately 15,000 patient-visits per year. This experience clearly demonstrated the difficulties that homeless people have in gaining access to health care services, and the consequent health and social problems that they experience.

In this chapter I will identify those who currently comprise the homeless population and will present an overview of their health status. Case studies from my own experience will be used to depict some of the complex (and often preventable) psychological, social, and health predicaments of the homeless. Finally, I will address some of the existing barriers to quality health care in this population and suggest approaches to overcoming them.

WHO ARE THE NEW HOMELESS?

The image of America's homeless has changed considerably over the past few decades, as have the names used to refer to them (Brickner et al. 1990). The stereotype of a "homeless person" used to be the inhabitant of skid row, referred to by historically evolving names such as hobos, tramps, drunks, winos, inebriates, bums, vagrants, derelicts, bag-ladies, or street people. The term *skid row* was derived from early Seattle's saloon-lined streets, down which logging teams slid their loads to the mill (Morgan 1962). It accurately described the downhill course of the health and lives of the (mostly alcoholic) men who resided there. "Skid row" areas were not unusual in most major cities in the decades following World War II. The standard skid row inhabitant then was a white male, alcoholic, approximately 55 years of age, who resided in a single-room occupancy hotel or on the street (Vanderkooi 1982).

Today, the typical homeless person is much younger; nationwide, the homeless population has a median age of 33 years. There has been a shift from isolated alcohol dependence to co-dependency (alcohol and drugs) and multidrug abuse, including crack cocaine and heroin (Stark 1987). There is also an increasing percentage of ethnic minorities in the homeless population. Although the racial makeup of the poverty population varies widely between cities, on the average the split is 47% white and 53% nonwhite (38% African American, 12% Hispanic, and 3% American Indian) (Brickner et al. 1990). In Chicago and other major cities, the proportion of homeless who are African American approaches 80%. This overrepresentation reflects city demographics as well as educational and socioeconomic status.

Another group of people who were previously labeled "mentally ill" and institutionalized are now labeled "homeless" and reside on the streets. As a result of the 1960s revolution in psychiatric medical management, the community mental health movement, and civil rights advocacy for the mentally impaired (Brickner et al. 1990; Lamb 1984), hundreds of thousands of patients were deinstitutionalized from state mental health hospitals (Pepper 1987). Community resistance, inadequate federal subsidies, and general economic hardship have prevented comprehensive programs that were intended to provide psychiatric/medical care and housing for these patients from materializing (Dowart 1988; Zusman et al. 1988). The asylum function has largely been taken over by homeless shelters and, in some situations, the local jails (Belcher 1988; Carter 1991). This situation was highlighted by the killing of an elderly New York City woman by a mentally ill homeless man in January 1993. The incident prompted state officials to send a team of psychiatrists, social workers, and nurses into New York City's homeless shelters in search of potentially dangerous psychiatric patients who belonged in hospitals.

Increasing numbers of women, youth, and families are joining the ranks of the homeless as a result of economic collapse (Baldicci 1990; "Homeless Need Humane Policies" 1990). Families are perhaps the fastest growing segment, and in Chicago they represent about 37% of the total homeless population ("Homeless Need Humane Policies" 1990). A large percentage of homeless women have left home because of domestic violence and frequently must seek medical care for associated injuries (Carter 1991; Chicago Institute on Urban Poverty 1990). Most homeless women with children are unemployed, and their search for employment is often hindered by a lack of adequate child care services. In addition, many lack adequate education and job skills to obtain well-paying jobs. Homelessness itself prevents them from being able to seek employment because of the stigma attached to it, and women are often afraid to give phone numbers or addresses of shelters to potential employers. Many are unable to work night shifts owing to shelter curfews that admit people on a daily basis and may have designated sign-in times each day. Although two-thirds of women with children in shelters receive public assistance, it is usually inadequate to provide affordable housing and food for their families. In one Chicago-area study, as many as two-thirds of homeless public aid recipients were made homeless because of reductions in their welfare benefits or simply a "lost" check. Another third lost permanent residency because of rent increases, and many become homeless when the building where they reside is condemned (Carter 1991; Chicago Institute on Urban Poverty 1990).

Homeless youth represent another growing sector, and it is estimated that there may be as many as 2 million nationwide (Council on Scientific Affairs 1989). This number includes youth ages 21 and under who have run away from home, been kicked out of the home, or whose home situation was lost when they outgrew the age limit for foster care. The youth group is often ignored when the health problems of the homeless are considered, perhaps because they infrequently seek medical attention. Although their health problems are similar to those of the general adolescent population (including skin disorders, nutritional abnormalities, and sexually transmitted diseases), they are exacerbated by the condition of homelessness.

People who live in single-room occupancy hotels or in "marginal" housing arrangements should also be counted among the new homeless population. Their patterns of morbidity and mortality are similar to those of people living on the streets (Brickner 1985). Nationwide, as our major cities become gentrified, residents of these hotels are displaced to the streets at an increasing and alarming rate (Kolbert 1989).

HEALTH PROBLEMS OF THE HOMELESS

There are complex theories regarding the cause-and-effect relationship between chronic diseases and the living situations of those who suffer from them. Are homeless persons ill more often because they lack a stable living environment and shelter, or are they homeless as a result of chronic illness, disability, and depletion of funds due to high medical care costs? In any case, there has long been an association between chronic disease and homelessness and poor living conditions, with prevalence rates of chronic disease considerably higher among the homeless than in the general population (Bogue 1963; Savitt 1978).

Tuberculosis, mental disorders, and respiratory diseases were the most common chronic disorders in the late 1950s and early 1960s. Today, hypertension, arthritis and other musculoskeletal disorders, dental problems, peripheral vascular disease, neurological disease, gastrointestinal disorders, eye disorders, chronic obstructive pulmonary disease, and genital urinary tract problems have been added to this list (Brickner et al. 1990). AIDS and tuberculosis have increasingly become significant contributors to illness in the homeless (Bloom and Murray 1992; CDC 1992c). Illnesses related to substance abuse are also commonly the reason that homeless persons seek medical care.

The case studies presented in the following section provide a close look at three major problems (substance abuse, AIDS, and tuberculosis) and demonstrate the complex interrelation of health and social problems in the homeless.

Substance Abuse

Next to nonspecific "aches and pains," illnesses related to substance abuse are the most frequently cited reasons for homeless patients' clinic visits (Brickner et al. 1990). Although alcohol abuse continues to have a higher incidence among the homeless than the general population, it is no longer the sole intoxicant of choice (Stark 1987). Crack cocaine, heroin, and speed are becoming increasingly popular and are often mixed with each other and alcohol. The following case of a co-alcohol and drug-dependent man with a psychiatric illness shows the unique complexities of providing care for homeless patients with these conditions.

SG, a 29-year-old African-American man, came to our clinic for admission to the residential alcohol rehabilitation program. He was unemployed and resided in a single-room occupancy hotel. He had a fifteen-year history of alcohol abuse and regularly used intravenous drugs. SG appeared to be withdrawn and complained of profound depression for many years. His melancholy moods were broken intermittently by "high periods." Two years ago he had attempted suicide, yet had never received psychiatric care. A psychiatric referral through the clinic resulted in the diagnosis of a bipolar (manic-depressive) disorder, and he was started on medical treatment (lithium carbonate).

When he returned to the clinic four months later, he was enrolled in a different residential treatment program and had been sober for two weeks. SG had discontinued psychiatric followup and treatment, and was still using intravenous drugs. His mood swings had become pronounced, and he complained of muscle aches, fatigue, nausea, and loss of appetite. He was diagnosed with acute hepatitis (due to the hepatitis B virus) and hospitalized. At hospital discharge he had no residence to which he could return and was readmitted to our residential alcohol treatment program.

Psychiatric care was reinstituted, and SG remained sober, drug-free, and in the residency program for the next four to five months. When he left the program, he was again lost to all followup care. He reappeared after a six-month hiatus and was living in a men's homeless shelter. He was experiencing frequent mood fluctuations, drinking, and using intravenous drugs. He was counseled regarding high-risk behaviors and HIV transmission. SG confessed to sharing dirty needles, was sexually active, and promiscuous. When he last visited the clinic, he was living on the street, reported persistent drinking and drug use, and had symptoms suggestive of a sexually transmitted disease.

SG's alcohol/drug abuse and mental illness are characteristic of many of today's homeless. Alcoholism and drug abuse are diseases characterized by "a tendency to relapse." Those with a history of these illnesses are continually at risk of relapse, and one-half to two-thirds will have at least one relapse within the first couple of years, independent of the method of treatment used.

The chemically dependent homeless are particularly difficult to treat given (1) limited public resources, (2) lack of successful drug abuse treatment programs, (3) few options incorporating prolonged recovery strategies, and (4) the many psychological and social problems associated with homelessness. Even if treatment is successful, sending a sober person back to life on the streets re-exposes her to the same stressful environment that initially contributed to the substance abuse. Clearly, there is a need for increased community resources for all substance abusers, and especially for the homeless.

AIDS

AIDS demonstrates the complexities of the cause-and-effect relationship between chronic disease and homelessness. AIDS is the primary cause of death in persons aged 22 to 44 years old who reside in major inner cities; because homeless people fall into this demographic category, AIDS has now become a critical health concern for them (New York Department of Public Health 1986). One theory suggests that homelessness itself with unemployment, disaffiliation, an inadequate support system, and lack of a stable living arrangement predisposes people to AIDS high-risk behaviors such as drug use, prostitution, and promiscuity. An alternative theory suggests that major disability resulting from AIDS illness causes impoverishment and an increase in the homeless rate. With frequent loss of jobs and/or private health care benefits (Brickner et al. 1990), many AIDS patients are forced into poverty in order to qualify for Medicaid and public assistance. The number of homeless persons with AIDS nationwide is not known, and estimates vary widely. Since many of them live on the street or in abandoned buildings, accurate numbers are difficult to ascertain. Estimates from nine cities suggested an AIDS incidence of approximately 230 per 100,000 (0.23%) homeless in 1986

(Brickner et al. 1990). In 1988 it was estimated that there was a 13 to 14% incidence of AIDS among the New York homeless population (5,000 to 9,000 persons). Estimates of HIV infection among the San Francisco homeless range from 5% to 21% depending on the subgroup screened and the diagnostic criteria used (i.e., HIV positivity versus ARC versus AIDS) (Brickner et al. 1990).

While "education" has been a key element in nationwide AIDS prevention efforts, it has not been effective in changing the behavior patterns of the homeless (Brickner et al. 1989). For this group, basic priorities are obtaining food and shelter rather than limiting high-risk behavior. In addition, access to TV or the printed media may be limited, and in some situations there may be a limited ability to comprehend or comply with educational information for a variety of reasons. The following case illustrates some of the problems associated with AIDS and homelessness, highlighting the need for effective prevention strategies.

When I met DT, a 19-year-old white teenager, she had been followed at the clinic for two years. She complained of wanting "to get pregnant" and reported one unsuccessful pregnancy (miscarriage) at age 13. Since then she had failed to conceive despite frequent episodes of unprotected intercourse. DT's past medical history included intravenous drug use (for three years), and she was currently using heroin daily. She had a history of hepatitis B and sexually transmitted diseases, including gonorrhea, herpes, and chlamydia. Other habits included heavy alcohol consumption, cigarette smoking, and marijuana use. At that time, DT lived with her parents and two siblings, had dropped out of high school after one year, and was unemployed. She was involved in a monogamous relationship with her boyfriend, who also used intravenous drugs. She was counseled regarding her high-risk behaviors, referred for drug rehabilitation, and advised against pregnancy.

Five months later DT came in for treatment of a local abscess, and she reported continued drug use. Her medical problem was treated again, and she was counseled regarding high-risk behaviors. Seven months passed before her next clinic visit. Still using drugs, DT requested a pregnancy test that was positive. Screening prenatal labs revealed anemia, inadequate immunity for rubella (German measles), a positive test for syphilis, and a negative HIV test. She was referred to a high-risk obstetrics clinic and was not seen again for a year.

On her return, DT stated that while in prison six months ago, she had delivered a healthy baby. She was presently on parole, drug-free, and in a work-release program. Her boyfriend was incarcerated, and her mother cared for the infant. The reason DT had presented to the clinic this time was to obtain "another opinion" after having been recently informed that her baby had AIDS. She expressed confusion and disbelief, as her prenatal HIV test had been negative. Yet, DT confessed to using intravenous drugs until the sixth month of the pregnancy. As expected, her repeat HIV test was positive, and she was referred for drug and HIV counseling.

Two weeks later the clinic was informed that DT had resumed her drug habit, as documented by a routine urine screening test. Her sporadic visits to the medical clinic continued over the next year. At the time of her last encounter she had "jumped parole," was living on the street with her boyfriend, and continued to use intravenous drugs.

This case offers one view of the difficulties, frustrations, and unfortunate consequences often encountered in attempting to change high-risk behavior with limited resources. Nationwide, there is a deficiency in AIDS education and drug treatment programs for the homeless. Effective drug treatment and rehabilitation programs are essential for the prevention of HIV infection. In addition, strategies to reach this population must include going into areas where the homeless congregate, discussing and providing information regarding safe sex and free condoms.

Some drug treatment programs consisting of methadone maintenance combined with HIV counseling have been found to be effective in decreasing the rate of HIV infection (Abdul-Quades et al. 1987; Brickner et al. 1989). Research has also shown that persons with stable housing arrangements are more likely to remain drug-free after treatment (Brickner et al. 1990). Therefore, housing must be recognized as a primary need in the prevention of HIV infection in the homeless population.

Treating the clinical spectrum of HIV infection can be a formidable task for those caring for the homeless. Many patients have coexisting medical problems; many are skeptical regarding the health care system and do not seek medical care until late in the course of the disease. Patients often present to clinics or emergency rooms without revealing their positive HIV status. The combination of a lack of background information, atypical presentations of disease pathology, poor general health status, and lack of access to regular followup care can make early, accurate diagnoses and proper treatment enigmatic for the most skilled clinician. Furthermore, many complications that would normally be managed in an outpatient setting result in prolonged hospitalization for homeless patients due to inadequate conditions for convalescence, including housing, nutrition, and supportive services (Small et al. 1988).

Tuberculosis

In the early twentieth century, tuberculosis (TB) was the number one cause of death in the United States. In the late 1950s a U.S. Public Health Service survey reported a tuberculosis death rate thirty-seven times greater for skid row men than for men in the general population (Bogue 1963). Nationally, with the advent of public health programs and effective antibiotics, the number of TB cases reported annually declined steadily between 1953 and 1984. The decline represented a 70% decrease in incidence rate from 84,304 cases or 53 per 100,000 in 1953, to 22,255 cases or 9.4 per 100,000 in 1984 (Reider et al. 1989).

As a result of poverty, homelessness, drug abuse, and HIV disease, there has been a resurgence of tuberculosis since 1984. In 1991 the annual incidence rate had risen to 26,283 cases or 10.4 per 100,000. Given the previous rate of decline, the Center for Disease Control calculates an excess of over 39,000 cases in the past seven years.

Despite the unprecedented recent increases, TB cases remain clustered in certain populations. Factors describing populations at increased risk include poor nutrition, HIV infection, older age, sex (men are at higher risk), and birth in a country with a high TB prevalence rate. Place of residence is a risk factor as TB has always been found to spread in overcrowded environments. In the current epidemic, transmission has been documented in homeless shelters, drug treatment centers, and residential AIDS care facilities.

Race (as it defines socioeconomic status and geographic area of residence) is also considered a risk factor. In 1992 almost 70% of all active cases of TB in the United States (and over 85% of cases in children under 15 years old) occurred in ethnic minorities. Between 1985 and 1991 there was an increased incidence of 72% in Hispanics, 26% in non-Hispanic blacks, and 32% in Asian/Pacific Islanders. During the same time period there was a decline in cases reported among non-Hispanic whites and Native Americans.

In addition, new drug-resistant strains of tuberculosis have emerged that are rapidly progressive and have a high mortality despite treatment. These new strains have occurred primarily because of patient noncompliance with therapeutic regimens (Dooley et al. 1992; Snider and Roper 1992). The following case illustrates some of the epidemiological and management problems in caring for homeless patients with tuberculosis.

JR, a 57-year-old homeless Hispanic man, was presented to the clinic after being discharged from the county hospital. He spoke little English but carried a discharge summary sheet with the following diagnoses: (1) chronic alcoholism, (2) reactivation tuberculosis, (3) scabies (parasites), (4) cellulitis, and (5) a history of frostbite. Prior to hospitalization, JR had lost 15 pounds but had been otherwise without symptoms of pulmonary infection. His admission chest X-ray had been suggestive of reactivation tuberculosis. Sputum smears for TB were negative, and culture results were pending at time of discharge. JR was given a supply of standard TB medications and referred to our clinic for supervision of therapy and followup. He soon failed to appear for daily medication. Six weeks later, the clinic was notified that the tuberculosis cultures were positive, indicating that he had active disease. Attempts to locate JR at local shelters and detoxification centers were unsuccessful, and the Chicago Tuberculosis Control Board was notified. The next contact with JR was one year later. Again, he had been referred to the clinic following a hospitalization, during which he had been treated for a foot laceration. Although he had lost his discharge summary, his containers of tuberculosis medications indicated that he was still being treated. This time he was admitted to the residential unit of our facility for medical supervision. JR reported for daily medication for six weeks until he went out on pass one afternoon and did not return; residents reported seeing him at a local liquor store.

This pattern of alcoholic relapse, loss to followup care, noncompliance with medication, and sporadic hospital and clinic visits with reinstitution of therapy continued over the next two years. JR's tuberculosis remained inadequately treated.

The homeless experience "double jeopardy" in regard to TB. Not only are they at a high risk of developing TB, but once they develop it, homeless conditions make it unlikely that they will receive curative therapy. TB control is challenging in the homeless because of issues such as concomitant substance abuse, poor nutrition, lack of incentives for treatment, and need for shelter and a place to convalesce.

Control of tuberculosis in patients in group living situations is further complicated by the (previously discussed) high prevalence of HIV infection in this population. Numerous epidemiological studies have confirmed the strong link between HIV and TB infection (Dooley et al. 1992; Murray 1989; Snider and Roper 1992).

Detection and treatment of TB in the homeless have been most successful when treatment programs are tied to housing and food programs (Brickner et al. 1990; Reichman et al. 1979). Close cooperation between local TB control boards and caregivers can assist in ensuring continued treatment once an individual leaves a shelter or fails to make a followup appointment. Better methods of screening, giving preventive medications, and ensuring compliance and followup need to be devised for preventive programs to succeed.

ROUTINE HEALTH MAINTENANCE AND PREVENTIVE CARE: VIRTUALLY NONEXISTENT IN THE HOMELESS

The emergency health care system, where the homeless frequently receive care, offers little in terms of continuity of services, long-term followup, or preventive services. The lack of proper preventive services and delayed treatment of early disease frequently result in the need for more costly and extensive health care services. The costs are high not only monetarily, but also in terms of human suffering and reduced quality of life for the homeless patients. In this section, I will discuss several preventable health conditions that are overrepresented, yet inadequately addressed in the homeless population.

Immunization efforts have historically reduced vaccine-preventable diseases in children, yet there have been recent cuts in the funding of childhood immunization programs (Edelman 1987). Studies of children in Boston and New York City revealed a marked delay in the immunization rate of homeless children as compared to children that were domiciled (49% versus 12% and 27% versus 8%, respectively) (Alperstein et al. 1988; Wise et al. 1985). Adults who were not infected or immunized during childhood are also at increased risk of certain infectious diseases and their complications (CDC 1990b). In addition, the lifestyles, poor nutritional status, and increased incidence of chronic disease among the homeless make them particularly vulnerable to contracting preventable diseases.

Measles, a vaccine-preventable disease, which experienced a resurgence in 1989, has been targeted for complete elimination by the year 2000. In 1990 over 27,000 measles cases were reported in the United States, the highest number in over a decade. Over 75% of these cases occurred in individuals who were unvaccinated or inadequately vaccinated. In children under 5 years of age, the measles incidence in 1991 for Indian, Hispanic, and African-American children was, respectively, nineteen, six, and four times greater than for non-Hispanic white children (CDC 1992a).

Selective implementation of immunization programs has neglected certain groups. For instance, prematriculation immunization requirements (PIRs) were instituted on college and university campuses to ensure adequate levels of immunity among the college student population (American College Health Association 1983). Yet there has been no similar "mandatory" immunization policy to prevent disease in the vulnerable homeless youth and young adults in this country.

Each year hepatitis B virus (HBV) infection occurs in an estimated 300,000 persons, and approximately 4,800 persons per year die from HBV-related cirrhosis and liver cancer (CDC 1990a). Because transmission of HBV occurs through exchange of body fluids (similar to HIV transmission), it is of particular concern among today's homeless population, which is younger, sexually active, and comprised of increasing numbers of substance abusers. Recently, there has been a 76.9% increase in hepatitis B infection among the heterosexual population and 77.1% among IV drug users (Alter et al. 1990). Special immunization efforts are clearly needed to prevent the spread of HBV infection, and they must be extended to the homeless as well as the general population, in view of their prevalence of high-risk behaviors.

The high incidence of the common cold and other respiratory conditions among the indigent and homeless has been well documented (Bogue 1963; Savitt 1978). In the 1950s the death rate of skid row inhabitants due to respiratory disease and pneumonia was well over ten times the national average (Bogue 1963). At our clinic, respiratory infections (primarily viral upper respiratory tract infections) were the most common acute problems causing patients to seek medical attention. Other studies have also reported high rates of influenza and pneumonia (Brickner et al. 1990). Although immunization awareness has recently increased, influenza vaccination rates remain low (approximately 30%) in most high-risk populations and in those with minimal access to care (CDC 1992b).

Heart disease continues to be a primary cause of death in the United States (CDC 1989). One review of indigent patients admitted to a major inner city hospital with a diagnosis of myocardial infarction found mortality rates to be 12.7%, compared to 8% in the general population (Castaner et al. 1988). Risk factor screening and treatment efforts made available to the general population in the 1980s have not reached the homeless population for a number of reasons, including the focus on other more crucial medical and social concerns. Hypertension, the most common chronic problem in the country, was the second most common diagnosis (behind alcohol/substance abuse) in our clinic. Hypertension screening programs developed over the past twenty years have significantly reduced the morbidity and mortality rates due to cardiovascular, cerebrovascular, and renal disease (Mosner 1983). Again, the homeless population remains largely untouched by these programs. Hypertension has a higher prevalence in the African-American population (Pratt et al. 1989); with increasing numbers of African-American homeless, there is an additional need for aggressive outreach, screening programs, and a patient-oriented hypertension treatment approach. The case presented next reveals the difficulty of treating hypertension in homeless situations.

NW, a 52-year-old African-American man with alcoholism and hypertension, had been sober for over a year when I first encountered him at the clinic. His blood pressure was poorly controlled (150/106), and he had "run out" of medication three days ago. His previous treatment regimen was reinstituted, he was given enough medication for one month, and he was advised to continue alcoholism counseling. He was compliant with his scheduled followup appointments and medications, resulting in well-controlled blood pressure for the next three months.

Then NW had an alcohol relapse; he presented to the clinic intoxicated, complained of stomach irritation, and his blood pressure was elevated. Medical treatment was reinstituted, and although he was referred to an alcohol detoxification program, he did not comply.

He missed several appointments before returning to the clinic. Again, he smelled of alcohol and had been out of medication "for a while"; his blood pressure was 178/110. He was treated in the clinic, and medications were once again restarted. This pattern of missed appointments and noncompliance persisted for six months while he continued drinking. He was sober, intermittently, for only five months of the next two-year period.

This case demonstrates that even when preventive services are available, circumstances associated with homelessness and concomitant conditions (such as alcoholism) often limit their effectiveness. Effective new strategies that address preventive health issues are needed. Other preventive health care services, such as glaucoma screening and routine cancer surveillance (including Pap smears, mammography, colon and prostate cancer screening), are often lacking as well. These preventive services are often overlooked because of lack of continuous care, or are simply not considered worth doing because of difficulties in followup (Woolhander and Himmelstein 1989). Cancer mortality rates are significantly higher among indigent populations with poor access to care. This is in part due to the lack of early screening; other contributing factors are increased stress and unhealthy lifestyles (including smoking, alcohol abuse, and low-fiber, high-fat diets) (Saunders 1991).

Barriers to Care

Providing humane, accessible, and quality medical care for the homeless population can be a formidable task for health care workers, as evidenced by the four cases presented in this chapter. In each of these instances, merely addressing the medical problems of the patients was not enough to effect a change in health status.

The homeless sick are totally dependent on the services of free clinics for care because they lack Medicaid coverage. They often do not have Medicaid coverage because they cannot qualify for benefits without an address or place of residence. In addition, the majority have difficulty in obtaining, completing, and posting the complicated paperwork required of Medicaid applicants, and few hospitals or clinics will accept homeless "charity" patients on a nonemergency basis. Other barriers include distance from shelters or temporary residences to the medical facility and lack of money for transportation, as well as lengthy emergency room and clinic waits. Curfew times at shelters and designated meal times at drop-in centers may further restrict accessibility to health care. Given these choices (food and shelter versus medical care for an ailment), it becomes easier to understand why homeless persons frequently wait until symptoms are severe before seeking medical care (Filardo 1985). Consequently, health care is administered in the emergency room (Brickner et al. 1990).

Once a person has obtained medical attention, an impression is formed about the health care system. All too frequently, homeless patients perceive their interaction with health care providers negatively and are unwilling to return for followup care. In addition to extended waiting periods, the health care providers may not be as sensitive to the feelings and emotional needs of homeless patients as they are to those of insured or paying patients. Patients speak of being treated rudely and with callousness, of their physicians' inability to understand their complaints, and of their inability to understand their physicians. Many patients do not understand the value of early medical intervention in treating disease, do not recognize the early warning symptoms, and do not make the association between certain behaviors and poor health. In addition, the health care provider may not understand the cultural background of the homeless patient. These educational and cultural differences, as well as a lack of sensitivity to the plight of the homeless, frequently result in poor relationships between the patients and their health care provider.

Difficulties associated with medication use are further obstacles to providing health care to the homeless. If prescribed medications are obtainable, they are frequently lost or stolen on the streets. Some homeless shelters have rules forbidding drugs of any kind and confiscate even prescription drugs from shelter residents. Medications requiring refrigeration (i.e., insulin) or special instructions create a special dilemma. Homeless people frequently have difficulty adhering to medication schedules, for example, every four to six hours or every eight hours. Not everyone has a watch or access to a clock to determine the time for medications. Medications prescribed to be taken with or after meals present a problem when meals are erratic or absent, and if taken without food may cause complications (i.e., gastrointestinal irritation with anti-inflammatory drugs or tetracycline). These factors contribute to making drug levels in the blood difficult to control (i.e., seizure medications and anticoagulants). All four cases clearly show that addicted patients often continue their habits while receiving medication. Concomitant treatment of drug and alcohol abuse is a difficult, yet necessary, part of any medical management plan.

The side effects of certain medications need to be considered when discussing noncompliance. For example, in a homeless hypertensive patient with no access to bathroom facilities, an increasing frequency of urination due to a diuretic can create an additional stress. Drowsiness or fatigue due to certain antihypertensives can cause difficulty when a person is sleeping on the street or dependent on a shelter bed. Nonpharmaceutical treatments are practically impossible in the setting of homelessness. Even with adequate treatment of infectious diseases, re-infection is common among patients in communal living arrangements (Bogue 1963; Brickner 1985; Brickner et al. 1990; Savitt 1978). Lack of an adequate place or ability for convalescence, as well as overall poor nutritional status and personal hygiene, may prolong the recovery course and worsen the prognosis of most illnesses. Lack of continuity of care and inadequate support systems or advocacy programs for homeless patients profoundly affect clinical effectiveness in all areas of medical management.

Providers caring for the homeless face many unique challenges. Feelings of frustration are common in the most dedicated practitioners, as their patients' social and psychological problems are often counterproductive to whatever medical care can be offered. Much time is spent completing routine physician's forms for entitlements, rehabilitation programs, shelters, or job applications. Because the homeless generally have unkempt appearances, low educational achievements, and many suffer from depressive disorders, communication is often arduous. After years of exposure to such patients, it is not uncommon for the staff to adopt some of the same behaviors (Brickner et al. 1990).

As would be expected, provider "burnout" or fatigue is common. It can adversely affect the quality of care provided as well as the health and quality of life of the provider (Shannon and Saleebey 1980). As exhaustion and frustration become pronounced, negative feelings may develop toward both the practice and the patients. This may take the form of trivializing patients' complaints. Practitioners may use medical terminology incomprehensible to the patients and fail even to attempt to educate patients regarding their illnesses. If burnout is severe, clinical decision making may suffer, and providers themselves may embrace unhealthy lifestyles (i.e., excessive smoking or alcohol consumption). Personality conflicts, incompetence, and unreliability of fellow workers (including frequent tardiness or missed days from work) can contribute to burnout.

Preventive measures can and should be taken to prevent fatigue among health care providers. Setting realistic treatment goals helps to ease feelings of futility. These goals should be in line with the existing psychological and social framework of the patients' lives. Keeping an open level of communication in the workplace and access to problem-solving forums is vital to the providers' intellectual well-being. Professional affiliations should be maintained, continuing education courses attended, and foremost, time should be scheduled away from direct patient services (Moulder et al. 1988).

People often have preconceived ideas that all homeless/indigent persons are drunks, lazy, or malingerers, and therefore "not entitled to" routine standards of care. There have been arguments that expanding the number of treatment facilities available will not improve the health-seeking behavior in this group because they "do not want help." However, studies have documented this population's willingness to take part in their health care if presented with acceptable options (New York Department of Health 1983–88). As important as expanding access to services, however, is the need to improve the sensitivity of the health care providers treating the indigent. The health care providers that they encounter are usually white, well educated, and middle class, often adding to their uneasiness in seeking medical care. Some of this reluctance could potentially be alleviated if the ethnicity of the health care providers better reflected the population being served (see Ferguson, Chapter 11, in this volume).

CONCLUSIONS

I have identified several new features of "the homeless" as they exist today, and have used case studies to demonstrate some of the special health concerns and problems of attempting to provide them with adequate medical care. Recent problems include co-alcohol/drug dependence, cultural variability, and increased number of psychiatrically impaired, and increasing numbers of homeless families (women with children). I have outlined diverse obstacles to quality care, including patients' reluctance to seek care, the attitudes of health care providers and the health care system as a whole, inability to comply with medical therapy, and a lack of rehabilitation programs. Most commonly, however, the health care problems in this group result from lack of access to preventive and basic health care services—the same services that modern medicine is capable of providing to those who can afford them.

The past decade has seen a magnification of the drug problem affecting all levels of our society, the escalation of the AIDS epidemic, an increase in the numbers of unemployed, and the emergence of homelessness as a major social, political, and health issue. With over 37 million Americans uninsured or underinsured (representing a 45% jump since the early 1980s), masses of people are descending on the emergency rooms of public hospitals and the scattered public clinics. Many without adequate coverage are now in need of high-cost care due to lack of routine and preventive medical services. The federal and local governments have been unable to underwrite the increasing financial burdens. The result has been patient overload with severe crowding of emergency rooms and public hospitals, further eroding the poor's access to primary health care services and thus creating a vicious cycle.

Certainly, many confounding variables negatively influence the effectiveness of care provided to the indigent and homeless. That we allow such financial waste in our health care system is unacceptable. The costs of job training, outpatient alcohol/drug treatment programs, and preventive hypertensive and psychiatric treatment are far less draining on the system (and more humane) than repeated emergency room visits or days in the hospital. The fact that vaccine-preventable diseases continue to take their toll and that certain segments of our society are devoid of virtually any preventive medical services is not only a public health hazard, but a national tragedy.

The poor health status of the homeless population reflects a much larger national problem in access and delivery of health care services. Increasingly, health care and modern medicine are being considered a privilege, reserved only for those with financial access to it. The problems facing America's homeless will remain largely unchanged, until access to quality health care for all socioeconomic-economic groups becomes a national priority.

Commentary by Christine K. Cassel

The professional who works with homeless patients confronts the moral question: "How far does responsibility extend?" Some feel responsible only for those people who appear in their office as patients, and even then only for those diagnostic and therapeutic recommendations related to physiologic disorders, and not to social problems that the patient may experience. But the philosophy of public health implies the physician's responsibility to reach out to the community, to recognize community hazards, and to interact with the political and social processes needed to improve the health of the public.

There is ample evidence that for any given medical condition, a person with inadequate income or education is likely to have a much worse outcome for that disorder, or to be at a higher risk for contracting diseases such as diabetes, hypertension, coronary heart disease, and many kinds of cancers. Physicians alone cannot create justice in an unjust world, but they can be important members of a community striving to improve the living standards for all its members. Meanwhile, people who are the unfortunate victims of social inequities or who are vulnerable to the inherent risks of chronic psychiatric or behavioral disorders do get sick and may appear as patients. Woods's article extensively reviews medical issues likely to occur in individual people who are homeless, as well as major public health issues that occur in homeless populations. She describes the dramatic change in the profile of homelessness that occurred over the 1980s and 1990s: from primarily white male alcoholics to a much more diverse group of men, women, and children with a greater proportion of people of color and a much higher percentage of people with chronic mental illness. The health problems they suffer are often related to alcohol and substance abuse, to lack of access to preventive care, and to exposure. Thus, a physician has to be prepared to treat everything from bacterial endocarditis and delirium tremens, to tuberculosis, AIDS, venereal disease, frostbite, malnutrition, hepatitis, and measles, as well as chronic diseases endemic in our society, such as heart disease, hypertension, and diabetes. She gives excellent practical advice on the barriers to traditional medical care in homeless people. For example, compliance with medication is difficult if the patient has no way of keeping track of time for multiple dosage medications, is at constant risk of having medication stolen, or sleeps in a shelter where even prescription drugs are forbidden. Diuretic therapy can be extremely difficult for a person who doesn't have easy access to a bathroom. These, and other social considerations, must be included in treatment plans if care is to be structured in a useful way.

Ethics issues are most strongly posed in the social problems complicating the care of these patients. If a homeless man has problems with frostbite related to exposure to cold and wet environments, would it not make more sense medically to get that person housing, rather than to figure out ways of getting him appropriate foot care? Here I believe Woods's chapter embodies a fundamental question for all health professionals and in particular, for medical ethicists. Most of biomedical ethics has distinguished between bedside clinical decision making and issues of social justice and resource allocation. The clinical issues raised by the care of the homeless show us that it is an illusion that these two can be so cleanly separated. From a moral perspective, it seems impossible for a physician who is truly concerned with the health of a homeless patient not to address the problems that led to that person's homelessness, whether it be inadequate mental health services or inadequate low-income housing in the community. Inadequate housing in particular is not a traditionally defined medical problem, but it shows us the implications for medical ethics of our understanding of the increasingly tight links between socioeconomic realities and health.

PART 3
ETHICAL RESPONSIBILITIES AND THE MEDICAL PROFESSION

11 The Physician's Responsibility to Medically Underserved Poor People

Warren J. Ferguson

INTRODUCTION

Ethical discussions of rights and access to health care often focus on government and corporate policies. Rarely, however, do these discussions examine the choices and responsibilities physicians must face daily in delivering primary health care to the disenfranchised. Although a myriad of issues influence the practicing physician's sense of duty and his or her decision to care for the poor, the limited capability of generating income by serving poor people, though real, is often overemphasized. Just as important, many physicians are uncomfortable interacting with people whose language, culture, sexual orientation, and socioeconomic status are different from their own.

In this chapter, first I will argue that physicians and their organizations must take responsibility for understanding attitudes and values that shape their delivery of health care to the underserved. Second, I will present vignettes of actual discussions with physicians who work with underserved populations. I will emphasize how personal views about the poor can either maintain or reduce the distance between physician and patient. Finally, I will discuss the implications of physician responsibility for medical education and the socialization of the physician.

THE RESPONSIBILITY OF AUTONOMY

Although physicians are under severe public scrutiny in an increasingly restrictive practice environment, their autonomy is still well established within the U.S. medical system. Doctors are free to set up practice in any geographic location and to accept patients at their discretion. The greatest challenge to their autonomy may ultimately come from the inequitable distribution of medical personnel across the country. Most physicians would agree that the lack of access to health care is a serious social problem, and many provide some care to the disenfranchised. Yet, they are also overwhelmed by the enormity of the situation and are confused about what their individual role should be in finding a solution.

Philosophers and medical ethicists may be able to guide physicians through the anxiety of their moral uncertainty. Edmund Pellegrino, for example, upholds autonomy, but believes that the profession also has an ethical responsibility to ensure that all segments of the population have access to health care. He notes that "fulfilling such ethical imperatives is sure to cause discomfort for the doctor as well as some loss of privileges and even of remuneration. However, unless concern translates into action, restrictive legislation to achieve these ends seems certain" (Pellegrino 1987, p. 59).

The real threat to autonomy then is the profession's own inflexibility and lack of action in responding to a societal need. When the potential of an imposed systemic change in the delivery of health care threatens physician autonomy, the concern for equity in health care takes a back seat to physicians' freedom to contract with whomever they choose. Without changes in physicians' attitudes and values, however, their autonomy will most likely have to be restricted in order to address the inequities in access to health care. A solution by the profession will be difficult without acknowledging the ethical dilemmas that individual physicians face in delivery of service to the underserved.

Pellegrino places this weighty responsibility of identifying ethical dilemmas on the shoulders of the profession as a whole, and delegates to the individual physician a narrower role (Pellegrino 1987). He states that each physician must establish some hierarchy of values and priorities that will define his or her individual and social ethical postures. By necessity, the physician's first-order priority is moral integrity in dealing with the patients he or she treats. The second-order responsibility is in helping shape policies that bear directly on the health of the larger community. For the majority of physicians, the line between these priorities is at best quite fuzzy. For physicians in rural towns and inner cities, where the demand for health care outweighs the supply, the moral dilemmas in choosing to exclude certain groups or individuals from care are stark and daily realities. Often overworked, these autonomous physicians "in the trenches" have no forum in which to examine their decisions. Traditional ethical discussions provide little guidance, because, as Leon Kass points out, "in ethics, the search for clarity, consistency and coherence has limited its scope. Little time has been spent on what genuinely moves people to act—their motives and passions; that is, their loves and hates, hopes and fears, pride and prejudice, matters that are sometimes dismissed as non-ethical or irrational because they are not simply reducible to logos" (Kass 1990, p. 7).

The majority of physicians seem to care deeply and have some sense of responsibility for the health care of the disenfranchised. While there is little economic incentive to work in poor communities, the economic factor has been overemphasized and used as a smokescreen to avoid facing the painful reality of the humanness of the physician. The fact is that physicians often shy away from members of society with language, culture, sexual orientation, and health habits different from their own. As David Hilfiker puts it, "If a patient cannot articulate his history, has a fourth-grade education, compounds hypertension with alcoholism, cannot afford laboratory evaluation or medications, is unable to return for consistent follow-up because of problems at home, and cannot afford a place to live, we who are trained to treat diseases will feel at sea" (Hilfiker 1987, p. 3156).

Historically, the profession has reinforced this distance between the physician and the poor patient. For example, physicians care for the disenfranchised in hospital clinics where care is discontinuous, rather than incorporating these patients into their private practices. In urban areas, the care of the indigent is often delegated to the house officer in charge of teaching services or to the outpatient clinic.

The editors of the *Journal of the American Medical Association (JAMA)* and the *Journal of the American Bar Association (JABA))* suggest that every physician and attorney provide at least fifty hours of free care each year to help alleviate the unequal distribution of health care and legal services (Lundberg and Bodine 1987). Unfortunately, this suggestion accepts and reinforces the existing distance between poor people and professionals. The implication of the suggestion is that physicians should deliver free care at a site separate from their usual practice. After completing free service at a clinic, the physician's obligation to those patients is over, but in private clinics the physician's obligation is to provide continuous care. If a physician were to incorporate free care into his or her private practice, there would be no means of limiting the free care to fifty hours per year. What happens when a physician has already fulfilled his or her fifty hours and an uninsured patient requires continued management of a chronic disease such as diabetes? Such neatly packaged suggestions do not do service to the complex ethical dilemmas facing physicians who want to provide service to poor or uninsured people.

THE UNASSIGNED EMERGENCY ADMISSION AND FOLLOWUP CARE

Many poor and underserved patients who have no personal physician receive their health care in hospital emergency rooms. Hospital physicians are assigned to them on a rotating basis. Once viewed as a privilege of staff appointment, physicians in communities with large underserved populations now view such service as a chore. Although relationships may be established during hospitalization, many physicians think that their duty to care for poor emergency patients extends only to the end of hospitalization. In contracting with the hospital—not the patient—they abdicate their responsibility to provide continuous care to poor patients.

Without continuity of care and adequate followup, the patient will likely return to the emergency room with the same problems. However, attempts to call the same physician for readmission typically result in an angry assertion that "the patient is not my patient. That was a service admission." The patient is then seen by another physician who may not be familiar with the patient's medical and social history. A cycle of emergency illness and discontinuity of care thus ensues.

The autonomous physician's freedom of contract has superseded responsibility to sick people. Perhaps even more disturbing is the physician's apparent unfairness in choosing to continue care for some free service patients, while refusing to care for others. Who are the "lucky" ones? Often, they are individuals who had no previous need to see a physician and are simply seeking treatment for an acute illness. The physician takes a liking to them, views them as a value to the practice, and thus offers opportunity for followup. They are the patients for whom the physician feels compassion and hope, a sense that they can be helped; they deserve to be helped. The unlucky patients, on the other hand, are those with a "social" illness such as alcoholism where lack of compliance and personal hygiene is anticipated and judged to be disruptive to the physician's practice. Usually, they are individuals with a culture, race, language, or sexual orientation that precludes a sense of comfort or identification for the physician. These differences between patient and physician can be more significant barriers to equal access to health care than the ability to pay.

ACCESS TO PERINATAL SERVICES

In this section, I will present a scenario depicting how two groups of physicians—obstetricians/gynecologists and pediatricians—respond differently to the needs of uninsured patients in a community of poor Latino immigrants with limited access to employment and an alarmingly high rate of infant mortality. These immigrants live in a small city thirty miles from a major metropolis. Although the only general hospital in the area is located in this city, the majority of physicians on staff maintain offices in the surrounding wealthier suburbs.

Although the gynecologists and obstetricians on staff do not accept Medicaid, the hospital maintains a free prenatal clinic. All ob-gyns are expected to help staff the clinic and provide health care for the indigent, caring for women in labor and handling gynecologic emergencies for women without doctors. This arrangement pleases neither patient nor physician. Patients experience long waits at the clinic as well as discontinuity of care. Physicians, moreover, loathe being on service call, finding it burdensome to maintain their own practices while at the same time donating care to the clinic population.

The state initiated a study to investigate the high infant mortality rate.

Research confirmed what was obvious to health care providers and to the community: the majority of prenatal patients received inadequate prenatal care. In an attempt to facilitate access to such care, the state established a dialogue with community physicians. Physicians presented a number of explanations for inadequate access. They complained that the reimbursement schedule for Medicaid was inadequate and that the billing system was too inefficient for them to consider accepting Medicaid patients. One physician stated that if the state would provide Blue Cross/Blue Shield for Medicaid recipients, he would be happy to care for all comers. Subsequently, Medicaid reimbursement for obstetric services was made more lucrative.

Unfortunately, however, reimbursement for gynecologic procedures was not increased. Medicaid guidelines mandate that physicians cannot accept Medicaid patients for one type of care and yet exclude them from other services. Therefore, the ob-gyns still refused to take Medicaid patients. The following year infant mortality had risen even further, and more meetings were held. At these meetings, physicians noted that difficulties in reimbursement remained. Other problems were raised having nothing to do with Medicaid. One physician was deeply concerned about his ability to communicate with Latino patients because he did not speak Spanish. Citing history-taking as the most important part of care and noting that relationship-building was key to avoiding malpractice, he was disinclined to open his practice to Latinos. Another physician remarked that Latinos frequently missed their appointments and that this would affect his efficiency. All felt strongly that the hospital clinic was working well and was therefore more effective than private practice for delivering care to the Latino community. They also felt that the state and the hospital had the responsibility for recruiting Spanish-speaking ob-gyns rather than taking it upon themselves to learn Spanish. In addition to the real and obvious economic difficulties, cultural and linguistic differences posed a deeper, subtler, and more divisive barrier to health care. The problem of access was not resolved after childbirth. Pediatricians also refused to accept Medicaid patients. When a local health center closed its doors to new patients, ob-gyns had no place to refer infants born at the free hospital clinic.

Although pediatricians and ob-gyn physicians had similar problems with Medicaid reimbursement, their responses to these problems were very different. Both physician groups honored their contractual agreements with the hospital to care for individuals without physicians. The ob-gyns fulfilled their obligation by volunteering at the hospital clinic, whereas the pediatricians—concerned about the continuity of care in a clinic system—opted not to work in a pediatric clinic. Instead, they made arrangements to see the babies for free in their private practices. The pediatricians clearly felt a responsibility to go beyond their contractual relationship with the hospital. They were willing to acknowledge the importance of their individual relationships with newborn babies and their parents and to continue those relationships. Nonetheless, they still struggled with other important barriers to access, including language and transportation difficulties. Several ethical values underlie the pediatricians' sense of responsibility in caring for children, apart from their cultural and economic differences. First, children ought not to be held accountable for lacking insurance. Second, children are an important investment in the future of society, and as such, pediatricians ought to be committed to reducing the alarming infant mortality rate.

The ob-gyns' arguments for maintaining the clinic system of care also require comment. Putting aside issues of reimbursement, let's examine their attitudes toward cultural and linguistic differences. In response to communication difficulties, the hospital employed a translator for the prenatal clinic; that is, physicians did not consider it their responsibility to learn Spanish. Although a translator narrows the gap, it is not the optimal solution to ensure quality communication. Direct communication is necessary for a complete and accurate medical history and is critical to the development of the doctor-patient relationship.

It was my impression that aside from language, the ob-gyns felt uncomfortable with the cultural differences between themselves and their adult Latina patients. There was a discernible belief that patients should work harder to better themselves, that they should speak English, and that they should be employed rather than be on public assistance. Thus, the unspoken value was that the patient had to prove herself worthy of quality health care.

VALUES, ATTITUDES, AND THE PROCESS OF MEDICAL EDUCATION

The last decade has witnessed striking changes in the funding of medical education. The majority of medical students are now forced to take out massive loans, often leaving them with debts in excess of $100,000. Consequently, there is an ever increasing focus on the costs and benefits of medical school. Never before have students been so aware of the salaries and malpractice rates of various specialties. Such considerations greatly influence a student's specialty choice and have perhaps contributed to the steady decline of student interest in such relatively low-earning specialties as primary care. Moreover, decreasing support for programs aimed at expanding services to the poor, such as the National Health Service Corps, has further reduced student interest in working with the underserved. While this focus on the economics of medicine is worrisome, even more dramatic are the changes in student attitudes and values that have arisen over the course of their medical education. In a superb and careful study of the socialization of house officers and medical students, Terry Mizrahi has shown significant personality changes in students—from idealistic, humanistic, and compassionate to hedonistic, cynical, and judgmental (Mizrahi 1986).

Fortunately, medical educators have reacted to this research with calls for radical change in the education of physicians (Department of Health and Human Services 1988). Courses on communication, ethics, and values and attitude clarification are now part of some medical school curricula. Moreover, the expectations of house officers in terms of work hours and workload have undergone substantial change. Some faculty physicians act as role models by including poor patients in their private practices rather than relegating them to the house officer in the hospital clinic. While these reforms are encouraging, they merely scratch the surface. Most medical students and residents still receive the majority of their training in teaching hospitals. Yet hospitalization can rob a patient of his or her dignity—people are too sick to be happy, well kept, and grateful. Hence, students and house officers rarely see patients at their best, that is, following recovery, and thus never reap the full rewards of their efforts.

Medical education further reinforces a depersonalized experience for the patient by encouraging compulsiveness, competitiveness, and autonomy. While tremendous effort goes into the pedagogy of diagnosis and treatment, this molding process is not accompanied by an interest in the student's own feelings and reactions. Thus, it is no surprise that hospital training is accompanied by tremendous swings in personality and values (Mizrahi 1986).

The constant reinforcement of obsessive-compulsive behavior, hard work with little reward, repression of feelings and attitudes, and the often sarcastic and cynical coping culture of medical training chip away at any humanistic values medical students and house officers may have once held so dearly. The dehumanizing process of medical education along with the economic burden of paying for one's medical education has a profound effect on the physician's sense of responsibility to care for underserved people. Add to that a physician's socioeconomic distance from the disenfranchised patient, together with the infrequency of contact during periods of wellness, and the result is often the perception of the poor as lazy, pathetic, stupid, manipulative, unappreciative, and noncompliant.

THE STRESSES OF PHYSICIANHOOD

The costs of medical education are rationalized by the rewards at the end of the tunnel. Students and residents are told repeatedly that the emotional and financial payoffs of the profession will be well worth the hardships of training. While this promise of success is often realized, the individual physician is usually overworked and overstressed. This is particularly true for the rural or urban physician working in underserved communities where the demand for service outstrips the supply.

The notion that physicians are perfect and the value that the profession places on autonomy discourage supportive discussions among colleagues of the stresses of practice. The physician's socialization to be perfect causes a number of stresses: reluctance to accept nurturing; the necessity of excluding some patients from care; and the difficulty in finding time to fulfill family responsibilities. Perfection is an unrealistic and unhealthy goal. As Samuel Gorovitz puts it, "Perfection is elusive in every sphere of life" (Gorovitz 1982, p. 110).

The stresses of the business aspects are also important. One friend describes intense pressure from his accountant to stop accepting Medicaid patients. Another physician, starting a practice in a poor, rural community, confides that a growing accounts receivable and an inability to cover costs have given him a new appreciation for the concerns of private-practice physicians in poor communities. In this climate, it is easy to understand why physicians shy away from discussing their responsibility to poor people.

TOWARD MORE EFFECTIVE ROLE MODELING

I have considered the physician's responsibility to poor people in a system that strongly emphasizes physician autonomy, and I have argued that in such a system, the profession must take responsibility for improving access to the poor. Beyond general policy-making, however, it is clear that this issue must also be considered by the individual physician. The majority of physicians face ethical dilemmas of serving poor people daily. I have illustrated this point through a scenario involving treatment of the disenfranchised. In this example, we have seen that issues of reimbursement, while certainly important, are often overemphasized, masking physicians' attitudes and values toward racial, sexual, and cultural differences between their patients and themselves. Finally, I have shown that both medical education and traditional private practice contribute to the existing maldistribution of delivery of medical services.

The experiences of medical students and house officers in teaching hospitals should be used to develop teaching materials that raise the moral dilemmas of serving poor people. There must be a safe setting for apprentices to share these experiences, including their feelings, struggles, and ineptitudes in dealing with people different from themselves. It is here that students can understand that a woman first seeks obstetric care in the third trimester not out of negligence but because she may lack transportation and child care. It is here that students can learn about the multitude of community resources for treatment of alcoholism. It is here that a resident can vent the frustration of being awakened by a mother at three in the morning because she's worried that her child is constipated. It is here that students can admire the dedication of a single African-American woman to her children, of a Latino family to their debilitated grandparent, or a gay partner to a loved one with HIV. It is here that the student can be awestruck when hearing of the escape of a Vietnamese family by boat to a new life. By shaping the experiences of physicians in training and giving them the tools to evaluate their own moral context in relating to the poor, we can facilitate an understanding of the breadth of the issues at hand. As training terminates, physicians should ask themselves a number of questions as they choose both where and what kind of medicine they will practice, which have important implications for meeting the needs of the underserved. If one opts for private practice, will office location and contracting with insurers act as barriers to the care of the underserved? Will choosing an HMO limit one's capacity to care for the underserved? Does selecting a community health center include the support services and work schedule that will facilitate a long-term commitment to the underserved?

The practicing physician has a tremendous opportunity to make an impact on the maldistribution of health care in this country. In addition to taking a leadership role in policy-making, Lawrence Kleinman has suggested a specific framework for how physicians might care for the poor. He suggests that physicians think like advocates; that we recognize that our institutions, our practices, and indeed we ourselves constitute much of the health care system; that we recognize the worth of making local efforts; that we develop a broad perspective that recognizes society as an integrated whole; and that physicians allot a minimum percentage of practice to care for the medically indigent (Kleinman 1991). These suggestions, though compelling, must be accompanied by a cautionary word on the overextension of the physician, mentally, physically, and emotionally. Nonetheless, it is the responsibility of physicians to have the courage to examine, and where necessary to change, the attitudes, values, and beliefs that separate us from underserved populations. Such action by individual physicians will be necessary if equity in access to health care is to be achieved.

Commentary by Neal Baer

Why do the poor so often receive substandard health care? Because they can't afford better care. Millions of uninsured children and adults must rely on Medicaid and the beneficence of beset public clinics and emergency rooms for their care. Not only is this kind of care often demeaning, with endless waits, a new doctor at every visit, and an indomitable bureaucracy that can thwart and discourage the patient, but also it is inefficient and sometimes life-threatening. What's more, poor people seek treatment later than people with insurance and are therefore sicker when they enter the medical system.

To argue that the cost of health care for the poor is the cause of our health care crisis is simplistic. Other factors, particularly the voracious demand for high-tech treatments, the lack of preventive health care, the cost of drugs, and the exorbitant salaries of some medical subspecialties all play into the calculus of exploding costs. And the reasons *why* the poor cannot afford health care beg for us to address what may be intractable problems of unemployment, racism, sexism, and the exigencies of a global economy on the skids. And yet, when it comes to an individual case in which a single-parent mother cannot afford a medication for her child, the bottom line is cost. She can't afford it, and her child pays the price.

Warren Ferguson asks how physicians can provide medical care to "people whose language, culture, sexual orientation, and socioeconomic status are different from their own." And that question has thrown physicians into an ethical quagmire: How to serve the poor and get paid (reasonably well) at the same time. Many physicians bristle at the idea of pro bono service, arguing that they've paid their dues in medical school and as residents. Yet, physicians must remember that their education, no matter how expensive, was largely subsidized by taxpayers (including their patients). Moreover, that they were able to attend medical school speaks for the advantages they had (good schooling, supportive parents, good health), which may not have been available to others less fortunate than they.

Ferguson argues that the lack of an economic incentive for working with the poor has been overemphasized and that cultural differences may be partly to blame. Some physicians feel inadequate in dealing with patients who speak another language or have different views about compliance. Still others cite the bureaucratic tangle of dealing with Medicaid for reimbursement. Some bemoan the patient's lack of incentive to meet scheduled appointments, and others complain about the inadequacy of treatment facilities. What can one make of these reasons? Basically, it's tough working in underserved areas with little support and often without necessary supplies and equipment, and doctors can contrive many excuses for not making the effort. It may be a challenge that many doctors simply aren't up to, and the pay is not as good as in the suburbs.

Part of the problem of the lack of interest in caring for the poor may also stem from the education and socialization of doctors. Ferguson points out that medical school is a highly competitive place where compulsiveness, rote memory, and autonomy reign supreme. Add to that a cynic's awareness of malpractice costs, debts often in excess of $100,000, and what promises to be an increasing competition for specialty residencies, and you have transformed idealistic and compassionate students into physicians who repress feelings and attitudes and often come to see the poor as "lazy, pathetic, stupid, manipulative, unappreciative, and noncompliant."

Physicians are thus caught in a "damned if they do, damned if they don't" syndrome. If they take the challenge and responsibility for caring for the poor, they face stress, possible burnout, and significantly lower salaries than those of their peers. If they turn their back on the poor, they are abdicating part of their responsibility to serve the needs of the ill; and few will quarrel with the fact that the poor have the greatest needs. Moreover, more and more doctors are being viewed by the public as adversaries in obtaining quality health care. By neglecting the poor, doctors are certainly not helping their cause. What, then, can doctors do?

Ferguson stresses that medical schools must take the lead in helping students to share "their feelings, struggles, and ineptitudes in dealing with people different from themselves." Here are some ways that medical schools are trying to help students to understand the needs of the underserved.

—Some schools offer a year-long course in which students practice history-taking during their first year and discuss such issues as access to health care, alcoholism and drug abuse, domestic violence, and working with various ethnic groups and people of color. Part of the course includes making home visits, visiting urban health centers, and shadowing primary care physicians.

—Students at some medical schools must consider the ethical and policy implications of treating the poor by using a case study approach. For example, students review a case in which a pediatrician sees a large number of patients with high lead levels in their blood. What is one to do? Throw up one's hands and say, "This is a terrible problem, but there's nothing I can do to change these children's living situations"? Rather, the physician should investigate what policies are being undertaken to ameliorate the problem and then act to find a solution, be it testimony before a legislature, contacting a reporter, or working on a campaign to test children at risk and educate families about what they might be able to do.

—Some schools require ambulatory care or family practice clerkships to introduce the student to primary care fields.

Medical schools must accept responsibility for assuring adequate training of every student in providing care to the poor and in understanding his or her fundamental responsibility to serve the medical needs of *all* people. Government support of a national health corps also will be beneficial, as will policies that make it easier for specialists to offer primary care, say once a week, while they maintain private practice.

Many physicians treasure their autonomy, but it is now very much threatened. If doctors fail to address the needs of the poor, they will ultimately be forced to make changes, which may not be to their liking. By serving the poor in some capacity, doctors will not only improve the lives of these patients, but will also be able to maintain some of their autonomy, which is crucial for enjoying this beleaguered but still deeply satisfying profession.

12 Access to Medical Care: Do Physicians and Academic Medical Centers Have a Societal Responsibility?

Patrick Dowling

INTRODUCTION

The core question is simple: Should we view health care services in the same way as we view other commodities in our society; that is, should health care be left solely to market forces, the mechanism by which most goods are allocated in this country? Since we allow such essentials as transportation, shelter, clothing, food, and, to an extent, even education to vary widely according to an individual's means, can health care also be suited for the marketplace? Or is it intrinsically wrong to make a commodity out of something so essential for life? In this chapter I will review the historical involvement of the U.S. government in health care to illustrate that health care is regarded as a special societal good, as opposed to a typical commodity. I will then posit that physicians as well as institutions share ownership of this public good (medical knowledge) with society, and therefore it can be subjected to restrictions according to societal needs. I will conclude that such requirements should not be viewed as an unfair abridgment of the individual physician's or institution's rights, but rather as consistent with the fair allocation of resources.

HISTORY OF U.S. GOVERNMENT INVOLVEMENT IN HEALTH CARE—HEALTH CARE AS A RIGHT?

Although health care access was not specifically addressed in the Constitution, the Bill of Rights, or in early federal and state laws, the U.S. government has been involved in providing access to health care for poor groups since the early decades of the republic. By reviewing history, we can understand how access to health care developed gradually as a special societal good. The first legislative involvement of the federal government in the provision of health care services was the 1798 Act for the Relief of the Sick and Disabled Seamen. Although the act provided for improved health care to merchant seamen and members of the armed forces, the goals of the law were primarily of a strategic and economic nature; health services were secondary to the more immediate social priorities of developing the country's shipping capabilities and improving the readiness of the armed forces (Stevens and Stevens 1974). The interests of our early federal leaders, as expressed in their legislative actions, represented a policy quite different from our present concern for individual welfare and improved access.

Following the original Public Health Service Act in 1798, the concept of the right to at least some level of health care has been an expanding and pervasive theme in the United States. Though not initially supported by the federal government, this concept was first recognized at the local level through the establishment of city- or country-sponsored public hospitals in our major urban immigrant centers. Most of these hospitals—like Bellevue in New York and Philadelphia General—were originally founded with multiple functions, providing social needs as well as minimal health care through almshouses, workhouses, houses of correction, infirmaries, and asylums (Dowling 1982).

A century ago, medicine alone could do very little beyond providing ease and comfort; it was placebo-based and rarely curative. Therefore, it was not surprising that society showed very little interest in providing medical care to the poor because that simply meant the provision of yet another amenity. Since the government was already providing food and shelter in these institutions for the poor, it felt no responsibility to provide further amenities. Furthermore, since all the major improvements in the health of the population that did occur at the turn of the century could be attributed to improved public health practices in sanitation, housing, and working conditions, the case could not be made for universal access to medical care (Rosen 1977).

As the twentieth century progressed, however, technological advances occurred in medicine which clearly led to improved outcomes. As a result, differences in access to medical care began to be viewed as unfair inequalities. For example, at the end of the nineteenth century most of the sick poor in large cities were institutionalized in local almshouse infirmaries along with paupers and petty criminals. When more effective medical care became available, sick people were separated from criminals. While this segregating action was beneficial from a health care standpoint, this governmental intervention did not occur for the sake of social justice (Freed 1976). Rather, it was simply a result of more effective medical care. Therefore, the nation's increased interest in the general provision of some medical care can be directly attributed to medicine's improved ability to help people as opposed to changing social doctrines and societal attitudes toward health care (Fried 1976).

A shift in political thought and public health care policy did occur later, but only after the medical profession's claims of special competence were accepted and laws regulating medical practice were enacted (Starr 1982). The post–Depression era is an excellent example of this shift, for it was marked by both significant medical advances and major pieces of social legislation. The resultant government programs suggested that health care was beginning to be widely viewed as a unique social good and that society had a moral obligation to provide for its equal distribution. During this period, the country funded a variety of services, including an expanded Public Health Service, hospitals for veterans and Native Americans, and special programs for the elderly, poor, disabled, and mothers and infants. All these programs tended to confirm the notion that health care was indeed a "special" commodity in our society (Friedman 1991).

During and immediately following World War II, modern medicine spawned numerous technological inventions that improved the diagnosis, treatment, and prevention of disease. With these new developments came a greater focus on health care as a right both nationally and internationally.

The United Nations' Universal Declaration of Human Rights of 1948 stated that "everyone has a right to a standard of living adequate for the health and well being of himself and his family, including food, clothing, housing, medical care, and necessary family services" (Browlie 1981, p. 26). In the United States, the 1952 President's Commission on Health Needs of the Nation came close to endorsing the UN declaration when it concluded that "access to the means for the attainment and preservation of health is a basic human right" (President's Commission on the Health Care Needs of the Nation 1953, p. 3).

In the interim years since the commission's 1952 report, our nation has modified its view. The more recent President's Commission for the Study of Ethical Problems in Medicine and Biomedical Research (1983) did not declare health care a basic right, but instead concluded merely that "society has an ethical obligation to ensure equitable access to health care for all" (President's Commission for the Study of Ethical Problems in Medicine and Biomedical and Behavioral Research 1982, Vol. 1, p. 4). It retreated from the basic human rights claim, stating that "such a right is not legally or constitutionally recognized at the present time nor is it necessary as a foundation for appropriate government actions to secure adequate health care for all" (Vol. 1, p. 32). Yet every industrialized democracy except the United States and South Africa has recognized health care as a legitimate basic right (Callahan 1990). This philosophical shift, however subtle the wording, from health as a "basic right" to health care as an "ethical obligation" can be linked, I believe, to the technological advances, effectiveness, and rising costs of medical care which occurred in the thirty-year interval between the two reports.

At the time of the 1952 report, the concept of a right to medical care attained respectability in what Charles Fried terms the "intermediate or perhaps Golden Age" of modern medicine (Fried 1976). During this period, multiple therapies (such as antibiotics and vaccines) became widely available and made a significant impact on preventing childhood diseases, restoring health, and prolonging life. Since these numerous treatments were relatively inexpensive, major health care legislation of the 1960s—Medicare and Medicaid—which extended care to vulnerable groups, was designed and passed at a time when it was affordable.

By the late 1970s medical technology had advanced to a much higher level. For the first time new tools were made available through research in cellular and molecular biology to treat chronic degenerative, malignant, and genetic diseases, as well as new infectious diseases. Because of the expense that was often associated with only marginally improved outcomes, the cost-benefit ratio of providing comprehensive health care became increasingly unfavorable and at times prohibitive. For example, in 1965 U.S. citizens spent $42 billion, or 6.0% of the GNP, on health care (Donabedian et al. 1980); by 1992 total outlays were projected at $800 billion, or 13.4% of the GNP (Fein 1992) Now, as we proceed further into the "Golden Age" of medicine, historical, philosophical, and legal arguments for a right to health care have been superseded by economic concerns.

HEALTH CARE: A MARKET COMMODITY OR A RIGHT?

Is Health Care Special?

After reviewing the history of health care in this country, I believe that this nation accepts the ideal of health care as a special social good, distinct from other market commodities. Most of us agree that all people should have roughly equal opportunities to achieve the most universally desired goods in life, and since illness and disability represent major unpredictable barriers to such opportunity, it follows that health care should be distributed in accordance with medical needs (Menzel 1990). Unfortunately, this simple conclusion does not bring with it any simple suggestions for change from the current system.

According to a *New York Times* (July 29, 1991) article, a consensus does exist in this country supporting the right to a minimum or decent level of care for all based on its relationship to equality of opportunity. Since our society has accepted the notion that an ethical obligation exists to ensure access to basic care, the question becomes: Have we as a just society done this? Although there are no current national standards that define a minimal or decent level of care for all age groups, we can observe, based on various accepted public health measures and current disparities in health among various groups, that this nation has not ensured basic care for all. It is known, for example, that the young, poor or near poor, as well as ethnic minorities, are disproportionately represented among the nation's 37 million uninsured. Lacking either public or private insurance, these citizens are less likely to have their children immunized, seek early prenatal care, have regular blood pressure checks, and are much less likely to seek early care for chronic and serious conditions (Hafner-Eaton 1993).

The issue of access is not limited to merely the inability to pay for services when available. Although millions face financial barriers, others, particularly in rural areas, have difficulty because of the absence of services. Both facets of access are closely linked to the availability of primary care services and to the response of the medical education system to meeting the country's needs. Since millions lack insurance and two-thirds of our nation's 3,100 counties are designated as federal professional shortage areas for primary care physicians, it is clear that not all sectors of our society are enjoying access to a minimal level of care called for in a just society (Schroeder et al. 1989; Verby et al. 1991).

Provider Responsibility and Liberty

The maldistribution of physicians both geographically and within specialties has been described as an "epidemic of metropolitan-based subspecialists" (Hill 1991). Who is responsible for treating this epidemic? Can we as a nation require physicians to provide care in certain geographic areas and to all economic groups, or is this remedy forbidden because it conflicts with physicians' rights to practice solely in accordance with their own preferences?

Lance Stell argues that such a compulsory requirement would be unjust because she believes that one cannot sacrifice the right of a minority—physicians in this case—to the interests of the majority even if it results in a greater net advantage for society (Stell 1982). Thus, in her view, one cannot restrict a physician's freedom of choice even in the interest of equality of opportunity for the underserved majority. Two values—individual liberty versus equality—are at odds here. To resolve this classic debate, we must weigh the rights of the individual physician against those of society. Stell believes that the physician has a right to serve where he or she pleases and in which specialty, and ought not be subject to national or societal needs. On the other hand, the patient has a right to basic health care necessary for equality of opportunity. If most physicians choose to practice in affluent areas, then patients in poor communities may be denied full equality of opportunity for life chances because they do not receive health care. Since the preservation of freedom of choice is meaningless without the preservation of health and access to quality care, the question then becomes, Are the rights of individual physicians so sacrosanct that the improvement of the health status of a large group of people must be sacrificed for them? Do physicians simply have a micro responsibility to provide care to some individuals, or do they, in fact, have a macro or societal obligation as special gatekeepers for a unique social good that is a prerequisite for equal opportunity? More specifically, does the physician's obligation "to do no harm" to patients on a micro level translate to a macro obligation to ensure the just distribution of health care to all since the absence of such does harm?

While the role of government should not be minimized, the major impetus for change must come from the health care institutions and providers themselves. As Norman Daniels has noted, social and moral obligations do not provide health care; institutions and people do (Daniels 1985). A just health care system depends on providers who are adequately trained and appropriately distributed both geographically and across the various specialties. It is also important to understand that access to medical care alone, especially in face of poverty, will not necessarily guarantee good health outcomes because other social services—housing, education, employment—also impact one's health (Starfield 1991).

Medical License—Private or Public Good?

Daniels argues that health care is indeed a unique social good intrinsically linked with equality of opportunity (Daniels 1985). If we accept his claim, the question then becomes whether or not providers of this unique good have a special responsibility regarding its allocation. To answer this question, we must determine whether having a medical certificate and license is a private good that belongs solely to the licensee, or a public good that ought to be used in accordance with some basic societal needs.

Governmental support of medical education in this country is widespread. Medical education is largely paid for by public funds through direct capitation dollars to medical schools, federal research and training grants, and public insurance monies that go to teaching hospitals where medical students and residents train. In 1993 the indirect and direct Medicare medical education passthrough to teaching hospitals alone exceeded $4 billion (Budetti 1993). Once physicians finish their training, which has been heavily subsidized from medical school through residency, they have access to hospitals that were built largely with federal funds, or municipal tax-free bonds, and are supported by public funds as community or governmental institutions. Even though many students complete their medical training with significant educational debts, the vast majority of their education has been funded through significant public investment and cooperation. Upon the completion of this subsidized educational course, physicians are certified and granted licenses by states. This process provides them with monopoly control over this unique good.

Teachers and police officers are similarly trained at public expense and certified by states. Yet upon graduation, these individuals do not have free access to practice in community institutions, such as public schools or public safety departments, unless they arrange a specific contract with those institutions. Indeed, most citizens who elect an occupation or profession recognize that the market economic system does not necessarily allow an open choice of both a particular job and location. Yet physicians generally have virtually unlimited access to public institutions such as community hospitals where they can practice their trade even if a surplus of physicians exists in that community. Other health care providers, such as nurses, would not have such access to institutions unless they were hired by the hospital. And if the nursing department at one hospital was fully staffed, they would not be hired. Finally, physicians are paid directly by third-party payers which are funded either publicly (Medicare or Medicaid) or privately through insurance companies based on the premise of tax-free health insurance employment benefits.

Individuals in fields other than medicine face limited choices that are influenced by the market, yet their need to choose is not typically viewed as a restriction of freedom. Daniels has described this independence of physicians as a "historical accident" that is much more visible in the United States than elsewhere (Daniels 1981) He states that physicians here have been much more independent of institutional settings for the delivery of their skills than most other U.S. workers, and even physicians in other countries. He notes that a college professor cannot simply decide that there are people who need to be taught, and then begin to teach. Rather, the professor must accept whatever jobs are available in colleges and universities. The professor's freedom to practice a publicly credentialed trade is limited by the needs of the university system. This is not true in medicine.

Furthermore, it has been repeatedly demonstrated that medical practice does not follow the traditional economic laws that govern supply and demand. From 1963 to 1978 the federal government spent over $3 billion to expand the number of medical schools and graduates in the United States. While this policy resulted in a 50% increase in the number of physicians by 1974, the specialty and geographic maldistribution worsened as the percentage of family and general practice physicians declined from 27% in 1963 to 16% in 1976 (Lewis and Sheps 1983). It is now down to 13% of total physicians (Starfield 1992). The free market theory predicts that physicians will elect to go into specialties and geographic areas marked by a shortage of supply. But in 1990 the federal government documented that 2,000 of the nation's 3,100 counties were officially shortage areas for primary care physicians (Politzer et al. 1991). The "trickle down" approach to physician distribution did not work. The lack of a coherent social policy to ensure access, coupled with generous public funding and autonomy, has resulted in the uneven quality of care, unfavorable mix, and distribution of physicians and substandard indices of population health. Physicians have elected to enter the financially rewarding specialties of medicine and to practice in affluent metropolitan areas, leaving the entire country short of primary care physicians, particularly in inner-city and rural areas.

The country is now faced both with numerous shortage areas and the relatively new phenomenon of "overdoctored" communities. If health care were a traditional market good, this situation would be only temporary, and not the growing inequality it has now become. The market would not support the excess. But physicians have been able to insulate themselves from the market pressures that normally affect income, fees, specialty choice, and locations because they are able to generate "demand" by ordering tests and performing procedures beyond that which is medically desirable. Because nine-tenths of hospital bills and three-quarters of doctor's fees are paid for by third-party payers, competition doesn't work (Lee and Lamm 1993). We seldom shop for what we don't pay for directly. And in health care it is often the physician doing our shopping for us.

Medical schools and teaching hospitals have also been insulated from traditional market forces. Most graduate medical education is supported by more than $4 billion in medical education funding to teaching hospitals as part of the Medicare program (Budetti 1993). As such, teaching institutions are also somewhat insulated from direct market pressures. Since they receive significantly higher reimbursement for procedures performed by subspecialists, they continue to train subspecialists and financially benefit from them, even though a surplus exists. As a result, the country's needs for primary care providers are not being met.

The fact that both individual physicians and academic medical centers are protected from traditional market forces is a salient argument that health care is indeed a unique or special good, a result of medical knowledge that is produced and financed largely by public funds. Furthermore, because the practice of medicine involves professional licensure by society, other principles can impact the manner and requirement of its distribution. Since the state grants individual physicians a monopoly by virtue of its licensing power, should it not be able to make demands that take precedence over individual liberty? As such, the physician in a just society becomes a trustee of a public good—medical knowledge—but society retains ownership, and society can decide where to locate practitioners. This does not represent involuntary servitude or an abridgment of the physician's individual constitutional rights because a contractual agreement exists between potential physicians and the society by virtue of the subsidized medical education. Moreover, it should not be viewed narrowly as a restriction on the individual's liberty, but rather as a realization that considerations of justice—in this case, social equality as it pertains to access to a basic level of medical care—require the prioritization of resource allocation. It is recognized that physicians as citizens have societal obligations. There is no constitutional right to use public money (in this case, medical education, which is the result of public funding) for the private pursuit of happiness.

The same argument can be extended to academic medical centers, including medical schools and major teaching hospitals. Since they, too, are insulated from traditional market forces, benefit from both substantial federal subsidies to educate physicians as well as nontax status, and are accredited by state and national bodies, they are not the exclusive owners, just as physicians are not, of the knowledge and services that they possess or finance. Society has a claim to shared ownership and can make a legitimate claim on those institutions to meet the needs of indigent patients and the health care personnel needs of the nation. Thus, institutions of medical education and training do not have an unlimited right to use their resources as they alone decide. At the macro level, justice is concerned with the fair allocation of resources, and fairness can justifiably constrain the freedom of institutions (McCullough 1991).

CONCLUSION

More than sixty years ago a privately funded commission composed of economists, physicians, and policy experts met to formulate a policy on health care in response to growing concerns in the 1920s about its costs and distribution. This group, based at the University of Chicago and known as the Committee on the Cost of Medical Care, issued its report entitled Medical Care for the American People in 1932 (President's Commission on the Health Care Needs of the Nation 1953). Noting the maldistribution of physicians both geographically and by specialty, it concluded that "there is a need for geographic distribution which more closely approximates the medical requirements of the people" and "there should be effective controls over the number and types of practitioners trained, and their training should be adjusted so that it will prepare them to serve the true needs of the people" (Lewis et al. 1976, p. 20). The committee failed in its attempt to generate a consensus for reform. While it has taken sixty years for such a consensus to develop, it is finally clear that the overwhelming majority of the nation agrees that access to health care is an ethical and economic imperative (Hill 1991).

These recent changes in public opinion will result, I believe, in public policy changes that will confirm the unique nature of health care as a public good. The nation is moving to fulfill its moral obligation in the provision of universal access and a decent level of health care for all. Clearly, this will require some reduction in the variety of personal choices available to physicians as well as academic medical centers, both of which have benefited greatly from past policies. But such restrictions are fair and do not constitute an abridgment of fundamental liberty. Rather, they signal the maturation to a more just society—one in which liberty denotes the freedom of all from the injustice of preventable and treatable disease.

NOTE

The author would like to thank Beckie Strode for helpful comments and manuscript revision, and Mari Morse for manuscript preparation.

Commentary by Stephen Miles

Patrick Dowling maintains that the United States has long recognized the specialness of health care and articulated the idea of a right to health care early in the eighteenth century. He finds support for this premise in the generous public support for medical education, the insulation of physicians from market pressures, and the special programs for the medically needy. This special status, he argues, is the foundation for creating public moral obligations on physicians to locate in poor areas. In my view, the moral respect for health care in the United States is centered on respect for the good of healing, rather than on respect for the moral claim of solidarity with those who are sick. Re-centering the moral premise of the health care system is necessary to health care reform in the United States.

Health care in the United States is a remarkable paradox. The world's most costly system of health care provides the least secure access of any developed nation. Fabulous tertiary care hospitals exist in blighted urban environments whose residents lack reliable access to basic health services. Physicians receive enormous respect even though they may not always deserve this respect.

A young woman is beaten; her arm is broken. In despair, she takes an overdose of a prescribed medication. She is taken to a world-famous university medical center less than ten blocks from the ghetto she lives in. After the medicine service treats the life-threatening emergency overdose, the orthopedic surgeon refuses to provide the internal fixation of her arm because she is medically indigent. (Miles 1992, pp. 2561–62)

Such wrongs suggest a fundamental moral problem. Our society values the act of healing as more morally compelling than solidarity with those who need to be healed. Healing is a good thing to do. Institutions and persons who heal deserve to be honored for their virtue. Accordingly, the United States bestows resources and respect on its healers. Our nation bestows a seventh of its wealth on healing. Physicians are well trained, well equipped, and well paid. Unfortunately, until recently this moral value for healing has been centered on the healer rather than on social solidarity with those who are sick.

This peculiar moral centering accounts for many of Dowling's findings. National resources support an elite set of providers and institutions without a national policy to secure care for all. We reward providers in glutted markets, and we tolerate astounding health disparities between rich and poor. Secure access to health care in the United States, to a much greater degree than in other developed nations, is proportional to nonhealth status. It is related to the status of a full-time job in a larger corporation or to the social merit of having served in the armed forces. It can be diminished by divorce. Insurers legally charge women more for insurance even though women have more needs, fewer dollars to pay for insurance or buy health care, and often are the sole support of children and children's health care. Children have access to health care in proportion to the status of their parents, rather than in proportion to their need. Medicare for the elderly is our most recent addition and the major exception to status-based secure access to health care.

Fortunately, our society's understanding of the moral center of health care is shifting as the paradoxes and irrationality of our nation's health care system are recognized as problems. I doubt, however, that we can directly translate our nation's grants to healers into a duty to those who need healing without relocating the moral center of health care.

In 1840 a French observer, Alexis De Tocqueville, noted a more promising cultural root from which the United States might grow an equitable health care system:

When an American asks for cooperation from his fellow citizens, it is seldom refused. I have often seen it spontaneously given with great good will.... If a great and sudden calamity befalls a family, the purses of a thousand strangers are at once willingly opened and small but numerous donations pour in to relieve their distress.... Experience quickly teaches them that although they do not routinely require the assistance of others, a time almost always comes when they cannot do without it. [A] covenant exists ... between all the citizens of a democracy when they all feel themselves subject to the same weakness and the same dangers; their interests as well as their compassion make it a rule with them to lend one another assistance when required. (De Tocqueville 1945, pp. 185–186)

The United States cannot base a just health care system simply on respect for healing. Health care reform must be grounded on a recognition of our common and morally compelling need to care for each other in order that we may be healed.

13 Experiences as a Black Medical Student

Michael Hebrard

Young African-American men and boys today are in a major funk. We're dropping out of school and into gangs, and the result holds dire consequences for our health. Whereas school only serves to remind us of our second-class status, street gangs give us the opportunity to identify with one another's fears and frustrations concerning poverty and the struggles that come with the territory of living in the "hood."

The senseless acts of violence and murder which characterize gang life are, in my opinion, an expression of the inability of African-American males to see hope in the future for a more positive and constructive lifestyle. Too damn many of my brothers have a much greater fear of living life, with all of its responsibilities, than they do of dying. And we all know that people who believe they have nothing to lose are very dangerous—to society and to themselves.

Understanding the sources of violence among African-American youth doesn't lessen the hurt I feel in my heart when I hear of another friend who has died in "cold blood" at the hands of another gang member or the police. This hurt is with me continually as I reflect on my future career in health care. I am a 27-year-old African-American man from Oakland, California, in my second year of medical school in the Midwest.

What kind of doctor will I be? What difference will I make? I continually reflect on the impotence of medicine in the face of the realities of everyday life in my community. And yet even acknowledging the inadequacy of medicine, the influences and experiences of my childhood provide compelling reasons, reinforcing my desire to become a health provider.

Since the time of my early childhood, I have been personally aware of problems of poor health and health care among African Americans. Growing up during the 1970s, I was aware of many people in my neighborhood community "skin popping" heroin and abusing other dangerous drugs as part of their regular diet of narcotic consumption. I knew many of these addicts very well as a child. I watched firsthand as their health declined in the natural progression of their frequent narcotic indulgence. I was 4 or 5 years old at the time, and my memories are vivid as they flash back to the scenes of rooms cluttered with junkies who were on the verge of suicide. Memories of such activities are hard to forget, and they recur when I see young brothers using crack these days. I know from personal experience that crack cocaine, heroine, and alcohol are some of the major agents contributing to the continuous and rapid deterioration of the African-American community.

It's obvious to me where the problems are. It's not so obvious to think about what kind of contribution this future physician might make to my community. Medical school does not provide a whole lot of answers for me. For an African-American male like me, medical school is a very strange, even alienating environment. There are infrequent shows of support from professors and other students, and hostility and racism are subtly present most of the time. Too often, predominantly white institutions (most medical schools) do not provide the kind of guidance and encouragement African-American students need. From my own experience I know in the absence of such support that it is easy to suffer from a lack of confidence, which then undermines the ability to maximize our innate abilities.

But I also know I have been lucky. I have had emotional support from some great people in my community who have made the difference in my life. In college I was "adopted" by an African-American physician and his ingenious wife, Michael and Beverly Charles. They nurtured me as if I was their own son, providing a source of positive energy and supporting my growing confidence to do anything my mind could conceive of achieving. Specifically, Dr. and Mrs. Charles helped me to develop greater academic discipline and organizational skills by reminding me to write out long- and short-term goals for the academic year. They also introduced me to other African-American professionals who had already successfully met the challenges I was beginning to encounter. My relationship with this wonderful couple continues to give me not only insight into my own personal power, but also a realization of the importance of giving back to the community as they unselfishly give to me.

My fiancee, Rachelle Vayson, provides the love and support that is paramount to my well-being and continued success in an otherwise hostile and negative institution. She has been there for me when times get rough, and even for nonminority students, rough times are what medical school is about. I remember last semester, for instance, when four exams were scheduled in one week. I couldn't find a study group of classmates where I didn't feel subtly unwelcome, and I was beginning to panic. A long-distance call to Rachelle assured me that someone cared for me as a person. In addition, she gave me some concrete suggestions about how to learn the material and enhance my confidence for the exam.

Through the Student Medical National Association (SMNA), I have extended my support systems beyond my hometown and developed friendships locally and even nationally. The SMNA provides minority students with academic, personal, and social support within a racially alienating environment. There aren't many African-American students enrolled in my school, but SMNA has maximized our cohesiveness by pooling our individual resources. We share class notes and learning and memory strategies to help each other survive the harsh assaults of medical school. Above all, our SMNA community service activities have kept us in touch with the real world and reminded us of our reasons for choosing medicine as a career.

One of the best ways to refresh my commitment has been to work with younger African-American students in junior and high school. Our SMNA chapter organizes a yearly "health career workshop" for kids to interest them in different areas of health care delivery, such as medicine, nursing, dentistry, and pharmacy. These workshops provide face-to-face encouragement for young people to pursue their dreams. We tell them, "Look, if we can do it, so can you!"

It has been so important for me to have role models—not distant paragons—but real people who struggle and falter, and keep going despite the sometimes harsh realities of life. By their example I find hope that I too may follow my dreams. As I continue to strive for success academically and personally, one of my major goals is to remain a viable and visible leader in my community so that I can be a role model to others. As acting chapter president of the SMNA, I have experienced many benefits from being a role model. Not only do I reconfirm my initial motivations to be a doctor, but this opportunity also challenges me to figure out what kind of doctor I will be.

Not long ago I spoke at a local junior high school about my "story," telling them about my path from street life to college and finally medical school. I can't say that I held their attention completely; the majority of the students were pretty disruptive. I ended the discussion by reminding each of them that they have a reasonable chance of future success, providing they continue to believe in themselves and seek help from dedicated role models. The room emptied quickly, but one young brother remained to talk. He asked frankly, "What can I do to change my life if I live in a war zone and all they do is gang-bang and sell crack?" I thought for a minute before saying a word. Then I offered him my experience and an implied invitation. I said, "I always try to find role models to help give me more options and ideas to do positive things for myself. I needed to see life does exist outside of semiautomatic weapons—maybe take a tour of a university campus and medical school, for instance." He knew what I was getting at because he replied with cautious acceptance, "Don't let me down, man." I know firsthand what he was saying; he was talking about the fragility of hope, and he was reminding me of my part in sustaining that hope—for him, for my community, and for myself. He is teaching me to be the kind of physician I want to be and is showing me the difference I can make.

Commentary by Chester Pierce

It was a privilege to read Michael Hebrard's experiences as a black medical student in a predominantly white institution. In the 1940s I entered the identical situation. Since then I have been a full-time worker in such institutions.

By Aristotelian notions, ethics speaks to what one does in a given instance, with a given combination of circumstances. Under this definition, a number of topics in the chapter merit commentary. In my view Mr. Hebrard dwells on something that is most special for African Americans and whites in terms of ethical responsibility. Majority members fail to recognize how limiting and frustrating it is for a minority person who is never ever acknowledged by his or her peers to be equal or who is never thought to be worthy or in need of group support. Mr. Hebrard's experience in being shut out of a study group illustrates this commonplace occurrence.

It reminded me of a story told to me by a black medical student at a leading university. Following an exam, a white classmate went from person to person in the lab, anxiously inquiring, "What did you get?" When he reached his black classmate, he said, "Did you pass?"

The vignette emphasizes the truism that white faculty, students, and administrators don't really believe African Americans are capable of excellence. When such ubiquitous and omnipresent judgments are acted upon, they become unethical. This diminishes the chance for harmonious ("good") human relations between blacks and whites.

Black readers should take particular notice of the "ethical" importance of role models. Dr. and Mrs. Charles, as well as Ms. Vayson, acted in such ways as to sustain, nourish, and strengthen a fellow human being. Such strength aided Mr. Hebrard as a student leader to serve as a valuable role model for other black medical students and at least one young black male from the community.

Perhaps the distillate from all this is something that can be serviceable for all of humankind regardless of racial persuasion. Simply stated, excellent ethics make excellent people, who in turn make excellent communities. Doctors, in their ceaseless quest to have more people live longer and live better, endorse the establishment of excellent communities. Therefore, it seems inarguable that the ideal physician is tireless in guarding, cherishing, and enlarging ethical responsibility. Mr. Hebrard has shown that racism is a factor in the physician's development and practice of ethics.

14 HIV Disease and Access to Care: A Crisis Within a Crisis

Renslow Sherer and David Goldberg

INTRODUCTION

The pandemic of Human Immunodeficiency Virus I (HIV I) is the most devastating public health crisis of our lifetime. AIDS, which is more appropriately called HIV disease, is challenging our public health and medical care institutions to be more responsive to the unique and rapidly increasing problems presented by the pandemic. Its challenges have initiated a revolution in health care (Mann 1990). One outcome of this revolution is a dramatic illumination of the serious deficiencies and inequities in the nation's health care, in particular those that constitute barriers to access to care.

From the beginning of the pandemic, access to a system of care was a serious problem for persons with AIDS and HIV disease and for persons at risk of the disease. However, early on, issues surrounding access were overshadowed by the social stigmatization faced by infected persons. Unimaginable worst-case scenarios were common in the early years. There were countless situations where employers fired persons with AIDS, doctors refused to care for patients, nursing homes refused to accept patients, landlords evicted residents with AIDS, and government agents denied entry into the United States of HIV-infected foreign citizens, making social pariahs of persons infected with HIV (Shilts 1987). In those dark years of fear and ignorance, many others simply tried to deny AIDS.

Today, AIDS and HIV disease are all too common, and access to care is a more widespread and pressing problem. While the horrors associated with stigmatization continue, the stresses which the magnitude of the pandemic has placed on health institutions will make access to HIV-related care a central issue for the duration of the decade. In this chapter, we explore the multifaceted issues related to access to HIV-related care. Our perspective is that care, services, and programs for HIV infection cannot be analyzed in isolation from other care provision. Providing access to HIV care ultimately means integrating HIV care into a complete health care system. This change will demand a radical rethinking and restructuring of how health care is delivered. For now, the urgency posed by HIV disease warrants our immediate attention, and deserves a careful description of the current status, problems, and trends in access to HIV-related care. (See also Thomas and Quinn in Chapter 7 and Williamson in Chapter 8 of this volume.)

TRENDS IN THE EPIDEMIOLOGY OF HIV

The sheer magnitude and rate of growth of the HIV epidemic is still its most alarming feature. Currently, more than 1 million persons have AIDS worldwide and more than 10 million are HIV-infected. By the year 2000, an estimated 20 to 30 million persons will be HIV-infected. The vast majority of worldwide HIV infections are transmitted heterosexually. In the United States, 6 to 8 million people will have HIV disease in the year 2000 (World Health Organization 1991). Several U.S. trends which were recognized in the mid-1980s persist today. Women are one of the fastest growing groups among persons newly infected with HIV. The proportion of women with HIV disease rose nationally from 2% in 1988 to 10% in 1991 (Chicago Department of Health 1991a; National Commission on AIDS 1991a, 1991b). As the number of HIV-infected women has grown, so has the number of infected infants and children. Injectable drug use, which has increased among both men and women, is the most common risk behavior in new cases of HIV disease in New York and other cities. Injectable drug use is also the most common direct and indirect cause in women; 71% of all female cases are directly linked to IV drug use (National Commission on AIDS 1991b).

HIV disease disproportionately affects communities of color. While the U.S. population is comprised of 12% African Americans and 6% Latinos, the overall U.S. data show that 29% of persons with AIDS are African American and 16% are Latino (National Commission on AIDS 1991a). In Chicago, as in many other large cities, the majority of new cases of AIDS and HIV disease are in men and women of color (Chicago Department of Health 1991).

The rate of heterosexual transmission continues to rise in the United States (Allen and Setlow 1991; Kreiss et al. 1990). Heterosexually acquired HIV disease rose from 1% in 1983 to 7% of cases in 1991. Heterosexually acquired HIV disease disproportionately affects communities of color, with eleven times the rate among African Americans and Latinos than among European Americans (Kreiss et al. 1990).

Homosexual and bisexual men continue to constitute the community most severely affected by HIV disease, accounting for 68% of cases. Although many successful efforts have been made to prevent the spread of HIV in the gay community, two disturbing trends have recently emerged. First, a significant return to unsafe behaviors has been documented in many cities (National Commission on AIDS 1991a), indicating erosion of prior successful prevention and education programs. Second, gay men of color continue to be infected at high rates (Conference of Mayors 1991). While there have been epidemiological shifts in the spread of HIV infection accounting for increasing proportions of infected women, children, injectable drug users, and heterosexuals, the gay community remains at high risk.

IMPACT OF THE EPIDEMIOLOGY ON ACCESS TO CARE

These data have many implications for the issue of access to care. Access may be seriously limited by the sheer volume of care and resources needed. For example, in New York City the demand for hospital beds and long-term care facilities overwhelmed the capacity of the system (Weinberg and Murray 1987). This situation is likely to be replicated in many urban settings as the infected population grows.

The recent rapid rise in HIV disease among women and families has reduced access in other ways. Eighty percent of women with HIV disease are African American or Latina, and the majority are medically indigent (Chicago Department of Health 1991a). Primary medical services were inaccessible for many in this population before HIV disease. Considering the context, in which multiple family members may simultaneously need care, may be debilitated, or may have died, care for women and children is further complicated by the need for specialized medical, pediatric, obstetric, and psychosocial expertise. The usual providers for these women and their families are unfamiliar with HIV needs, and are often disconnected from the existing HIV service continuum. HIV-infected women also face difficult decisions regarding pregnancy, occurring in a climate of increasing hostility and diminishing access to abortion services, especially for poor women (Chavkin 1990).

Injectable drug use as it relates to HIV disease poses other service and access problems. It is widely recognized that medical care must be linked with appropriate chemical dependency treatment in order to be effective. Yet in Illinois, only 8,000 treatment slots are available for an estimated 70,000 injectable drug users (Popkin et al. 1991). Nationally, an estimated 107,000 injectable drug users are on waiting lists for drug treatment slots (National Commission on AIDS 1991b). Even when chemical dependency programs are available for HIV-infected persons, they are likely to be fragmented from traditional health care. An injectable drug user may require medical care in one location, drug treatment, when available, in a second, and support services in yet a third. Yet the problems of drug-using HIV-infected persons seldom occur in isolation. For example, in Chicago, 23% of injectable drug users are homeless and 29% live in unstable housing (Popkin et al. 1991). The majority of injectable drug users at Cook County Hospital have three or more case management needs (Sternberg et al. 1991). Lack of services and fragmentation of existing services complicate care and restrict or inhibit access. This is a common experience in HIV care; the existing institutions and dysfunctional health care system have failed to address major health problems. The rise in HIV among communities of color further exacerbates long-standing inequities in access to health care services in these communities. For example, in Cook County, Illinois, the volume of ambulatory care required for the medically needy exceeds the capacity of the current system by over 2 million visits. The need is most acute in communities of color (Chicago and Cook County Health Care Action Plan 1990). Because communities of color lack a system of primary care, programs for screening and early detection of HIV infection will be difficult to develop. Even if HIV is detected, African Americans and Latinos face limited options for care in their communities.

As we learn more about HIV infection and its treatment, the health care system will have to respond to changing needs. Persons with HIV disease who are asymptomatic can now benefit from therapeutic interventions. Zidovudine (AZT) therapy has been shown to significantly reduce the number and severity of opportunistic infections in persons with fewer than 500 CD4 cells. Primary prophylaxis against pneumocystis pneumonia is indicated for persons with fewer than 200 CD4 cells. As many as 65% of asymptomatic HIV-positive people may qualify for these interventions (Vermund 1991). A recent study by the U.S. Navy found that of 2,800 asymptomatic working personnel who were HIV-positive, 65% had fewer than 500 CD4 cells at initial examination and therefore qualified for zidovudine therapy. Twenty percent had fewer than 200 CD4 cells and would qualify for primary prophylaxis against pneumocystis pneumonia (Vermund 1991). Prophylactic therapy demands extensive resources for both screening and treatment.

Until recently, services for people with AIDS have largely focused on opportunistic infections; that pattern is changing. Increasing numbers of lymphomas and carcinomas are occurring in HIV-infected persons, owing to the extended life expectancy of people with AIDS and the successful treatment and prevention of opportunistic infections (Andrulis 1991). The rising number of women with HIV disease has been accompanied by the finding of accelerated cervical neoplasia (Minkhoff and Dehovitz 1991). Thus, the resources needed now include, for example, additional oncologic and gynecologic treatment.

The holes in the U.S. medical care "safety net" which antedated AIDS left the principal burden of hospital and outpatient care to the public hospitals. HIV disease has worsened that trend. In 1988 public hospitals cared for 9,495 persons with AIDS—19% of living PWAs; this figure doubled from 1985 to 1988 (Andrulis 1991). In Chicago, Cook County Hospital provides primary care for 2,265 persons with HIV disease—38% of the total need in Cook County—and 20 new patients enroll in the clinic weekly (Moore and Weslowski 1992). Programmatically, the demand for HIV-related care at public hospitals has played havoc with clinical services striving to keep pace with the need. The rapid development of AIDS care teams is often a source of tension in public hospitals, where there are many worthwhile and needed clinical programs, and terrible problems of limited space and personnel. Staffs providing HIV care at public hospitals face ever increasing workloads and risk long-term burnout. The principal burden, however, is on the patients in public hospitals in the form of further overcrowding and longer waits for appointments, medications, and elective surgery (Moore and Weslowski 1992).

FINANCING OF HIV CARE

The cost of care for HIV-related disease has been estimated to be nearly $4 billion (Reillo and McMahon 1991), representing 0.7% of the total health care budget for 1989–90 (Moien and Kozak 1991). Because the number of cases has steadily increased, both the total HIV-related costs and the percentage cost of the health care budget have risen dramatically. For example, the number of hospital days for HIV-related care, and the attendant costs, rose by 75% between 1987 and 1989 (Moien and Kozak 1991). They are projected to continue to rise. The costs for HIV-related care in Chicago are expected to increase from $40 million in 1989 to $267 million in 1994, a rate of increase that far outstrips the rate of health care inflation (Salem and Lenihan 1991). A brief analysis of the financing of HIV-related care is important to the understanding of economic constraints and barriers to access to care for HIV-infected persons. Adequate funding of care will ultimately determine whether existing care options are accessible, whether institutions will provide care, and whether the level of clinical care keeps pace with changing therapies.

Health insurance status is customarily divided into the categories of private insurance, Medicare, Medicaid, self-pay, and other (mostly care financed by charity, special grants or programs, or the correctional system). In 1987 private insurance covered 17% of inpatient HIV care. This is a very low rate compared to the 46% of general hospital care that private insurance reimburses. Moreover, the care covered by private insurance was disproportionately concentrated in private hospitals. Private insurance covered only 7% of public hospital HIV care. The overall rate of Medicare coverage was remarkably low at 2%. While this is due in large part to the fact that HIV disease occurs mostly in people younger than 65, it also reflects the inaccessibility of full disability benefits to HIV-infected persons. Together, private insurance and Medicare accounted for only 19% of the total care for HIV-infected persons, compared to 76% for all hospital care (Andrulis et al. 1987; Sloan et al. 1988).

Medicaid was the main mechanism of insurance for HIV care, accounting for the insurance status of more than half of the HIV-related admissions, or an overall rate that was nearly five times that for all hospital discharges. Self-pay, a financially tenuous category, accounted for 17% of care, or more than twice the percentage of HIV-related care compared to hospital care in general (Andrulis et al. 1987; Sloan et al. 1988). These comparisons lead one to conclude that the financing of HIV care is relatively unstable compared to the financing of care in the health care system at large (Gage et al. 1991). Considering that the health care system has increasingly become financially constrained, resulting in worsening overall access to care, the instability of HIV care financing is worrisome.

At least two trends pose additional problems. There is a shifting emphasis toward testing, monitoring, and early intervention of anti-retroviral therapy together with other prophylactic therapies, discussed earlier. The projected national cost of such a program is $5 billion per year (Arno et al. 1989), more than double the current annual cost of HIV care. Early intervention will require allotment of enormous additional financial resources.

The second trend involves how care is being financed. Data from New York City, San Francisco, and Los Angeles (1983–88) have shown a drop in the rate of private insurance of between 28% and 48%, and a rise in the Medicaid coverage over the same period of 38 to 167%. This trend has been called the "Medicaidization of AIDS" and portends future stresses on financing the health care of persons infected with HIV (Green and Arno 1990). These stresses are likely to be disproportionately borne by the public hospitals and selected urban private hospitals (Andrulis et al. 1989; Levine 1990a). Low reimbursement rates by Medicaid contribute to the overcrowding of hospital clinics providing HIV care, can lead to interinstitutional transfers or "patient dumping," and may threaten the solvency of certain institutions. Medicaid is generally the insurance of last resort, and eligibility is determined by the states. There are vast state-to-state differences both in who qualifies for Medicaid and in the level of coverage extended under Medicaid. Thus, although Medicaid is the most common source of coverage for HIV-infected persons, it is by no means a source of "universal" coverage (Bartlett 1990).

There are several reasons why HIV-infected persons rely mostly on Medicaid or are medically indigent. These factors go beyond the issues that relate poverty and the acquisition of HIV infection. HIV-infected persons have difficulty maintaining their insurance (Bartlett 1990; Fife and McAnaney 1993). As the disease progresses, many persons leave their jobs. An estimated 50% of HIV-infected people stop working over a two-year period once they become symptomatic. By ten years into the symptomatic phase of the infection, all once-employed HIV-infected persons are no longer working (Yelin et al. 1991). Thus, debilitated individuals covered through workplace insurance benefits lose their insurance. There are programs for people to maintain private insurance coverage after a health-related job loss, but these require considerable out-of-pocket costs. They are unlikely to remain affordable throughout the course of the illness. A diagnosis of AIDS results in an income change from a mean of $17,500 to $7,125 (Crystal and Schiller 1991). The impoverishing nature of HIV infection results in what has been described as a "two-tier system" of care for HIV-infected persons who initially have private insurance. Care begins in the private sector covered by private insurance. As the disease progresses and HIV-infected persons become uninsured or covered by Medicaid, care tends to shift to the public sector (Mansell 1987).

HIV-infected persons have difficulty obtaining individual insurance policies. Insurance company practices serve to prevent HIV-infected or high-risk persons from obtaining individual policies. These practices include testing for HIV, questioning applicants regarding sexual orientation or history of intravenous drug use, or redlining based on an applicant's occupation or neighborhood. There is evidence that these practices are achieving their goals. The Health Insurance Association of America and the American Council of Life Insurance found that, while group policy expenditures for claims for AIDS care more than doubled between 1986 and 1987, the expenditures for individual policies remained constant (Bartlett 1990).

HIV-infected persons who are younger than age 65 qualify for Medicare based on disability. In order to qualify for disability, there must be an AIDS-defining diagnosis followed by a minimum five-month waiting period prior to the activation of the disability income. Disabled persons qualify for Medicare twenty-four months after beginning to receive their disability income. This twenty-nine-month interval between qualifying for disability and obtaining Medicare, during which time HIV-infected persons are likely to be on Medicaid or be medically indigent, is crucial for health care needs (Bartlett 1990).

There is a complex network for financing HIV care, with regional differences in patterns of coverage, shifting patterns for infected individuals over the course of the disease, and an increasing burden of care falling to the Medicaid system. Helpful programs (e.g., the U.S. AIDS Drug Reimbursement Program) have been added to this network and address some shortcomings (Horner et al. 1991). Yet between the increasing number of cases, lean government budgets, and the fact that HIV care is less profitable or unprofitable for the insurance and hospital industry, forecasts for the financial future of HIV care are troublesome. Unless there is a dramatic and deliberate reversal of the dominant financial trends, we may see declining access and greater inequity for HIV-related health care.

DISCRIMINATION

No discussion of access to HIV-related care would be complete without an analysis of discrimination against HIV-infected persons. Discrimination is a mechanism for creating and maintaining social hierarchies. It manifests itself through apathy and neglect, denial of basic rights, and outright violence toward a subordinated group. The strength of the reaction is determined in part by the perceived threat and the degree to which control must be maintained. Because HIV infection largely affects distinct groups that are already socially marginal, HIV-related stigmatization has been nourished by prevailing prejudices. As one author has written, AIDS "provides many people with a metaphor for prejudice—a convenient hook on which to hang their hostility toward out-groups" (Herek and Glunt 1988, p. 889). Because many of these prejudices are ingrained in our nation's psyche, and because they have powerful proponents even when only a minority of the population holds these prejudices, they affect attitudes and the course of public policy. Discrimination ultimately affects access to care and so needs to be addressed.

Early in the course of the HIV pandemic, when the cases were most heavily concentrated in gay communities, many people considered AIDS as retribution for homosexuality (Kegeles et al. 1989). Responses included a virtual news blackout on the subject (termed by one author as "a collective yawn over the story of dead and dying homosexuals" (Shilts 1987, p.191)), victim-blaming, proposals to quarantine or tattoo infected persons, and a rising tide of personal violence against gays (Blendon and Donelan 1988; Herek and Glunt 1988; Kegeles et al. 1989; Shilts 1987). As the infected population of intravenous drug users grew, thereby affecting a growing number of African Americans and Latinos, the idea that HIV infection was punishment for deviance was reinforced (Kegeles et al. 1989). Disdain for injectable drug users served as an acceptable form of prejudice against African-American and Latino communities. In minority communities, the legacy of racism and the abhorrence and fear of drug abuse led to an initial near-paralysis of political and service self-organization for prevention and treatment of HIV disease (Dalton 1989; Friedman et al. 1987).

Women were initially forgotten in the pandemic. As the number of infected women grew, public attention focused on women as HIV carriers to men and infants rather than as a group with different manifestations of disease and health care needs (Anastos and Marte 1989; Treichler 1988). Interest focused on preventing transmission to economically secure men from prostitutes and to infants from their infected mothers. Other issues related to preventing and caring for HIV infection in women were seldom raised (Anastos and Marte 1989). In the sexist eyes of much of the public and the health care community, women were reduced to "mothers and whores" (Carovano 1991).

The common link in each of these responses has been described as a viewpoint that seeks to limit the scope of the infection by a policy of containment-coercion (Kegeles et al. 1989). The response in the containment-coercion approach is biased and punitive against the socially marginal. It tends to be dispassionate toward suffering and hysterical in overemphasizing risks. The attitudes are exemplified by a statement in 1985 by Margaret Heckler, then U.S. secretary of Health and Human Services. She said, "We must conquer [AIDS] . . . before it affects the heterosexual population and threatens the health of our general population" (Dalton 1989, p. 221). AIDS had to be stopped at the border of mainstream America.

The containment-coercion approach has been countered by eliciting the voluntary cooperation of people through prevention and education (Kegeles et al. 1989; Sherer 1990). The prevention-education approach is founded on the fundamental public health principle of respect for the public. As clearly expressed by one author, "Advocacy of voluntary approaches stems not from ideology but from the facts of the case: since private behavior is at issue, the most effective policies will be those that enlist the cooperation of those at greatest risk, thus optimizing both human rights and the health of the public" (Osborn 1988, p. 446).

Recently, the containment-coercion approach has been applied to policy issues concerning HIV-infected health care workers. Proponents of the containment-coercion ideology have advocated routine testing of health care workers for HIV, with either public notification of the results or mandatory relief of duties of HIV-positive individuals. Such an approach views health care workers as carriers of transmission, and seriously overstates risks (Hammell and Sherer 1991). In part, this policy is a means of putting on the defensive vocal advocates of the prevention-education model who work in health care. It is part of an ongoing ideological struggle over the shaping of society and the health care system. The fact that such a policy goes against well-founded public health care knowledge and practice is irrelevant to those in the containment-coercion camp.

The ideology of containment-coercion has shaped negative attitudes toward HIV-infected persons and undoubtedly affects these persons' quality of and access to care. Physicians are more likely to blame a person with HIV for their illness than they are a person with leukemia. They are more likely to believe that AIDS patients deserve their illness and that they are socially dangerous (Kelly et al. 1987). Physicians in internal medicine residencies also tend to blame AIDS patients for the disease. This trend is stronger when the patients are minorities, gay, or intravenous drug users. In one study, 36% of physicians reported that they planned to structure their practice so as not to care for HIV-infected persons ("Many Plan to Avoid AIDS Care" 1990; Kelly et al. 1987). A group of hospital directors has ranked the social value of AIDS patients, placing infants with transfusion-acquired AIDS at the top of a value hierarchy, and black, gay, drug users at the bottom ("Many Plan to Avoid AIDS Care" 1990).

These patterns of discrimination have been reflected in research institutions. Drug trials, an important mechanism of access to restricted therapies, tend to overenroll relatively socially advantaged HIV-infected persons through restrictive entry criteria (Milano et al. 1991). Women, people of color, and injectable drug users have been consistently underrepresented in such trials. Their participation has been concentrated in 11 of 107 AIDS

Clinical Trial Group trials and at a minority of the sites (D'Eramo et al. 1991). Thus, the generalizability of some studies is rendered questionable. Good science has been impaired by cultural, social, and institutional biases.

The national HIV-related establishment has been slow to recognize gynecological conditions as HIV-related and therefore as case-defining. HIV-infected women have been found to have refractory yeast vaginitis and pelvic inflammatory disease and to have aggressive cervical cancers (Hawkins and Handley 1992; Minkhoff and Dehovitz 1991). Until the end of 1992, these conditions were not defined as HIV-related, according to criteria of the Centers for Disease Control. Thus, women were less likely to be properly identified and treated, and therefore less likely to obtain appropriate services and entitlements. Case definition among women is not merely a biological event, but reflects biased social norms (Anastos and Marte 1989).

The social fabric of the United States is woven in part by threads of racism, patriarchy, homophobia, class hierarchy, and xenophobia. Each of these threads tends to make an "other" of individuals who are not of the socially predominant race, sex, sexual orientation, class, or nationality. Their collective negative impact on health has been demonstrated for a wide variety of conditions from infant mortality, to cancer survival, hypertensive heart disease, and access to preventive services. These issues are of vital importance for the care of HIV-infected persons. Because HIV infection is additionally associated with the fear of contagion, the public and some health care workers have tended to see the "other" as a social danger. Discrimination is never entered on death certificates as a secondary cause of death, but surely it has contributed to who dies, when, and where from HIV infection.

RESEARCH ON ACCESS TO CARE

Research has begun to specifically examine the question of whether care is uniformly accessible to all HIV-infected persons. One marker of access is whether standard therapies are equally available to all persons requiring them. Zidovudine and pentamidine have been studied as markers. In one study, for example, men were three times as likely to have been offered AZT as women, whites were nearly twice as likely to have been offered AZT as nonwhites, insured persons were twice as likely to be offered AZT than the uninsured, and nonusers of injectable drugs were more than twice as likely to be offered AZT than injectable drug users (Stein et al. 1991). Data from a second study showed that those receiving AZT lived six months longer than those who did not (Hidalgo et al. 1990). Thus, demographic factors shape the care offered and received, and contribute to survival.

A second type of study examines whether demographic variables predict patterns of disease. Since 1988, there has been a shifting pattern of AIDS-defining diseases among homosexuals and bisexuals. There has been a downward trend in the rate of pneumocystis pneumonia and increases in the rates of candida esophagitis, Cytomeglovirus (CMV), retinitis, and lymphoma. This altered pattern is likely a result of prophylaxis of pneumocystis pneumonia. A similar trend has not been found among injectable drug users, indicating that changing therapies have not effectively had an impact on this population (Ciesielski et al. 1991).

A third type of access study examines service utilization according to demographic factors. Inpatient service utilization is greater for African Americans, injectable drug users, persons with a history of pneumocystis pneumonia, and those not regularly taking AZT. While gender did not independently predict utilization, African-American women were found to have significantly higher hospital utilization (Merzel et al. 1991). Another study compared persons using emergency departments to those receiving traditional primary care. Persons using the emergency departments were more likely to be women, people of color, and substance abusers, and were less likely to be on AZT (Buskin et al. 1991).

Together, these studies suggest the existence of barriers to access to care that are based on such factors as color, gender, substance abuse, and use of and access to AZT. Health care is not equally available to all HIV-infected persons. The patterns by which access is denied for HIV care are similar to the patterns for other diseases, health indicators, and populations (Schiff et al. 1991). While HIV disease has unique aspects, the access issues are not wholly specific to HIV disease. Rather, they reflect the current organization of health care. Thus, solutions to access to care for HIV-infected persons must be grounded in solutions to access for the whole of society.

MODELS OF CARE

Recognition that HIV disease poses critical medical and social problems has led to the development of numerous innovations in health care. Comprehensive model programs have been developed using multidisciplinary teams of providers, ancillary psychosocial support services, residences for homeless persons with AIDS, case management approaches to care, community-based services, and integration of volunteers into the care team. Needs for services for women and children, abortion, dental care, experimental therapies, same-site chemical dependency treatment, and primary medical care have brought innovative models of care and novel linkages between providers.

Prevention, education, and outreach programs have successfully taken their messages to the streets, finding culturally appropriate and effective means to reach diverse persons at risk, be they gay, African American, Spanish-speaking, women, or injectable drug users (National Commission on AIDS 1991b; Wofsy 1990).

Another innovation resulting from the HIV epidemic is the development and research of new treatments for HIV and its complications. An extraordinary and unprecedented public debate began early in the pandemic and continues today on the need to significantly reduce the time required to evaluate new drugs and to expand the enrollment in these trials to more broadly include all populations affected by HIV disease (Shilts 1987). This remarkable self-empowerment was led by activist-minded persons with AIDS and their advocates, and has clearly led to significant changes in the way new drugs are developed and brought through clinical trials (Mann 1990; Milano et al. 1991). In addition, an explicit attempt is in progress to expand the access of clinical trials to include more women, people of color, children, and injectable drug users.

Here again, innovative model programs have offered an alternative means of care, in this case organizing clinical trials. Community-based research organizations in San Francisco and New York began their own clinical trials out of dissatisfaction with the pace and bureaucracy of the National Institutes of Health (Milano et al. 1991). These efforts led to two national community-based systems of clinical trials—the Community Programs for Clinical Research on AIDS (CPCRAA) and the Community Based Trial Network—which offer clinical trials in existing community-based primary care settings. The trials have simpler designs, with research endpoints that are commonly used in clinical practice (Lackman et al. 1991). The results of these efforts are promising, and they appear capable of readily enrolling large numbers of study subjects. It is clear that quality clinical research can be conducted in settings that accommodate the patient and physician alike.

The most ambitious and comprehensive response to the HIV epidemic in the United States is the Ryan White Comprehensive AIDS Resource Emergency (CARE) Act, which was passed by the Congress in the spring of 1990 (Ryan White CARE Act 1990). This act was the culmination of an extraordinary effort by a broad political alliance of AIDS advocacy groups, community organizations, health care providers, and many others concerned about the need for a comprehensive federal response to the service needs of persons with HIV disease and their families and loved ones. A total of $900 million per year for five years was authorized for this bill.

The explicit intent of the legislation was to provide support for primary medical care and services for persons with HIV disease nationwide, with particular emphasis on the medically and socially underserved. It includes essential health services such as case management, medical, nursing, and dental care, mental health, developmental and rehabilitation services, substance abuse services, nutritional services, and home and hospice care. In addition, it provides for essential support services such as transportation, attendant care, homemaker services, day or respite care, and benefit advocacy provided through public and nonprofit private entities. Services that are adjunctive to the provision of health care for individuals with HIV disease, including housing referral services and child welfare and family services (including foster and adoption services), are also provided.

These services are to be integrated into a network. For example, linkages and cross-referrals to existing counseling and testing sites, both public and private, are required. Access to available local clinical trials is required for all who enter the care system. Access to substance abuse treatment must be made available to clients with chemical dependency, and, where possible, these should be linked with primary medical care. Services for women and children must be linked to day and respite care. Home health and hospice programs must be provided for the severely ill and must be linked to support and respite care for the family and caretakers. And transportation and informational outreach must be included in the overall continuum of care.

More than any other health legislation in memory, the AIDS CARE Act was developed by persons affected by the disease and their caretakers. We learn from this comprehensive approach to service provision that the design of public health policy should be and can be responsive to the expressed needs of those affected by disease and their caretakers. The AIDS CARE Act has served an invaluable role in defining the true care needs of communities that have been devastated by HIV disease. Furthermore, it has acknowledged the importance of participation of affected communities in the planning of the service provision programs. It has offered a measure of hope to cities and states, and particularly to care institutions that are community based or in the public sector, which have been hard hit by the growing service needs. With the AIDS CARE Act, a legislative solution was proposed to the long-recognized problem of access to medical care and services for the medically underserved.

While it is too early to assess the outcomes of the CARE Act, a few preliminary observations can be made about its potentially serious limitations. The available resources will fall far short of the identified need. For example, a conservative estimate of the need for HIV services in Chicago in 1991 totaled over $10 million, yet only $3.2 million was available (Chicago and Cook County Title I Planning Council 1991). Local governments are required to maintain current funding levels for AIDS services under the act, yet most cities, states, and local governments are experiencing serious budget shortfalls. Finally, much of the allocation for the CARE Act is money already committed to existing federal AIDS programs, such as the drug reimbursement program and the home health and hospice program. The need for support for these programs is rapidly escalating. Through 1990, $80 million was spent on the drug reimbursement program, and $18.6 million was set aside for the home health program (Horner et al. 1991; McCarthy and Soliz 1991). In the future these programs will compete with other service programs of escalating need, such as primary care and case management. Thus, the promise of the continuum of services embodied in the CARE Act will be significantly compromised from the outset by escalating and competing needs and insufficient resources.

The AIDS CARE Act may fall short of its goal for broader, systemic reasons. Health care in the United States functions amidst enormous access problems. Thirty-seven million Americans are uninsured (Short et al. 1989), and one million families are denied health care annually for financial reasons (Woolhandler and Himmelstein 1989). Publicly supported programs have faced consistent reductions in benefits for more than a decade. Numerous inner-city hospitals have lost accreditation or have closed, leaving fewer resources available for care for the urban poor (Gage et al. 1991). In this context, the AIDS CARE Act is an attempt to construct a model system on a crumbling infrastructure. While some aspects of the legislation will undoubtedly enhance access, others can only fail unless the pressures on urban care centers are alleviated. The goals of the CARE Act—continuity of care, broad and accessible comprehensive service, health care in concert with support services, prevention linked to community care, and access to clinical trials—should be embraced. These concepts need to be incorporated into reforms that move the health care system toward a national system of primary care and support services, with local control, into which HIV care will logically fit. The time may be near when the problems and solutions to access to HIV care help forge a program to resolve the general health care access crisis. Otherwise, HIV care may degenerate into just another aspect of our dysfunctional, chaotic, fragmented health care system.

CONCLUSIONS

The revolution in health care, catalyzed by HIV disease, has helped expose the access-to-care crisis in the United States. HIV disease has not created the crisis; rather, it has dramatized and heightened existing problems. Enormous forces have rallied, with compassion, insightfulness, and political persistence, to solve aspects of the access crisis for local as well as national issues. With each solution, additional concerns have emerged and have been rapidly pushed to the fore by the continued growth of the pandemic. Today, we stand at a crossroads. In one direction is the warning that existing programs could be overwhelmed if our collective will fails in the struggle to provide access to care. In the other direction is the hope of generalizing experiences, continuing to develop novel models of care, and providing universal access for health care by forging a national health system. The National Commission on Acquired Immune Deficiency Syndrome has recognized this historic juncture. In its analysis and recommendations, national and local planning for HIV care stands hand in hand with universal health care coverage (National Commission on AIDS 1991a). If our national conscience chooses indifference to the suffering, the future will be bleak. If, however, we confront the suffering, we can solve the problems before us. The benefits will touch us all and will ensure better health care for future generations.

Commentary by David McBride

Until recently, the dominant focus of Western medical ethics has been on the rights of the individual. Priorities in the field centered on such issues as defining life and death, informed consent, and protection of human subjects in research. However, in the past decade or so the large segment of the nation's population who lack any or adequate health care has become a central issue in the field of medical ethics. This chapter by Sherer and Goldberg yet again challenges medical ethicists to lend their ears and expertise to the latest, most imperiled social groups underserved by the U.S. health care system: those citizens and other world citizens who have HIV disease.

The authors discuss the HIV disease crisis in both quantitative and social policy terms. By the year 2000 they estimate that between 6 and 8 million people in the United States will have HIV disease, and some 20 to 30 million worldwide. HIV disease victims are not receiving the health care resources they need and are, in fact, losing treatment avenues due to public and private health financing inequities. Sherer and Goldberg show that because HIV disease has become viewed largely as a problem of already marginal social groups and racial minorities, political support for improving the medical and social plight of HIV disease victims has been exceedingly weak.

Between 1980 and 1983 President Reagan commissioned groups of leading ethicists and health care experts to explore the current ethical dilemmas in U.S. medicine and behavioral sciences. The commission addressed equitable access to care and established that the idea that all should receive the highest level of care was impractical. The financial status of our nation's people is just too variable, and medical resources are too limited, it stated. It proposed the more practical standard of "an adequate level of care" (President's Commission for the Study of Ethical Problems in Medicine and Biomedical and Behavioral Research 1983).

But what has the adequate-level-of-care ethic to say about (1) extralegal discrimination—discrimination identified by social groups that experience the victimization; or (2) the traditional resistance by the medical care establishment to national health insurance? Sherer and Goldberg emphasize that involvement in social movements to end discrimination and to provide universal health care is imperative if we are to address the AIDS crisis in ethical terms.

Sherer and Goldberg do not expect their work to produce any sweeping federally sponsored remedies for the social groups most victimized by HIV disease. Since 1970 most U.S. presidents and Supreme Court civil rights decisions have eschewed federally initiated and enforced remedies for historically victimized social groups such as impoverished blacks and Native Americans.[1] For these groups illegal economic exploitation and government-sanctioned institutional inequities reach back over a century. By contrast, the suffering and death of AIDS victims have occurred only in recent years. AIDS researchers must recognize that administrations and courts, uninterested in equality for social groups who have been historic victims, are also prone to neglect AIDS victims within these groups. Hence, Sherer and Goldberg posit not just an ethics of social obligation, but an ethics of social struggle.

NOTE

1. See, for instance, the analysis of the turnabout of the *Brown v. Board of Education* public education policies by J. H. Wilkinson III, *From Brown to Bakke* (New York: Oxford University Press, 1981).

15   Genetic Screening: Toward a New Eugenics?

James E. Bowman

INTRODUCTION

Genetic screening programs have been in vogue for twenty years, and still there are many lessons to be learned from the successes and failures of screening for Tay-Sachs in Ashkenazi Jews and especially for sickle hemoglobin in African Americans. With the advent of cystic fibrosis testing, and the potential for the prediction before birth and in early life of a variety of cancers, and cardiovascular, neurological, and psychiatric disorders, the entire population of the United States (not just Jews and African Americans) has become a target for genetic testing. These recent developments in genetic understanding, as well as the great potential of the human genome project, require critical discussion of related ethical, legal, and social concerns, including issues of confidentiality, autonomy, fairness, and justice.

Why have screening programs? An answer often given to this question is that noncoercive genetic testing programs provide important information, allowing affected individuals to make informed decisions about reproduction. For many people, however, genetic testing would seem to require, or at least imply, action; otherwise, why have a screening program? Furthermore, many people find it unlikely that federal and state governments and foundations would allocate so-called scarce health care monies—totaling millions of dollars over the past twenty years—merely to educate the public. Screening for genetic disorders and genetically transmitted disease implicitly calls for a reduction in the number of affected children.

Although genetic information may be important to scientists and others in positions to appropriate and use the knowledge, genetic information may constitute a low priority for those who live on the edge of a health disaster because of poverty and an inequitable health care system. Consider the following scenario: A destitute and distraught mother in Chicago was informed that her infant (after death) had been screened as part of a state-mandated hemoglobin screening program and found to be a carrier for hemoglobin C, a completely innocuous condition. Several weeks earlier, the same hospital had turned the infant away with a treatable illness. Would this medical center reject the child of affluent parents in the middle of the night? No, of course not; but the hospital would be able to produce reams of paper to justify the dumping of poor infants in an overcrowded public hospital many miles distant—a daily occurrence in the United States. For poor women in an unjust health system, paternalism is alive but justice is barren. Mass genetic screening of populations, particularly for sickle hemoglobin, crystallizes the difficulties and pitfalls of genetic education, testing, and counseling programs in the context of an inequitable health care system.

This chapter discusses some of the ethical issues surrounding genetic screening. I will use the history of sickle cell screening of African Americans to illustrate the interrelationships of paternalism, justice, injustice, and autonomy. First, I will review the evolution of sickle cell screening in the United States from the 1970s to the present, including two recent sickle cell screening projects. Second, I will discuss the threat of a new eugenics in the face of current violations of informed consent and autonomy in sickle cell screening projects. Finally, I will defend the need for scientific inquiry, even if abuses do occur.

SICKLE CELL SCREENING IN THE 1970s: MISINFORMATION AND INJUSTICE

Sickle hemoglobin testing was initiated in the early 1970s following the commercialization of a solubility test for sickle hemoglobin by a major pharmaceutical company (Bowman 1977). Unfortunately, the test did not distinguish between sickle cell trait and sickle cell disease, although it was advertised to do so. The test was widely available, and mass screening for sickle hemoglobin was often led by black organizations, guided by the mistaken belief that sickle cell trait was equivalent to sickle cell disease. Using the solubility test, the Black Panther organization in Chicago, for example, screened over 5,000 black schoolchildren in Chicago. They informed parents and the community that 10% of the children had sickle cell disease and that those who were affected would be dead before age 20 (Bowman 1977). Because the disease had been neglected and because it affected only blacks, black community organizations began to raise accusations of genocide.

Educational brochures rarely mentioned that sickle hemoglobin is also prevalent in populations (such as Greeks, Southern Italians, Arabs, Southern Iranians, and Asian Indians) other than Africans and their descendants. These brochures—some even emanating from the National Institutes of Health—were replete with misinformation, the most serious of which was the equation of sickle cell trait with sickle cell disease. For example, in a news release entitled "Background Information—Sickle Cell Disease," the then Heart and Lung Institute claimed that sickle cell disease is the most common inherited disorder in the United States and is present in more than

2 million black U.S. citizens. The institute should have said that 2 million blacks had the trait (Bowman 1977).

In addition, the erroneous belief that sickle cell disease not only was a major problem in the black community, but also had been neglected because it affected only blacks, led to political action to initiate mandatory testing for sickle hemoglobin. At least twelve states rapidly passed mandatory sickle hemoglobin screening laws, often under pressure from black community organizations. Many of these laws were restricted to the testing of blacks and targeted preschool children, schoolchildren, couples before marriage, and inmates of mental and correctional institutions. Major corporations, including banks, began selectively screening blacks seeking employment. Black flight attendants—who had just been admitted to these jobs—were screened for sickle hemoglobin, and those who tested positive were discharged. Major insurance companies raised rates as high as 25% on persons with sickle cell trait, even though it was well known at that time that the life expectancy of individuals with sickle cell trait was the same as those who did not have the trait. Sickle cell organizations proliferated—some legitimately concerned, others blatantly entrepreneurial—and vied with each other for funds. Most of them propagated misinformation that was already rampant in the black community (Bowman 1977; Reilly 1977).

As a result of community pressure and politics, the National Sickle Cell Anemia Control Act was passed in 1972 (National Sickle Cell Anemia Control Act 1972), expanded in 1976 (Omnibus Genetics Bill 1976), and amended in 1978 (Health Services Amendments 1978). The very title of the Sickle Cell Anemia Control Act was unfortunate because "control" of sickle cell anemia and most serious genetic disorders is possible only by adopting eugenics practices reminiscent of Nazi Germany. Regrettably, sickle hemoglobin misinformation infiltrated the first line of the text of the Sickle Cell Anemia Control Act, repeating the Heart and Lung Institute's claim that over 2 million blacks in the United States had sickle cell anemia. But neither the politicians nor the black organizations should be blamed; they were only quoting presumably reputable sources. Federal legislation led to support of community sickle cell programs, to the establishment of Comprehensive Sickle Cell Centers with education, testing, counseling, and research components, and to the funding of program projects that were limited to research.

National guidelines for education, testing, and counseling programs attempted to introduce sanity into chaos. The National Sickle Cell Disease Program and the Hematology Section of the Centers for Disease Control cooperated and set standards for appropriate hemoglobin testing by various electrophoresis techniques. They also discouraged the use of a solubility test as the primary screening device (Schmidt and Brosius 1972). Finally, the equation of sickle cell trait with sickle cell disease was unequivocally rebutted.

Unfortunately, however, many community groups and even federal programs, in attempting to adhere to guidelines, set unrealistic goals for population testing. Generally, about 15,000 to 20,000 individuals per year were targeted for screening, even though the personnel to care for the educational, counseling, and psychosocial needs of the target populations was not available. Numerical goals that amounted to about eighty-three clients per day, based on an eight-hour day, five days a week for twelve months were unattainable. Individuals and couples at risk for having children with sickle cell disease could now make informed decisions about reproduction. But since prenatal diagnosis was not available in the 1970s, what were their options? They were all somewhat distasteful: chosen childlessness (either through abstinence or birth control), donation of sperm by unaffected donors, or genetic roulette. These first-phase programs and guidelines were initiated before the 1973 *Roe v. Wade* Supreme Court decision, when abortion was legally available in only a few states, or abroad. So abortion was an impractical solution for women who did not want to risk having an affected child or who could not financially afford travel for abortion.

SCREENING IN THE 1980s: NEW ETHICAL ISSUES

Newborn Screening and Prenatal Screening

While the first phase of sickle cell screening targeted children and adults, the second phase (beginning in the mid-1980s) focused on newborn and prenatal screening. In 1985 Marilyn Gaston and her co-workers showed that implementing penicillin prophylaxis of newborns with sickle cell disease and continuing the regimen throughout childhood could ameliorate morbidity and mortality (Gaston et al. 1986). Some programs operate under the principle that the purpose of newborn screening is strictly medical, and that followup of carriers and of other members of the family will dilute the effort and compromise the primary purpose of the program. However, there are good reasons why newborn screening programs for sickle cell disease and for other hemoglobinopathies should encourage testing of other family members when either the disease or the carrier state is found in the infant. To ignore carriers is to miss undetected sickle cell disease in other family members and in future children. Furthermore, such a policy denies the parents' right to know and abrogates their right to choose prenatal diagnosis in a future pregnancy. Therefore, newborn screening for sickle cell disease should lead to programs of prenatal diagnosis. However, prenatal programs, in turn, lead to further ethical dilemmas, which I will discuss by reviewing two current studies on prenatal genetic screening.

Two Recent Prenatal Screening Programs for Hemoglobinopathies

The National Association for Sickle Cell Disease under Charles F. Whitten, president, developed a position on prenatal diagnosis of sickle cell anemia, which I will now summarize (National Association for Sickle Cell Disease 1990). The association recommended that at the first prenatal visit, all black mothers be tested to determine whether they are carriers of the sickle cell gene. (Note that Whitten's program emphasizes sickle hemoglobin, and not hemoglobinopathies, and only black pregnant women are screened.) Each mother who is a carrier should be (1) informed of the nature of sickle cell anemia, (2) counseled that the unborn child may have sickle cell anemia if the father is also a carrier, and (3) counseled that the father should be tested to find out if he is also a carrier. The partners should be informed that if both are carriers, there are techniques to determine if the fetus has the disease. They can then decide whether they wish to test the fetus and whether to terminate the pregnancy. A decision to terminate must not be a condition to obtain prenatal diagnosis, and if the partners elect to continue the pregnancy their decision must be supported. Postabortion counseling should also be offered if the partners decide to abort. Whitten's program did not mention the mother's options if the father is unavailable or refuses testing.

Let us now examine Peter Rowley and co-workers' prenatal screening program for hemoglobinopathies which I analyze elsewhere in detail (Bowman 1991). The first report outlined the design and overall results of the study (Rowley et al. 1991a); the second evaluated the response to genetic counseling (Loader et al. 1991); and the third analyzed counseling in terms of the Health Belief Model (Rowley et al. 1991b).

Rowley's prenatal screening program emphasized two points: (1) the proper goal of the pregnancy screening program is not to reduce the incidence of hemoglobin disorders, and (2) counseling should be nondirective: couples should be allowed to make decisions based on relevant information and their own reproductive goals. Community prenatal care providers from obstetricians in private offices, to public health care providers, to health maintenance organizations participated in the research project. All pregnant women were screened for hemoglobinopathies at the first visit. The provider was given the option of obtaining informed consent for hemoglobinopathy screening, but only one of nineteen participating centers elected to inform its patients. The others asserted that they had their patients' implied consent for relevant diagnostic tests. Patients who tested positive were notified by telephone or by certified U.S. mail. Patients who were carriers were informed that their health would not be affected but that the fetus could have a serious disorder should the partner be a carrier. Genetic associates experienced in counseling for hemoglobinopathies counseled the women without charge, and all laboratory services including DNA analysis were free; however, the project did not cover the cost of amniocentesis. Women who tested positive were offered counseling, but prenatal diagnosis was offered only to women whose partners agreed to be tested and were found to be positive. Couples also had to agree to counseling regarding risks, as well as options.

Rowley's research asked four questions: (1) Does a woman make a special visit to receive an explanation of her test results? (2) Does she want her partner tested? (3) Does the partner come for testing? (4) Do couples at risk choose prenatal diagnosis? The results of the study were as follows.

Of those who came for counseling, 50% were not living with the father and 62% were single. Significantly, 75% of pregnancies were less than eighteen weeks duration. Of 810 positive pregnancies, 68% of the women returned for counseling. Of 453 women counseled during the first screened pregnancy, 86% wanted partners tested and 55% had their partners tested. In seventy-seven pregnancies found to be at risk, twelve women were too late in their pregnancy to be offered prenatal diagnosis; in another twelve pregnancies, the condition for which the fetus was at risk was considered too mild to offer prenatal diagnosis. The mild risks were hemoglobin C disease (HbCC) and hemoglobin E disease (HbEE). (No mention was made of HbE/beta-thalassemia, which is not mild.) Prenatal diagnosis was offered in the remaining fifty-three pregnancies and accepted by twenty-five couples.

Ethical Issues in Prenatal Screening

Rowley and co-workers raised a number of important ethical issues: Should only high-risk populations be targeted for screening? Does screening result in increased abortion in black communities? Is informed consent practical? Should women whose partners are unavailable be offered prenatal diagnosis?

First, who should be screened? Should programs for prenatal testing for hemoglobinopathies include only populations at high risk, such as blacks, peoples of Mediterranean origin, Middle Easterners, Asians, or Southeast Asians? Apparently not. The first paper pointed out that 7% of the subjects with sickle cell trait were not black, and 22% of the beta-thalassemia trait individuals were neither Mediterranean, black, nor Asian. The authors concluded that these findings indicated the need for prenatal screening of all women, rather than only those of high-risk groups. States, such as Georgia, that selectively screen only those identified as African American in newborn screening programs may wish to take note of Rowley et al.'s reports.

Second, will prenatal programs for pregnant women in black communities result in a significant number of abortions of affected fetuses? Or is abortion so anathema in the black community that prenatal diagnosis for sickle cell disease will more commonly be rejected? Are there population differences in the acceptance of pregnancy termination? Rowley and co-workers found that black women often declared that they would not terminate a pregnancy for any reason, while Southeast Asians more frequently accepted pregnancy termination. These findings were in keeping with a survey (Rowley 1989) of prenatal diagnostic services for sickle cell disease at twelve sickle cell centers in the United States, which aimed to estimate the total number of prenatal diagnoses performed and the number of terminations when the diagnosis was positive. The induced abortion rate for fetuses with sickle cell anemia was 39%, and 23% for hemoglobin SC disease. Interestingly, however, induced abortion is proportionately far more frequent in blacks than in whites in the United States (National Center for Health Statistics 1990). Among whites there were 17.5 abortions per 100 live births in 1973 and 30.0 in 1987. Blacks were classified in an "all other" group but possibly constituted the vast majority. In this population there were 28.9 abortions per 100 live births in 1973, and in 1981, 55.7. Perhaps further studies are needed on the acceptance rate in African-American women of abortion for genetic disorders, for it would be odd if black women abort unaffected fetuses at a higher rate than white women, but forgo aborting fetuses with sickle cell disease.

Third, is informed consent practical when pregnancy testing is moved from the genetics testing center to the busy obstetrician's office? There is considerable evidence that the screening of pregnant women and other adults will detect a significant number of individuals who do not know that they have sickle cell disease, and Rowley and co-workers found similarly unsuspecting patients. Accordingly, pregnancy screening for hemoglobinopathies offers both reproductive and crucial medical information. Thus, if obstetricians do not screen for hemoglobinopathies, they could be at risk for medical malpractice if a pregnant woman with sickle cell disease is overlooked and suffers complications from the disease. Furthermore, there have been many successful "wrongful birth" lawsuits against obstetricians and other health workers who fail to inform or counsel, or who use improper techniques to detect genetic variation disorders in members of high-risk groups (Capron 1979; Shaw, 1984).

Rowley and co-workers understood that busy obstetricians have neither the time nor luxury to provide genetic counselors—even if they existed—for every patient at the initial screening. Nevertheless, informed consent and confidentiality safeguards should be part of the design of genetics programs and incorporated into medical decision making. As genetic tests have the potential to invade the privacy of the individual and the immediate family, pregnant women should be able to refuse tests that may affect them adversely. For example, genetic screening may raise unwelcome questions of paternity. Or insurance companies and employers could take measures that protect their own interests but punish the patient.

Although obstetricians cannot practically provide genetic counselors, informed consent must be part of any genetic screening program. One alternative to the busy obstetrician's office is community education programs and projects. The papers of Rowley and co-workers are significant because they raise issues that form a bridge between the era of testing for rare and selected high frequency genetic disorders and future testing for literally hundreds of genetic markers in busy physicians' offices. Michael Kaback and John O'Brien (Kaback and O'Brien 1973) emphasized the importance of a period of community education before implementing genetic screening programs. This approach became an integral part of federally funded sickle cell disease programs (once the chaos subsided): education, testing (with informed consent), and counseling were integrated into community screening programs. Perhaps, if genetic education becomes an important part of the curriculum in schools, future testing subjects will be aware of their options long before they are confronted with genetics screening programs. At any rate, proper education of the community—an admittedly difficult task—may obviate some disadvantages of testing without informed consent by health care providers.

Fourth, should women whose partners are unavailable or refuse testing be offered prenatal diagnosis? The National Association for Sickle Cell Disease/ Whitten report did not address this issue, but the program did emphasize partner decision making. On the other hand, Rowley and his co-workers terminated the options of approximately one-half of the pregnant women: of 463 black women counseled during pregnancy, the partner was not tested in 209 instances, and therefore, prenatal diagnosis was not offered. Nevertheless, if a black woman has the sickle cell trait, and if her partner is black, the odds are about one in forty that she will have a child with sickle cell disease—more commonly sickle cell anemia (hemoglobin SS), hemoglobin SC, or hemoglobin S/beta-thalassemia. A recalcitrant or unavailable father in the Rowley and co-workers' program subjects a woman to a high risk of having a child with sickle cell disease that she may not want. Ironically, prenatal diagnosis, however, is commonly performed for many disorders with much lower frequency. Should not the pregnant woman be allowed to make a choice? Is not her autonomy compromised if she can receive prenatal diagnosis only when accompanied by a man? Should a genetic counseling program implicitly conceal important reproductive options simply because one partner is not available?

Unfortunately, current screening programs do not offer prenatal diagnosis to women if the male partner is unavailable or refuses testing. Lamentably, federal and community sickle screening programs ignore an escalating out-of-wedlock birth rate in the black community (Bowman 1983). Undoubtedly, and understandably, out-of-wedlock births are cautiously dealt with by geneticists, though not by social scientists and the media. Genetics programs are usually constructed on the testing of couples before marriage and on the basis of the classical description of the family; the real world of out-of-wedlock births is ignored.

The research findings of William Julius Wilson, a sociologist at the University of Chicago, provides insight into this phenomenon (Wilson 1987). Wilson's group investigated out-of-wedlock births in the black community. Not only has the incidence of premarital conception increased, but also the proportion of premarital pregnancies that were legitimated by marriage has decreased. Accordingly, out-of-wedlock births today constitute a much greater proportion of total births than they did in the past. Interestingly, Wilson asserts that the black out-of-wedlock birth ratio has increased precipitously, not because the rate of extramarital births has significantly increased, but because both the proportion of women married and the rate of marital fertility have declined. Furthermore, the decrease in the proportion of all women who are married and living with their husbands reflects both a sharp rise in separation and divorce rates, and a considerable increase in the percentage of never-married women. These figures have been particularly striking for black women: the proportion of women married and living with their husbands decreased from 52% in 1947 to 34% in 1980. Wilson also showed that the proportion of never-married black women increased from 65% in 1965 to 82% in 1980 for those aged 14 to 24, and from 8% to 21% for those aged 25 to 44.

Finally, Wilson indicated that the jobless rate for black males also contributed to the out-of-wedlock birth rate, because black women see little advantage in marrying a man who has little prospect for contributing to family support. A program that depends on the cooperation of unavailable fathers, then, places the pregnant woman who does not wish to have a child with sickle cell disease in an untenable position, compromising her autonomy.

On the other hand, if all the burden is placed on the woman as to whether or not to abort an affected fetus, she could be more susceptible to coercion if she were alone in making the decision. Family, community, and other pressures can be more directive; the victim, the pregnant woman, is vulnerable and likely to be blamed for her condition during a time when she can least sustain social pressure. The choice is between autonomy or paternalism.

PUBLIC POLICY AND THE THREAT OF A NEW EUGENICS

Issues of Justice in Public Policy

Paternalism, a denial of autonomy, and spurious justice mar today's genetic screening programs. Communities are bombarded by genetic education, testing, and counseling programs. Advertisements in newspapers, magazines, radio, and television offer adolescent and adult screening, including prenatal diagnosis—all supported by public funds. However, public funds for pregnancy termination have been denied, and under the Bush administration, clinics were prohibited from informing poor mothers of their reproductive options. (This policy was reversed by President Clinton in 1993.) An editorial in the *New York Times* ("The Importance of Dr. Sullivan" 1988) pointed out that 4 million women—mainly poor women—who depended on federally supported family planning clinics were denied access not only to abortion, but also to medical information that could keep them from becoming pregnant. The editorial asked how a physician, forbidden under the regulations even to mention the word "abortion," could help a woman make informed family planning choices. "And how cruel that a poor woman can't be told that an abortion is a legal option—and given a referral if she requests one—compared with the woman who can afford a private doctor" (p. A22). The editorial concluded that the United States has two kinds of family planning counseling: one for the affluent, and one for the poor. Although the federal government denies women access to modern family planning, policies that could lead to censure or incarceration of pregnant women are prevalent (Hopkins 1991).

In addition to the ethical issues just discussed, the work of Rowley and colleagues also raises some crucial public policy issues. First, is a public policy rational that offers support for newborn screening, as well as prenatal diagnosis of hemoglobinopathies and other disorders, and at the same time renounces support for abortion of affected fetuses? Such a policy may not be rational, but it is the law. The Supreme Court has repeatedly upheld the denial of public support for abortion if the state so chooses (*Harris v. McRae* 1980) (*Maher v. Roe* 1973). Nevertheless, several states (for example, New York, California, and Oregon) do provide public monies for abortion. Poor women in most states are encouraged to participate in genetic testing programs that are supported by public funds, and prenatal diagnosis is offered. Thus, pregnant women are led to the brink and left on their own (Bowman 1983).

The Supreme Court (*Dandridge v. Williams* 1970) upheld legislation in the state of Maryland to limit the number of children for which the state would provide AFDC (Aid for Dependent Children). Thus, poor women in Maryland—and everywhere, if the states so decide—can either elect to have additional children who will become wards of the state or be restricted to the unsavory options of abstinence, sterilization, or abortion. Even if a poor woman meticulously practices contraception, contraceptive failure can be penalized. Unaffected children cost the state far less than children with sickle cell disease and other serious genetic disorders. And if the state—by indirect coercion—can place limits on the birth of poor unaffected children, it can also place limits on the birth of children who have serious genetic disorders. Thus, the specter of *Dandridge* may haunt us as health care costs escalate. There are many back doors to eugenics, but this one is real.

The consequences of even the most rational court decision also cannot be foreseen. The doctrine of the police power of the state was introduced in *Munn v. Illinois*, which confirmed the common law principle that the private interests of the individual must be subservient to the interests of the state (*Munn v. Illinois* 1876). No one could have predicted that the police power of the state would be used to sanction compulsory vaccination for a variety of communicable diseases, marriage laws, mandatory sterilization, mandatory newborn screening for genetic disorders, seat belt laws, prohibition of spitting on the sidewalk, and countless other city and state regulations. As Dan Beauchamp emphasized, the restriction of personal liberty or property to promote public welfare is firmly rooted in the republican soil of our political tradition (Beauchamp 1988). But this is a cause of concern, for the police power of the state is based on utilitarian ideals. Bernard Williams warns us that a minority population subject to discrimination would be foolish to subscribe to a utilitarian philosophy, which sacrifices the interests of the few for the greater amount of benefit of the majority (Williams 1985).

In an attempt to resolve some of the major objections to utilitarianism, John Rawls developed an important theory of justice based on the public interest (Rawls 1971). He examined a social contract mechanism, which was an outgrowth of previous social contracts as outlined by Locke, Rousseau, and Kant. Rawls argued that injustice is permitted only when it is necessary to avoid an even greater injustice. A just society not only is designed to foster the good of its members, but also is regulated by the public's definition of justice. Rawls acknowledged that perceptions of what is just and what is unjust are often controversial.

The extent of injustice in a society may be a more accurate measure of that society than an evaluation of justice. Judith Shklar explores the question, "When is a disaster a misfortune and when is it an injustice?" (Shklar 1990, p. 1). If, for example, a dreadful event is caused by the external forces of nature, it is a misfortune. However, if it is under the control of humans, it is an injustice. If an earthquake kills thousands of people, it is a misfortune, but also an injustice, because many of the people would not have died had the buildings been constructed properly. But proper building construction is often an indication of affluence. Thus, the consequences of the earthquake were the result of an injustice. Similarly, high infant mortality was once considered a misfortune, but today, in the United States, high infant mortality rates are an injustice because they can be reduced. In addition, poor blacks are differentially affected; this constitutes an even greater injustice. The death of poor children because affluent university hospitals turn them away is another example of the injustice of the federal and state governments, the medical establishment, and those who vote and pay taxes. And it is an injustice and a denial of autonomy when poor women are denied public support for abortion and thus indirectly coerced to have child after child with the risk of congenital abnormalities. It is an injustice that California has one of the best genetic screening programs in the country, including prenatal diagnosis and support for abortion, but denies prenatal care in county hospitals for poor women because of alleged budget constraints (Bowman 1991).

The New Eugenics and the Fear of Scientific Discovery

Technical advances in prenatal diagnosis make possible the selection of children without certain genetic and other congenital disorders. These discoveries, combined with health care budget constraints, produce fears of a scientific eugenics and an environment that emphasizes a more "rational allocation of scarce health resources"—a euphemism for rationing health services to the poor. Eugenics precepts have been with us since at least the time of Socrates, and represent society's attempt to restrict the production of individuals whom it deems unfit. The unfit have included people with severe birth defects or mental deficiency, as well as religious, ethnic, or racial groups different from those who are in power. Before the advent of new genetic technologies, distinguishing the perfect from the imperfect was a mixture of conjecture, prejudice, racism, anti-Semitism, and other bigotries. Now science can be more precise.

Margery Shaw raised new conundrums about paternalism, autonomy, and justice (Shaw 1984). She analyzed the prospective rights of the fetus and emphasized that recognizing fetal rights leads to certain parental obligations before conception. Shaw asserted that because having children is usually a foreseeable event, parents should consider the quality of the gametes that their children will inherit. Radiation exposure, chemical mutagens, and defective genes are important, and physicians and parents should take appropriate steps to ensure that children are not affected. Shaw also argued that the right to reproduce is not absolute, and, as an example, she cites state prohibitions against certain types of marriage.

Shaw goes further. She maintains that genes, like bacteria and viruses, are transmissible units, and she observes that the law can impose compulsory vaccination in order to prevent or control the spread of communicable diseases. Shaw compared genetic and infectious diseases: both are transmitted to others; both vary in their rate of "contagion"; both are unequally distributed among populations; and both vary in morbidity and mortality. She concludes that

as individuals and as members of the human community, we have the power, and the moral duty, to promote the health and well-being of our children. For the first time in human history we can begin to free ourselves from our biological constraints and shape a better destiny for future generations by promoting the goals of our forefathers to "promote the General Welfare, and secure the Blessings of Liberty to ourselves and our posterity." (Shaw 1984, p. 116)

Ironically, the quotation within Shaw's concluding statement is from the preamble to the Constitution. What might the mothers of slave children have thought of the justice of the preamble? Their children did not count then, just as poor children in the United States are expendable today. If Shaw's suggestions become public policy, there is no doubt that poor women and their families will be selectively affected.

Shaw's position is an example of the new eugenics. One of the most outspoken opponents of the old eugenics was the late Lionel S. Penrose, who, ironically, held a professorship at University College London named in honor of Sir Francis Galton, a pioneer of eugenics in the nineteenth century. When Penrose became Galton professor, he also became editor of the *Annals of Eugenics*. Much to the consternation of some geneticists, Penrose changed the name of the journal to the *Annals of Human Genetics*. Daniel Kevles succinctly summed up Penrose's disdain for eugenics:

According to some our true destiny must be to try to produce perfect genes, regardless of our social interests. . . . It is ultimately a matter of opinion but for myself, I would rather live in a genotypically imperfect society which preserves human standards of life than in one in which technological standards were paramount and heredity perfect. (Kevles 1985, p. 289)

Unfortunately, the specter of eugenics invariably leads to pleas for restrictions on scientific discovery. Science and pseudoscience have often been used as weapons against minorities, particularly blacks in the United States. Phrenology and IQ tests have been supplanted by genetic tests for several hundred disorders, before and after birth. With each new development, naysayers appear on television and inundate the world with instant scholarship. Meanwhile, scientists quietly make new discoveries, oblivious to the full impact of their work. The full potential of the wheel, fire, manned flight, and even nuclear energy, for example, was unimaginable to their discoverers. While these inventions have destroyed many lives, who would propose to discard these discoveries or not to use them? We live in a world with potential for scientific advances on every continent; thus, our prohibitions in the United States are mere feathers in a tornado.

Marc Lappé, for example, is deeply concerned that the discovery of bipolar disorders linked to DNA markers on chromosome 11 could be used to abort fetuses with bipolar manic-depressive illness. He queries, "Should we use the knowledge of the likely presence of such "deviant" genes to abort affected fetuses? Such a program would . . . potentially deprive us of great poets like Sylvia Plath or politicians like Winston Churchill, both of whom may have suffered from bipolar manic depression" (Lappé 1987, p. 5).

Later, Lappé postulated that uncovering genes that regulate human vulnerability to grave illnesses such as Huntington's chorea or Alzheimer's disease could increase the incidence of suicide or selective abortion, and he wonders what limits, if any, should be imposed on the acquisition of such knowledge. Lappé's remarks are well intentioned, and in his defense, as long as we have scientists like him around, eugenics will be challenged at every rising. But to succumb to Lappé's thesis would take us back to the days of Galileo, the Inquisition, or the suppression of genetics in the Soviet Union. Our country is preeminent in science in part because scientists and scholars fled to our shores after their own country denied them freedom of inquiry. Yes, there have been numerous abuses of genetic testing, and the prospects are even greater that each scientific advance in genetic testing and prenatal diagnosis will also fall prey to the abuse of charlatans. However, the acquisition of knowledge should not be sacrificed because of what some fool may propose, or even attempt. This thesis may appear to contradict my reservations about eugenics, but suppression of knowledge is the first step to decadence.

CONCLUSION

The faces and interrelationships of paternalism, justice, injustice, and autonomy are many. We must force ourselves to recognize them, particularly those that we relegate to our subconscious in order to protect our own equanimity. Many years ago, after living for six years in a country in the Middle East, friends visited us from the United States. We were walking down the street when suddenly a look of horror came on their faces. My wife and I asked why they were so upset. One of them replied, "Did you see that child with hundreds of flies on his face?" My wife and I had not noticed the child. This anecdote has two messages: first, how easy it is to ignore the plight of others; second, how unfair it is that health and physical well-being are not the birthright of us all.

Injustice is, of course, inevitable. Even with uniform or standardized health care, people will be served imperfectly because their needs are not the same. However, to admit that we cannot be fair in the allocation of resources is not the same as the deception that we cannot provide a base line standard of care for all. We have arsenals of weapons that can make this planet uninhabitable for all. Yet we subscribe to the shibboleth that health care resources are scarce in this the most affluent of countries. Universal health care is a policy and a moral affirmation that all major industrialized countries have—with the exception of the United States and South Africa. Still, universal health care does not mean equitable health care, for no matter what kind of society (communist, socialist, market, military, right-wing totalitarian, or otherwise), for the affluent there is always affirmative action in health care.

NOTE

The research for this chapter was supported, in part, by grant #HG 00641-01, National Initiative for Human Genetic Research, National Institutes of Health.

Commentary by Robert Murray, Jr.

Dr. James Bowman considers the paternalism and injustice of the current health care system and its relation to genetic testing and screening programs. He draws on his firsthand knowledge and experience of the errors that were made in genetic screening programs for hemoglobinopathies in the 1970s to show the interconnection of paternalism, justice, injustice, and violations of autonomy. He identifies a potential "new eugenics" based on the use of modern molecular genetic technology to produce better genetic specimens through negative eugenics. He then reviews two programs of prenatal diagnosis for sickle cell disease and related hemoglobinopathies. These programs demonstrate that prenatal diagnosis for sickle cell should include *all* women, because significant numbers of nonblack patients were found to be trait positive. Furthermore, Bowman notes that amniocentesis should be provided for all carrier pregnant women, even when the father of the fetus is unavailable for testing. His rationale is that the risk of having a child with sickle cell disease in such a situation is significantly greater than that for other indications—for example, Down's syndrome based on advanced maternal age, for which prenatal diagnosis is routinely recommended.

Bowman indicates that common conceptions of "parental obligations" and the need to control genetic disorders may undergird the application of this new eugenics, because they result in a disproportionate imposition of reproductive restrictions on poor black individuals. But while he decries the misapplication of genetic technology because of injustice and paternalism, he presents a strong argument against any restriction of the advance of genetic knowledge, even if it might mean negative or potentially harmful outcomes for people who have untreatable diseases, for example, Huntington's disease. He feels that knowledge must not be constrained or sacrificed because of the potential for harmful use.

Bowman's major emphasis is on the unethical application of the principle of justice as depicted by Rawls. Poor, black, and disadvantaged men and especially women are denied the benefits of the health care system as it is currently constituted; at the same time they are subjected to coercion and paternalism in genetic screening programs. Thus, their autonomy is denied or restricted in a variety of ways that do not seriously affect the members of the Anglo-American community. Without major reforms in the health care system, it will be impossible for members of the disadvantaged minorities to avoid being morally abused by programs of genetic screening and prenatal diagnosis. They can best be protected through a well-designed process of informed consent. Unfortunately, current programs of genetic screening and prenatal diagnosis are generally not designed with the special problems and ethical values of minority individuals in mind. The negative eugenic goals implicit in currently operating programs of screening and prenatal diagnosis promoted by public health agencies and justified by the new eugenics will have a disproportionately negative effect on the already disadvantaged segments of our society. This further compounds the injustice that already exists in our health care system.

The injustice and inconsistency of the health care system in the United States have been well known for many years. Unfortunately, the inequities in access and quality of care between Anglo and African Americans that have been recognized for years not only continue to exist, but also in some instances have worsened. It just does not make sense to deny access to certain basic health services, while at the same time requiring or encouraging participation in specialized programs of genetic screening, especially when the genetic conditions screened for are of fairly low frequency even in minority populations. Health care funding for routine prenatal care, for instance, would significantly reduce more common health conditions that currently constitute a significant health burden in the black community.

This kind of behavior violates not only the principle of justice but also the principle of beneficence. Furthermore, when additional harm is done to a disadvantaged and poor population through the introduction of negative eugenic programs (especially when they are disguised as something else), the principle of nonmaleficence is also undermined. For those populations who are most in need of help, it is imperative that a new program should, on balance, do no harm. I am in agreement with Bowman that genetic testing programs should be of lower priority than programs for basic primary health care and health care delivery (e.g., immunization, screening for and eliminating lead from the environment of children, prenatal care, and providing proper nutrition). I also agree that programs of prenatal diagnosis for hemoglobin disorders ought to be available to any black mother positive for a hemoglobinopathy carrier state, whose baby has a black father. This is not only consistent with the recurrence risks seen in other programs of prenatal diagnosis, but also will turn out to be cost-effective even if the relatively low rate of using the option to terminate affected pregnancies is taken into account (39% for sickle cell anemia and 23% for Hb SC disease).

On two points, however, I disagree with my distinguished and learned colleague. There is little doubt that when government and public health officials promote the expenditure of funds on a health program they expect a payoff in the form of a significant reduction in the frequency of affected individuals and a reduced amount of money spent in that category of disease. Yet this official attitude does not have to dominate or even constitute the primary goals of genetic screening programs. Even though the money may not be primarily appropriated for public and professional education, it is possible for directors to structure their programs so that the participants not only get the genetic benefits of the program, but also derive ancillary benefits in areas of more primary need. The outreach (mobile) sickle cell screening program of the Center for Sickle Cell Disease of Howard University, for instance, was federally funded to do hemoglobinopathy screening, and the major focus was on identifying individuals with sickle cell trait. However, all individuals were also offered free screening for two treatable conditions: high blood pressure and iron deficiency anemia. Adding these screening tests changed the balance of the benefit/harm ratio from negative to positive for the person screened. Mass genetic screening of populations need not be more harmful than beneficial.

I find myself leaning toward the position suggested by Marc Lappé who worries (with justification in my opinion) about the harm that might come about through the misapplication or premature use of predictive genetic information about diseases of late onset. I think it is an exaggeration to suggest, as Bowman does, that attending to the concerns of Lappé and others "would take us back to the days of Galileo, the Inquisition, or the suppression of genetics in the Soviet Union." The proposal is not to sacrifice the acquisition of this knowledge, but rather to introduce it in a public and medical atmosphere that will not sacrifice innocent people who have inherited a genetic disorder on the altar of scientific research. Instead, they should be made, on balance, the beneficiaries of the best that medical science and the health care system have to offer.

16 Women and Underserved Populations: Access to Clinical Trials

Sara Goering

INTRODUCTION

Lack of adequate access to health care for traditionally underserved populations (most notably poor ethnic minorities and women) is tied to a lack of medical research focused on their particular needs. The two problems are intricately related—each feeds on the other. Many of the factors that make access to health care difficult for underserved populations (including, for instance, lack of funding, geographical maldistribution of services, inadequate transportation, and cultural or linguistic differences and discrimination) also make it difficult to involve them as subjects in medical research. Although a majority of these barriers to health care could be overcome by balancing current socioeconomic inequities, a growing body of literature suggests that in at least some instances diseases themselves may be manifested differently among the races and sexes, requiring different kinds or levels of treatment. Thus, socioeconomic reparations alone will not remedy the health problems of underserved ethnic groups and women (Mullings 1984). Without research to assess the particular needs of these groups, access to the existing health care system might not significantly help them and in some cases could even be harmful.

Biological differences cannot account for all or even most of the current disparities in health and health care among the races or the sexes. Clearly, much of the inequity in the health care system stems from barriers to access that affect people according to social conditions associated with class, race, or gender. The inequity may also be the result of structural problems within the system. Any theory that attempts to explain ethnic and sex differences in rates of morbidity and mortality without acknowledging the influence of social and structural factors is inappropriate (Leary 1990). However, since most of the other authors in this volume stress structural and cultural barriers to health care, I feel it is appropriate also to consider some of the duties of the health care system to provide equal services where racial and sexual barriers go beyond what is strictly socially or politically imposed. Thus, while focusing on biological differences as the sole source of health inequity is mistaken, ignoring these differences when they do exist is equally wrong. In addition to addressing the problems associated with social conditions and economic barriers, we must address and be willing to accept certain inherent biological differences and their influences on health status. Perhaps the actual number of biological differences is relatively small, but ignoring the significant ones can be devastating. It simply makes sense to test treatments on populations representative of those who will be receiving treatment, rather than on a skewed sample population.

In this chapter I will show why restricting medical research to studies done with white, middle-aged men as subjects is inappropriate and unjust. I will point to several examples in which such conduct has led to worrisome results. I will also show how the current justifications for the exclusion of minorities and women in research are based on racism and sexism in the medical establishment, and suggest that steps be taken to remedy this situation. Finally, I will offer a word of caution regarding the segregation of races and sexes in research, for the potential for great benefits is tainted with the possibility of serious costs.

PROBLEMS WITH THE WHITE MALE MODEL

A growing body of literature reveals clinical studies in which ethnic and sex differences have a significant effect on the course and kind of treatment. Simply extrapolating data obtained from white middle-aged men is proving not to be the answer to settling these differences. Although they are an easily accessible population to procure as research subjects, white middle-aged men are not a truly representative population, and the seemingly less accessible populations pay the price of misrepresentation.

Techniques and treatments that have been studied on white middle-aged men in a controlled and closely monitored research environment are then unleashed on the much more diverse general population, most often without the security of the clinical setting. Patients from populations who experience difficulties in getting access to health care may be given a new treatment and never be heard from again, at least not by the same physician. Given that population differences in disease manifestation and treatment do exist, this is a dangerous method of treating underserved populations and may place them in even greater danger than the illness for which they believe they are receiving treatment. In what follows, I will give several examples as evidence of this problem. Clearly, the solution is to target more clinical studies on the particular medical needs of these populations, using members of the groups themselves as subjects.

Thus far, the issue of ethnic and sex differences in disease diagnosis and treatment has been addressed only in obvious cases, such as sickle cell disease among African Americans, Tay-Sachs among Eastern European Jews (Leary

1990), and breast and uterine cancer in women (although, strangely enough, Rebecca Dresser reports the existence of a pilot study to look at the effects of obesity on these cancers that was conducted solely on men) (Dresser 1992). Noteworthy population differences, however, go far beyond these most obvious cases. Consider the following examples.

Studies conducted on white men led the American Heart Association to suggest a diet for all Americans to reduce their cholesterol levels in order to decrease the risk of coronary heart disease. Although they recommended a general reduction in cholesterol intake, they targeted low-density lipoproteins (LDLs) in particular. Further studies, however, have suggested that, although high levels of LDLs are dangerous for men, they are far less threatening for women. In addition, women are much more sensitive to low levels of the so-called good cholesterol, or high-density lipoproteins (HDLs). This means that diets that recommend a general cholesterol reduction are potentially harmful to women (Purvis 1990).

In another study, African-American men with psychiatric problems traditionally treated with lithium, a drug tested and used successfully on white men, suffered excessive toxic reactions when treated with the drug. It was found that the African-American men as a group had less efficient lithium-sodium countertransport mechanisms than white men. The toxicity of the lithium treatment greatly increased the already high risk of renal failure for the African-American men (Cotton 1990b).

A number of studies have shown that Asian patients react more strongly than whites when treated with propranolol, a beta-blocker that reduces heart rate and blood pressure. While this variation was traditionally accounted for by generalized differences in body size and/or weight, new evidence shows that Asians as a group have a much faster metabolism for propranolol than whites and that a smaller percentage of the dosage is inactivated by plasma protein binding in Asians (Zhou 1989). On the other hand, data show that African-American hypertensive patients do not respond to beta-blockers as well as whites (Sirgio et al. 1986) and that the serum concentration of propranolol is lower in African-American patients than in whites who received identical doses (Walle et al. 1985).

While the list of studies showing significant differences between populations goes on, its length is not to be outdone by the number of studies continuing to ignore these findings. For instance, an NIH-funded study on the potential prophylactic effects of aspirin on heart disease was conducted entirely on men, although heart disease is the number one killer of women. One reason cited for the exclusion of women as subjects was the lack of available women physicians. (The study was conducted with physicians as subjects.) Others blame the extra time and money that would have been needed to complete the study to significance. (According to Paul Cotton, some say that heart disease "fails to kill enough of them [women] fast enough to make its study in females 'feasible' "; see Cotton 1990b, p. 1049.) Still others ascribe it to blatant sexism. (Consider Dr. P. L. Frommer, who doesn't think enough women would "be interested in participating and be content to go through the hassle of taking a placebo"; see Cotton 1990a, p. 1055.) The lack of women in the subject population of this study made it difficult for many doctors to personally prescribe the courses of action that are publicly suggested by organizations such as the American Heart Association. However, after an uproar about the unknown effects of regular aspirin consumption on women, another study was undertaken with female nurses as subjects, with the conclusion that aspirin does indeed reduce the risk of heart attack for women (Tavris 1992). The fact that these studies rendered similar results for both sexes should not be too quickly generalized to other disorders and treatments.

Recently, for example, concern has arisen about sex differences in response to HIV infection. In order to be considered for most clinical drug trials for AIDS, a person must exhibit "full-blown" AIDS, which includes a broad spectrum of illnesses related to HIV infection. Until recently, many women did not fit this description because their infections had progressed in a different pattern than that strictly recognized as AIDS, resulting in a new diagnosis, AIDS Related Complex (ARC) (Levine 1990b). If HIV affects men and women differently, resulting in varying groups of infections, we ought not limit our studies to the syndrome as it affects men. In 1993 the Center for Disease Control revised its classification system for HIV infection, in part to address these concerns (CDC 1992a).

Craig Svensson has investigated the exclusion of African Americans from clinical drug trials, focusing on studies published in *Clinical Pharmacology and Therapeutics* over a three-year period (Svensson 1989). He found that only ten of fifty published accounts of new drug trials included any racial data, and even in the study of antihypertensive drugs, an area in which differential racial responses to drug treatments have been well-documented, only about half of the researchers gave racial data. Of the antihypertensive studies that included subjects of different races, only one attempted to determine if there was a race-related response difference. Furthermore, in more than half of the trials in which racial data were available, the percentage of African-American subjects was less than the percentage of African Americans in the community and in the U.S. population. Apparently, African Americans were underrepresented in the clinical trials, and as Svensson notes, this "suggests that insufficient data exist to accurately assess the safety and efficacy of many new drugs in blacks" (p. 265).

JUSTIFICATIONS FOR THE EXCLUSIONS IN CLINICAL TRIALS

How do researchers explain this blatant and seemingly unethical exclusion of ethnic minorities and women in medical research? Their reasoning is varied and extensive, covering problems from financing and recruitment to problems with tight experimental control and subject safety. Svensson's study suggests that many researchers simply have not even considered racial health differences a pertinent issue in their research. In what follows, I will address these so-called justifications and show why none of them is truly substantial, and how most of them can be overcome.

Some of the researchers involved claim that using white middle-aged men is necessary because of the need to maintain tight experimental controls and to avoid confounding factors. Clearly, research done on homogeneous groups yields tighter, more exact results. Yet this is precisely the problem at hand. The tighter and more exact the results are, the less they can be safely generalized to the population as a whole. Since the population in general is not homogeneous, why should we take data from one of the homogeneous groups within it and apply it to all the other groups? Surely it would be safer and more beneficial to society as a whole to study representative groups from each population sector and thus to obtain tight and exact data specific to each population's distinct needs.

In defense of the exclusion of women in medical research, many researchers claim that the fluctuating hormonal cycles of women serve as confounding factors in clinical studies. However, as Dresser correctly questions, "Why is it female, but not male, hormones that 'complicate' research?" (Dresser 1992, p. 25). Why is it that white men must serve as the exclusive prototype? In addition, one wonders why, if the menstrual cycles of women may complicate the experimental results, women are then allowed and even encouraged to abide by the results obtained on men—results that take no account of the potential complications? The fact is, women have distinct hormonal cycles, and if complications are a possibility during clinical trials, then they are also a possibility after drug or treatment approval, when women may be taking a new drug outside the safe confines of the clinical setting.

Another excuse for not using women as subjects in clinical trials deals with the possibility that a woman may become pregnant while participating in the research. In such a case, participation in the experiment may cause complications with the pregnancy, miscarriage, or birth defects. This means that, in effect, "In the name of *potential* protection for *potentially* pregnant women and their fetuses, all women have lost the opportunity to improve and extend their lives" (Dresser 1992). This attempted justification ignores the fact that many potential women subjects may be beyond their reproductive years, not sexually active, or simply taking adequate precautions against pregnancy. To preclude all women from participating is to assume that all women are simply walking wombs who are unreliable in their contraceptive practices (Levine 1990b). This assumption is a bit ridiculous, particularly when some of the women concerned may be elderly cardiac patients who presumably are not planning pregnancies (Purvis 1990).

Even if we consider only sexually active fertile women who are in their reproductive years, it seems that we really ought to allow these women them-selves to make decisions regarding their participation in clinical trials. Most of the women in this group would no doubt prefer to be informed of the risks and hazards as well as the potential benefits, and then to choose whether to participate. We might also ask why sexually active fertile women of reproductive age are excluded while men of the same class are allowed, and in many cases encouraged, to participate. Drugs and other treatments that could potentially damage a woman's reproductive system or a fetus might very well also have a detrimental effect on a man's sperm (Becker 1990).

Problems associated with the recruitment of minority and women subjects are also often cited as reasons for their exclusion in clinical trials. There are at least several reasons for recruitment problems. First, these difficulties point to much greater problems within the medical system. For instance, a great disparity exists between the numbers of ethnic minorities and women, as compared to white men, studying in medical schools and working as med-ical researchers and physicians (Jonas and Sylvia 1988). Therefore, this com-mon subject pool for medical research is nearly devoid of available nonstandard (white male) subjects. The long-term answer is to get a more diverse population into the profession. In the short term, however, there are other solutions. Clearly, subjects will have to come from outside the medical system, and the solution to their recruitment will have to address the existing obstacles. Poor women, for example, may need help with child care and transportation in order to participate. This will undoubtedly involve extra financial burdens on the researchers and, in the end, on the taxpaying public, but as it has been pointed out, "The policy line thus far has been that [research on nontraditional subjects is] too expensive. But too expensive compared with what?" (Cotton 1990b, p. 1050). The potential payoffs are surely worth the associated costs.

Second, widespread distrust of the medical establishment was understand-ably strengthened after the Tuskegee study (in which African-American men with syphilis were deliberately left untreated in order to study the course of the disease; this study started in the 1930s and was not ended until 1972). Following this study, the National Commission for the Protection of Human Research Subjects of Biomedical and Behavioral Research released the Bel-mont Report, which warned against "vulnerable subjects . . . such as racial minorities . . . being continually sought as research subjects" owing to their availability in research-oriented university and public hospitals (National Commission for the Protection of Human Subjects of Biomedical and Be-havioral Research 1978). The commission was concerned that less advan-taged populations would become guinea pigs for treatments that would in the end be more readily available to the more advantaged groups who wer-en't involved in the risks and discomforts of the research. While this was and remains a serious concern, researchers may have overcompensated, translating it into a policy of complete exclusion of minorities and women from clinical studies. Today we must understand that ethnic minorities and women have much to gain from participation in clinical studies. As long as their participation is carefully controlled and not abused, they will be able to reap benefits that have for too long accrued almost exclusively to white men.

One potential solution to the recruitment problems is to start with community-based research that comes out of minority practices and clinics in underserved areas. Minority populations will presumably be more likely to trust community health care facilities and physicians than more distant and less personal health care providers. This would also alleviate some of the problems of transportation, accessibility, and linguistic or cultural differences and discrimination in the delivery of health care (see Schensul and Guest, Chapter 3, and Ferguson, Chapter 11, in this volume). However, potential conflicts of interest exist when the provider serves a dual role as researcher and physician.

Finally, there are the inevitable financial difficulties associated with intensified recruitment and more diverse research. These difficulties have been remedied in part by the recent NIH Women's Health Initiative—a ten-year, $500 million study involving three large-scale research projects on women's health issues (Palca 1991). This project was launched under the directorship of Bernadine Healy, after several years of NIH guideline revisions regarding the inclusion of women and minorities in research, and a General Accounting Office investigation into the rules, spurred by the Congressional Caucus for Women's Issues. The result is an enormous and lengthy research initiative for women's health issues. Significant financial backing for health issues specific to particular ethnic groups is needed before we can realistically feel that health care equity in clinical studies is being adequately addressed.

CONCLUSION

There are, of course, more problems on the horizon. Acknowledging inherent differences between the races and sexes may inadvertently cause a rise in racism and sexism. It may refuel the fires of the once livid nature/nurture debate, which will bring with it all the misconceptions about superior and inferior genetic abilities associated with eugenics. It may "serve only the interests of those eager to blame the disproportionate share of the burden of poverty and disease borne by minorities on inherent racial traits and genetic defects rather than on societal problems such as poverty, suboptimal health care, or a legacy of racial prejudice" (Osbourne and Feit 1992, p. 277). Differences in disease manifestation, treatment, and incidence among population sectors could lead to increases in discrimination and exclusionary hiring practices. Differences between the blood and kidneys of different ethnic groups could lead to white-only or black-only blood banks and organ donor lists, reminiscent of the segregated drinking fountains and restaurants of another era (Leary 1990).

On the other hand, failing to acknowledge the differences is also a form of racism, one that is alive and well today, and that is thus perhaps more important than the distant fear. Our society ought to be able to address the inherent differences among its population and embrace them, rather than instinctively labeling them as flaws. As Dresser has said, "Perhaps we have come far enough to recognize such differences without transforming them into tools for maintaining the traditional social hierarchy" (Dresser 1992, p. 29). The challenge is ours to move forward rather than to stagnate or return to the clearly unjust ways of bygone eras. An ethical medical establishment must ascertain the particular needs of all its patients and must find a way to allow them equity in access to treatment. One of the first steps toward this goal should be the inclusion of nontraditional groups as subjects of medical research.

Commentary by Richard Schmitt

Sara Goering cites evidence for biological differences between white men and other men, as well as between men and women, which significantly influence the effects of medications and required dosages. Even though that information is well known, clinical trials are still frequently limited to white men. Goering argues that that practice must, for ethical and medical reasons, be discontinued. These facts are disturbing. Goering asks that in future clinical trials the subjects be drawn from different groups, depending on the existing evidence that group differences exist in the effect of drugs, in the way they are assimilated, and the dosages needed for them to be effective. These are good suggestions, but how will we make sure that they are implemented? An answer to that question was not in the scope of Goering's chapter. I want to raise that question briefly, in order to bring out the sweeping political implications of her work. I will argue that medical care for the underserved requires a different kind of democracy.

Clinical trials are restricted to white men owing, in part, to pervasive race and gender prejudice, which often takes the form of ignoring all those who are not white males. In this case, once again white males are regarded as the paradigmatic human beings. Until that neglect, not to say, disrespect for men of color and for women is overcome, we cannot be confident that even clinical trials will take account of biological group differences. Even less can we be confident that the same prejudices will not affect medical care in some other way.

Two kinds of strategies can be employed to remedy the situation. The first tries to remove prejudice through education—it attempts to "sensitize" white males to the existence and needs of persons who are different from them. I am sure that such efforts have had some salutary effects in the remote and more recent past.

But reeducation leaves current power distributions unchanged. Those who are now in power remain in power and those whose medical care, for instance, suffers from relative neglect because they are not white men are still dependent on the good-will of those white men if they are to receive better medical care. That, in turn, depends on the efforts of those same white men to eradicate among themselves the rampant prejudice—often not even clearly understood, let alone acknowledged—against all others.

Obviously, a redistribution of power is needed. This particular case requires a redistribution of power which allows groups in the society to express their needs, for example, with respect to health care and, more important, which permits those expressions of need and interest to be heard *and* taken seriously. How would such a redistribution of power come about? We need a new and different conception of democracy from the one that is now dominant. According to that conception, democracy is competition for political, that is, governmental power. One version centers on the competition between politicians for political office (Schumpeter 1989), and another on the competition between powerful groups for greater access to resources distributed by the government (Dahl 1989). These conceptions of democracy implicitly accept the differential in power which ultimately underlies the facts observed by Goering. If democracy is competition for power, then there are going to be winners and losers. The winners will use their power at the expense of the losers, and thus racial and gender oppression appear perfectly compatible with democracy. If we are to redistribute power, we need to alter our conception of democracy to one in which the central goal is continually to equalize power differentials (Cohen and Rogers 1992).

The most popular and familiar form of such a new understanding of democracy demands election reform. Inasmuch as large campaign contributions buy access to the government and influence over government decisions that ordinary voters do not have, such proposals call for completely publicly financed election campaigns (Miller 1993). It is clear, however, that that is not sufficient. Election reform may change the extent to which money buys control over the workings of the government. Therefore, election reform moves toward equalizing power in some respects. But power is lodged not only in the government, but also in "private" groups such as corporations, trade associations, schools, and associations that lobby, educate, do research, and so on. In our present case, for instance, the government is only peripherally involved in the choice of subjects for clinical trials. The main actors are the researchers and their employers, universities, and drug companies. They have the power to ignore the needs of large groups of the population because most of them are private organizations.

The centrality of private groups to democracy was recognized long ago by the pluralists—who described our democracy as a competition for power among organized groups. That important insight was immediately distorted by the additional claim that what we have is a pluralist system. It is obvious, however, that many groups do not effectively compete for power. It is equally obvious that many citizens are completely disenfranchised because they are not members of politically effective groups at all (Eddins and Eddins 1983).

Besides election reform, an alternative conception of democracy needs a major public effort to help the unorganized organize themselves. This effort has long been advocated by Saul Alinsky and his followers, and was begun in the Lyndon Johnson years, though very timidly. A democracy that aims to equalize power needs not only to safeguard the civil liberties that we enjoy today—some more than others, to be sure—but also to protect the weaker groups against the depredations of the stronger. Weaker groups, groups that are barely organized, need protection against the local board of realtors or the local businessmen's associations. The early beginnings of such protection are, for example, the laws that govern employers' dealings with labor unions. The laws we have clearly do not protect labor unions sufficiently, but they suggest that legislation that regulates relationships between nongovernmental groups is possible and could be effective.

In addition, individual members need protection within the groups to which they belong against unscrupulous leaders or against majorities. Existing examples are regulations that protect union members against the depredations of union leadership. These, too, are not what they should be, but they suggest that it is possible to add to existing civil liberties that protect us against an overbearing government and others that protect us against overbearing institutions of a private kind.

Therefore, a stronger form of democracy must surrender the narrow limits we now set for democratic procedures: we think that democracy is appropriate today only in selecting political representatives, but not in schools, workplaces, or the family. The problems Goering brings to our attention can finally be resolved only if the research of universities or private companies is also open to democratic procedures where the persons affected by the research have an effective voice in planning and criticizing research projects.

The ultimate goal would be to transform democracy from a system where a limited number of people and groups compete for power to one where all participate fully. Short of hoping for a miraculous alteration of ordinary human behavior, we need to weaken the competition-for-power model of democracy by (1) giving public support for the unorganized to organize themselves—a suitable project for the "National Service Corps" that is once again under discussion; (2) regulating transactions between groups to protect the weaker participants; and (3) protecting the rights of group members against the groups to which they belong.

These suggestions may strike the reader as utopian. It is important to remember, however, that mass democracy with universal suffrage is a very recent—as recent as 1964—phenomenon in the United States and appeared to be utopian a hundred years ago. We must also remember an important contribution of people of color in the United States: they have always kept alive the utopian strain in our tradition, the hope that the seemingly impossible will become possible. This tenacious and uncompromising utopianism has brought about what liberation we have experienced in our lifetime. It is due to the struggles of women and of people of color that the United States holds out some hopes for living up to the promises of its founding documents.

PART 4

A PRACTICAL ETHICS
FOR REFORM:
COMMUNITY
EMPOWERMENT

17 The Evolution of a Community Hospital: Improving Access to Ensure Political and Financial Viability

Alma Roberts

Baltimore's collection of internationally renowned health care institutions is as impressive as that of any major city in the United States. Yet living in the shadows of these institutions are some of the most medically underserved and underinsured citizens in the state of Maryland. The Johns Hopkins Hospital system, one of the world's premier medical institutions, with its sprawling complex of facilities, focuses primarily on providing a broad spectrum of training and research opportunities for its faculty and student physicians, not on addressing the medical care needs of the poor and underserved populations in the city. Similarly, although the University of Maryland medical system is legislatively mandated to provide maximum access and care to the at-risk citizens of west Baltimore, it too has physician training at the core of its operation.

The tertiary care stratum of the Johns Hopkins Hospital system, the University of Maryland medical system, and the other specialty medical centers existing in Baltimore have not improved access, have not reduced morbidity and mortality, and have not translated research and technology into improved health status or even improved health care delivery for the low-income, disenfranchised, and largely minority populations of the city.

The disparity between institutional resources and improved community health is not unique to Baltimore; it is the norm in all urban areas. It is the crux not only of the access issue, but also of issues surrounding health care delivery generally.

In the early 1980s public hospitals became extinct in Baltimore and were drastically reduced nationwide. A secondary stratum of medical delivery evolved as a direct response to the very real gaps in health care delivery. Community hospitals emerged with mission statements that elucidate a commitment to increasing health care access and meeting the needs of their communities. These hospitals have attempted to develop services and programs that are patient-focused, and have made community service and outreach initiatives the cornerstones of their institutional marketing plans. Over the years, however, increased competition, decreasing revenues, and the cost of acquiring advanced technology have thwarted many of the "good intentions" of community hospitals. Furthermore, the emergence of managed care plans, which channel patients to the least costly providers and limit unnecessary use of medical care resources, has also altered the mission of community hospitals. Thus, even with the existence of community hospitals, gaps in care and care delivery still exist and the appropriate model for care delivery in an urban setting remains a discussion topic for conferences and workshops.

Yet there is a glimmer of hope for the disenfranchised, fragile, at-risk patients in Baltimore. One community hospital in the city has taken a slightly different tack in its evolution. It has evolved differently, not because its leaders have been visionary giants, but more because financial and political disempowerment left the institution limited options for ensuring its continued viability. The institution I write about is Liberty Medical Center. I do not point to Liberty Medical Center as the glimmer of hope simply because I am employed there, but because of what the institution is and what it can become.

Liberty Medical Center is a 282-bed community hospital located in west Baltimore. While the hospital is only six years old, it was created from a merger of two community hospitals with long, rich histories. One of these, Provident Hospital, was the state's only African-American-owned and operated hospital. This institution had been the conduit through which African-American physicians, nurses, and other providers of care to the disenfranchised populations of Baltimore linked arms with the community to try to make a difference in how and where health care was delivered. Eventually, however, the hospital succumbed to internal strife between management and medical staff, amid declining financial resources. Meanwhile, Lutheran Hospital, a subsidiary of the Lutheran Church, was caring for a predominantly white patient population that was only slightly more enfranchised than Provident's. Lutheran was plagued with difficulties, union issues, and a deteriorating physical plant. When the two hospitals merged, Lutheran moved to Provident's facility, and Liberty Medical Center was founded in August 1986.

The merger resulted in a hospital that took on all the burdens of the preceding institutions, but not all their strengths. Because Liberty Medical Center was housed in Provident Hospital's physical plant, people referred to it and thought of it as Provident. Rather than major financial assets from either of its parents, Liberty inherited a huge debt associated with Maryland's "bailout" of Provident Hospital. While Provident was a galvanizing point for the community, Liberty Medical Center was a constant reminder to the community of its dashed dreams. The new hospital represented another invasion and defeat at the hands of "white" people. While Provident had management and staff working in traditional employer/employee relationships, Lutheran brought a professional nurses union and the stresses and strains between staff and management that are associated with such a bargaining agreement. All of this made for a different organization, and waiting at Liberty Medical Center's doors when it opened were the sickest of sick patients—physically, emotionally, socially, and financially compromised.

The mission statement of the "new hospital," Liberty Medical Center, mirrors the mission statements of community hospitals nationwide. Liberty Medical Center is here to serve its patients and its community and to meet their needs. The statement envisions a broad scope of "community-responsive services" and increased access to affordable services. At the same time, the mission statement recognizes the necessity of maintaining a financially viable institution.

This is where Liberty Medical Center becomes even more unique. Liberty Medical Center has been asked to serve a population with a demographic profile resembling that of a Third World country and to serve that population with the least endowed coffers of any other hospital in the city of Baltimore. It has been asked to serve the largest population of HIV/AIDS patients in the state of Maryland; the largest substance-abusing and mentally ill population in the state; a population that is second in the state in cancer deaths and first in diabetes and hypertension mortality and morbidity; a population with one of the lowest rates for completion of high school, the lowest income levels, and the highest rates of crime and deaths due to violence in the state. It provides the largest percentage of care to nursing home patients of all hospitals in the city, and its care of Medicare and Medicaid patients is the largest proportion in the state.

Yet the regulatory environment in Maryland only marginally adjusts for Liberty's special patient mix. The Maryland Health Care Cost Review Commission rates it as one of the highest cost hospitals in the state without full recognition of the large amount of uncompensated care provided and its need to utilize more resources per patient for longer lengths of stay. The "powers that be" only marginally acknowledge the unique role of this community hospital to this special community. Liberty cares for the most fragile with the least resources. It has evolved in a relative state of disempowerment, alienated by its history from those segments of the community that could bring political and financial resources into the hospital, and targeted by regulators who are not culturally sensitive in a health care environment that has its priorities askew.

The glimmer of hope lies in the remainder of Liberty Medical Center's story. The institution not only accepts its role as "the community hospital in Baltimore City" but is basking in that special role. Not the least of the factors involved in this role was a series of strange "marriages" that were made early in the history of the center. Six years ago at its inception, the center's administration agreed to provide a select group of physicians with staff, supplies, and space for their private practices in exchange for their admissions. This provided a physician base and cash flow when they were much needed. At the same time, the hospital also entered into a contract with a Medicaid managed care plan to provide ambulatory and inpatient services to its members in space on the former Lutheran campus and in an ambulatory center on what was now Liberty's campus. The agreement was an exclusive arrangement, forcing Liberty Medical Center to relinquish opportunities to enter into similar arrangements with other Medicaid managed care plans. It did, however, provide Liberty with entry into the managed care market. In addition, four years ago, the institution expended scarce resources to begin looking to the future. A corporate development initiative was established to strategically develop programs and services that focused on patient and physician needs.

These three decisions proved to be the foundation for the evolution of Liberty Medical Center into a politically and financially viable community hospital. They resulted in the following set of features that continue to influence Liberty's evolution:

- The health trend that touts ambulatory community-based care as the focus for the future offers Liberty Medical Center an opportunity to capitalize on the program and service array it has assembled to respond to its desperate community.
- The hospital's leadership is culturally and personally sensitive, yet practical in its vision.
- The dawning of health care reform as a national priority, and urban health care issues as the most significant key to that reform, offers Liberty Medical Center a strategic position as policy and new initiatives are decided upon.

The story continues to evolve as of this writing. Liberty Medical Center has developed a strategic plan that is singularly geared to maximizing its political and financial viability through initiatives that increase care access for the disenfranchised. The hospital is slated to receive significant funding from the Maryland State Legislature to create an Urban Medical Institute that represents the vision of the current president and chief operating officer. It is a coordinated care model that will provide a series of preventive, educational, screening, counseling, and treatment programs aimed at addressing the highest priority health needs for the major pocket of underserved areas in Baltimore. Liberty has already invested $13 million in the development of programs to be included in the institute. With its emphasis on ambulatory preventive services, the institute is projected to generate significant new revenues for Liberty Medical Center while saving the state significant dollars.

The hospital has initiated a major physician bonding program that unites its medical staff with a community-based network that is currently very attractive to area managed care plans and draws on the experience gained from the hospital's prior managed care arrangement. This strategy directly addresses increased access for Liberty's service area.

The hospital has also initiated major efforts aimed at politically positioning its administration as the advocacy voice for urban health care and delivery. The hospital has successfully waded through a recent series of regulatory validation surveys that appear to have been a veiled attempt at forcing closure of the institution. Through this process, community, medical staff, board members, managers, and political representatives rallied to support Liberty Medical Center. The hospital's special position in the health care delivery spectrum of Baltimore and Maryland began to become clear to those most closely affiliated as well as to those administering the health care system in the state. Liberty has begun to develop tentacles that reach beyond its walls, into and beyond its community.

The challenge for Liberty Medical Center is to translate its special role as an advocate for and provider of care to the disenfranchised into sustained political and financial viability. Every program, every bed, every staff person, and every dollar must be dedicated to that singular focus.

Commentary by Nathaniel Wesley, Jr.

Alma Roberts provides an overview of the health community landscape for the city of Baltimore, describing how one hospital has made a commitment to caring for the people of that city. She is careful to point out that Baltimore is not an exception, but exhibits the problems of access to care and disparity of resources that exist in most major cities.

Understandably, the background on the merger of two inner-city hospitals to become Liberty Medical Center must be brief; however, such abbreviated background minimizes the tremendous community struggle that preceded the merger. The pains of that struggle are still evident six years later, as outlined in the chapter. Liberty Medical Center, housed in the Provident Hospital facility (one of the merger hospitals), still has the ghost of the past from its predecessor as it takes bold steps to become a new and different kind of community-based health organization. Creating a new mission statement for the hospital was a monumental task.

Roberts does not discuss the evolution from a governance or community consensus basis. However, it is obvious that, while the hospital organization has changed, the question of access is still a critical factor in assuring services to the community. The laundry list of morbidity is a long one and can be repeated in most major urban communities. The chapter points out the difficulty in convincing regulatory bodies that the high levels of uncompensated care delivery by the hospital should be a consideration in the statewide cost review program. The hospital is surrounded by those who are more politically powerful and financially stable, but it refuses to back away from its commitment to the entire Baltimore community.

The essence of the evolution that is addressed in the chapter is found in the three factors that have contributed to the hospital's success: (1) development of community-based ambulatory care programs; (2) hospital leadership that is culturally and personally sensitive; and (3) development of a strategic position in addressing urban health problems. The hospital feels so strongly about its commitment and ability to address the questions of access and unmet community need that it has proposed the establishment of an Urban Medical Institute. Some $13 million have already been invested in the programs that would become part of the institute, and state funding is being sought.

Roberts highlights a number of ethical issues. Key among those issues in the Liberty Medical Center history and mission are: (1) Who should determine the merits and community benefits to be derived from a merger of two hospitals? When should this be done? Should the community have something to say about the process? (2) Does public health policy constrain or expand access in a city like Baltimore? How far should political consideration go in addressing community health needs? and (3) Does the question of rationing play a role in determining the ability of a hospital to address community need? How does a small, inner-city community hospital face the problem of providing compensated care and also recruiting new physicians to continue care for those least able to pay for services? How does priority become established?

The advent of reform in our national system promises to address the issue of universal access. However, the problems will most likely not be entirely solved under managed competition proposals, because the same financial incentives will still be at work. The questions faced by the Liberty Medical Center are the same sort of questions that the Clinton administration must address in its effort to implement health care reform. Furthermore, the successes of Liberty Medical Center and other community-based hospitals and health centers must not be sacrificed or dismantled as the country goes about building a new health care system. Rather, successful community-based health care systems must be meaningfully involved in creating and implementing the new system.

18 Toward Successful Urban Perinatal Health Care

Brian Hertz

INTRODUCTION

Despite great technological advances in perinatal health care in the United States, perinatal morbidity and mortality rates continue to rise, with rates now exceeding those of many developing countries. The problem is most severe in socioeconomically diverse urban areas, which face high rates of teen pregnancy, sexually transmitted disease, and substance abuse (Wegman 1990). These and other social problems disproportionately affect perinatal morbidity and mortality among poor peoples of color (Gortmaker 1979) who also have less access to perinatal health care services (General Accounting Office 1978). Current perinatal care fails because it inappropriately and ineffectively applies technological fixes such as neonatal intensive care nurseries while inadequately providing access to preventive and primary health care services. How can this failure of perinatal health care be reversed?

Comprehensive perinatal services, which include educational and social support, have proven effective in reducing infant morbidity and mortality (McLaughlin et al. 1989; Olds et al. 1986). Ironically, low-cost primary care and preventive services (such as the neighborhood health center) are often less accessible than the more expensive neonatal intensive care nursery. Urban areas typically have the most advanced perinatal services in the midst of neighborhoods with the highest perinatal morbidity and mortality rates. A foundation of comprehensive primary and preventive services is a key component of successful, cost-effective health care reform. To this end, I will describe a successful comprehensive perinatal program in southeast Chicago at the Claretian Medical Center. Based on the Community Oriented Primary Care (COPC) model (Abramson and Kark 1983), Claretian provides a model for improvement of perinatal care and community involvement in decision making.

THE CLARETIAN MEDICAL CENTER

The southeast side of Chicago exhibits infant morbidity and mortality problems typical of many economically depressed, diverse urban environments in the United States. A number of southeast Chicago residents receive comprehensive perinatal services at Claretian Medical Center, a federally funded community health center. In addition to standard physician visits and nurse-administered prenatal classes, Claretian's team approach also provides health education, nutritional and substance abuse counseling, and dental care. Claretian extends comprehensive services through a system of patient tracking and referral. This system includes a liaison with a nursing school for home visits and transportation of clients, assisting patients with difficult social situations and enticing noncompliant patients to conform with medical recommendations. The program emphasizes continuity. It covers prenatal through postpartum care, and it includes presentations in schools, family planning counseling, and teaching young mothers to care for their infants. The health center attempts to provide a multilingual, culturally sensitive health care team.

Although Claretian's clients are not a random sample of southeast Chicago residents, they come from a population that otherwise has poor access to health care services. As a federally funded community health center, Claretian must accept patients regardless of their ability to pay. Claretian also accepts all forms of commercial insurance, has several managed care contracts, and provides a grant-funded sliding scale payment system for under- and uninsured patients that assists with the cost of office visits, procedures, out-of-office referrals, and medications.

Patients are referred to Claretian through several mechanisms, including formal overflow referrals from the city-funded Department of Health Clinics. Hospital referrals originate predominantly from two local hospitals and Cook County Hospital. Private physicians may also refer patients who lose insurance benefits. However, the majority of patients served at Claretian are referred from community agencies or by word of mouth.

Retrospective demographic analysis of Claretian patients by race and source of payment is consistent with the southeast Chicago community. Approximately forty-two percent of Claretian's patients are African American, 49% Hispanic, and 9% Caucasian. Breakdown by payment source was 62% Medicaid, 14% private insurance, 4% HMO, 17% uninsured, and 3% unknown. A large number of Claretian clients were of undocumented nationality. These predominantly Spanish-speaking patients from Mexico and Central America had limited alternative sources of health care, particularly in 1989, before Medicaid expanded eligibility criteria in 1990 to include undocumented patients.

Claretian provides perinatal services for more than 600 clients each year. These clients originate in six target communities served by two outpatient sites in the southeast Chicago area: South Chicago, East Side, Roseland, Pullman, West Pullman, and South Deering. Compared with these figures from the overall southeast Chicago area, Claretian's perinatal data reveal striking differences. Aggregate 1989 data from the Chicago Department of

Health for these six communities reports an infant mortality rate of 18.3 per thousand, whereas at Claretian, infant mortality was 2.9 per thousand. In southeast Chicago overall, the low birthweight percentage was 12.8; at Claretian it was 6.9. In southeast Chicago, 24.1% of the mothers were teenagers, while at Claretian, this figure was 22.2%. Both the Claretian percentage of low-birthweight neonates and infant mortality rates are significantly lower than those of the southeast Chicago area overall. These remarkable differences can be attributed to the comprehensive services offered by the center.

PERINATAL SERVICES AT CLARETIAN

The structure of Claretian's perinatal services has evolved over fifteen years. Currently, perinatal staffing and services overlap with other personnel and programs of the community health center's two outpatient facilities. Health providers include obstetricians, family physicians, pediatricians, and family nurse practitioners. Other staff include registered nurses, health educators, a substance abuse counselor, and dental and social services staff. The nursing school liaison and a mobile homeless health care program based at Claretian assist with off-site visits. Each patient is case-managed and is offered all appropriate services determined by an initial interview and followup tracking.

An example of Claretian's expanded perinatal services is the registration process. New clients are interviewed by a registered nurse. This extensive interview aims to identify prenatal risk factors, expanding on standard prenatal health and social risks to include known problems in the community, for example, clients without telephones or those who are homeless, or who engage in specific high-risk behaviors. Initial risk assessment helps ensure that appropriate referrals are made early on. At registration, clients also sign a contract that discusses their rights and responsibilities. The contract informs the patient about Claretian's services and explains the best way to take advantage of the 24-hour on-call system. The contract also attempts to promote healthy behavior.

An extensive prenatal education program is part of Claretian's expanded comprehensive service. For example, nutritional counseling in the patient education room uses a kitchen to teach proper preparation of infant formula and sterilization techniques. The patient education room is large enough for La Maze and other educational programs.

A family nurse-practitioner who has both administrative and clinical responsibilities coordinates educational, clinical, and administrative programs. She oversees perinatal staffing and works with primary providers to ensure a cooperative team approach, which is essential for success. In addition to developing prenatal risk assessment methods, the team has developed medical protocol guidelines to help ensure quality prenatal services. These include screening for gestational diabetes, anemia, and sexually transmitted diseases, including hepatitis B and HIV.

Comprehensive services emphasize continuity of care. For most patients continuity of care extends throughout their hospital stay. Physicians have hospital privileges at a nearby community hospital, South Chicago Community Hospital, and share call responsibilities. These comprehensive services—from community and patient education to risk assessment and prenatal and postnatal patient management—contribute to Claretian's lower rates of low-birthweight babies and infant morbidity and mortality.

THE COMMUNITY-ORIENTED PRIMARY CARE MODEL

Community health centers such as Claretian are mandated by federal grant regulation to orient services according to the principles of Community Oriented Primary Care (COPC) (Abramson and Kark 1983). COPC offers a model for developing health care systems that deliver effective and efficient health interventions. The COPC principles dictate that primary care practice should address accessibility, comprehensiveness, coordination, continuity, and accountability.

The COPC process includes four steps. First, it defines and describes the target population or community. Second, it systematically identifies major community health problems, and it creates a partnership with community members for selecting problems and planning interventions. Third, COPC builds in flexibility to modify the health care program. Fourth, it provides a mechanism to evaluate the impact of the system modifications and interventions.

The value of community-based services is apparent in dealing with problems of substance abuse in pregnancy. Traditional doctor–patient encounters often underdiagnose and ineffectively manage this difficult clinical problem. The community health center model starts with a comprehensive risk assessment, followed by appropriate referral to a trained substance abuse counselor on site at the community health center. This counselor can see clients at the same time as their physician visit, or, when necessary, refer a client to residential treatment in a selective and appropriate manner. Management can be flexible and cooperate with community-based and tertiary care services, guided by community-based tracking and surveillance.

CONCLUSION—LESSONS FROM CLARETIAN

Claretian's community health center is successful because it addresses the needs of patients and their community. In an ideal world, the health care needs of a community dictate appropriate health care services for all patients, including medical diagnosis, prognosis, and treatment. Epidemiological analysis can determine the health care needs of a community, and the choice of health care services will follow. Ideally, health care services would be guided by a normative, needs-based analysis. Unfortunately, our current health care systems are guided by market forces and professional autonomy.

A community health center such as Claretian can offer health care that addresses these expanded concepts of autonomy, because its governing board, made up of community people, helps determine what services will be offered. Their decisions are based on community experience and perceptions. The specific perinatal services offered by Claretian meet many of these needs. In addition, a small flexible administrative unit working with the community may be able to provide more comprehensive health services. Examples of this flexibility are the sliding scale fee system, which can bridge the gaps of limitations in coverage, or the ability to make contact with schools and shelters in the service area.

The preferences of an informed and empowered community guide appropriate health care services. In COPC, community involvement determines the selection of problems for intervention. Adequate communication, including common language and education on a community level, must coexist with the development of services. Addressing community needs requires cultural sensitivity. For example, in African-American and Latino cultures, community needs and preferences may take precedence over individual concerns.

Our current health care system has failed to ameliorate rising perinatal morbidity and mortality rates in sociologically diverse and economically depressed urban settings. To solve this problem, we must extend successful perinatal services, including appropriate use of medical technology, and expanding access to preventive and primary care to underserved peoples.

Community-based perinatal services offer advantages in meeting the needs of a socioeconomically diverse urban setting. Specifically, the COPC-designed health care system, such as Claretian's community health center, offers an organizational model that can improve access to and quality of perinatal care.

Commentary by Laurence J. O'Connell

In his brief, but full, description of a community health center in southeast Chicago, Brian Hertz lays bare a disturbing fact: perinatal morbidity and mortality rates continue to rise in many economically depressed, diverse urban environments in the United States. A sad convergence of social problems, coupled with a misguided medical response, accounts for excessive illness and premature death among poor newborns of color in a country that boasts of its superlative ability to treat imperiled neonates.

Hertz argues persuasively that today's high-tech "rescue medicine" should be replaced by a community-based approach that emphasizes continuity of care that includes public and patient education, early intervention through preventive and primary care, as well as prenatal and postnatal patient management. The inappropriate and ineffective application of technological fixes to a population that has been seriously compromised by lack of preventive and primary care often leads to poor outcomes. It is a case of too much, too late! Given the statistical, not to mention human, success of his program, Hertz's point would be difficult to refute.

Hertz takes us to the very heart of health care ethics. His chapter raises serious issues in social, clinical, and corporate ethics. Social ethics focuses on socially shared patterns of moral judgment and behavior. It examines social structures, processes, and communities in an effort to understand what constitutes right or wrong in a given social context. From an ethical point of view, there is something very wrong with urban perinatal care in the United States. Given the resources available in our society, it is ethically unconscionable that we have perinatal morbidity and mortality rates that exceed those of many developing countries. Clearly, the unjust allocation of health care resources, as well as many other social ills that fall disproportionately on poor peoples of color in our cities, constitutes an ethically untenable moral situation. There is an obvious need for reform that is sensitive to distributive and social justice.

The high rates of perinatal morbidity and mortality in our cities also raise questions in clinical ethics. It is ironic that highly trained clinicians routinely treat sick and dying neonates in urban, university-based intensive care nurseries, without attending to the underlying causes that stock the steady stream of infants. Clinicians have a moral duty to reflect on the relative effectiveness of their work. Although it may be more convenient, and in many cases safer, to work within an institutional setting, clinicians ought to reflect on their duties to the surrounding community. Why are so few clinicians out among those who need them? In the face of such high infant morbidity and mortality rates, might we question the moral judgment and pattern of behavior observed among health care professionals? Perhaps some soul searching is in order.

Finally, corporate ethics adds another perspective to Hertz's position. An institution's responsibilities vis-à-vis its local community are taken up in corporate ethics. As Hertz notes, "Urban areas typically have the most advanced perinatal services in the midst of neighborhoods with the highest perinatal morbidity and mortality rates." The responsibilities of a large health care institution cannot be separated from its immediate geographical location. It represents human capacities and competencies that ought to be shared with its immediate neighbors. A failure to assess and approach the needs of the local community reflects negatively on the ethical character of any not-for-profit health care facility. Of course, an institution can be overrun by those they find on their doorstep; but they must make a good-faith effort to provide all they can. The notion that a health care institution can be an island, existing in splendid isolation, is morally repugnant.

Hertz's illuminating piece on urban perinatal health represents a stimulating point of departure for many of the ethical problems that beset health care delivery in the United States today. It provides an invaluable gamut of concerns that naturally lend themselves to ethical analysis. This is a rich field where the concerns of ethicists and health care providers and practitioners come together on a common ground and find the incentive to work more collaboratively as the United States struggles to reform its health care system.

19 Interview: Lay Midwifery and the Traditional Child-Bearing Group

Evelyn C. White and Shafia Mawushi Monroe

Shafia Mawushi Monroe dispenses with the formalities the minute you step into the office of the Traditional Childbearing Group (TCBG). Actually, a visit to TCBG bears no resemblance to a "standard" medical appointment. There's no sterility, stacks of confusing forms, or impersonal staff members. Instead, there's a comfy couch, a pot of tea, and a wall filled with photos of smiling babies. Shafia and I had one of those long, loving, and laughter-filled conversations that black women used to have over the back fence while they hung the laundry on the clothesline.

Times sure have changed for black women. Our mothers may not have had executive suites or their own talk shows, but by and large, most of them had healthy babies. Their babies did not come into the world drug-scarred and trembling—[two] times more likely than white babies *never* to see their first birthday. Shafia Monroe has made it her business to improve the pathway for black children as they enter the world. We need to listen to this sister and support her as if our life depended on it. I began by asking Shafia how she became interested in midwifery.

SM: At fifteen my mother passed away and I moved in with an older woman and her family [in Boston]. She had three other children, and she was pregnant.

I lived with this woman in her house for about a year. I was very attracted to her pregnancy. I would rub her stomach and talk to her at night and shake the baby to feel it move. She said, "You know, you are really so good at this, you should consider being an obstetrician." So I ran it by my father, about being an obstetrician, and he said, "You know you had a great aunty who was a well-known midwife in Alabama." I bought a book on midwifery.

So at fifteen, I started reading more about it. Then at eighteen, I joined a group in Newton, [Massachusetts], called Homebirth Info Movement. I was the only person who was black. They were nice, but there was a cultural difference, and I didn't feel comfortable with them. Instead I got a job at Boston City Hospital as a nurse's aide. I was lucky, I got on the newborn nursery floor. As soon as the baby was born, back in the '70s, it went from the mother's body into a nursery. We're talking about second-old, minute-old babies.

EW: Just taken away like that.

SM: Yes. But there was an advantage to working in the nursery. During my year there I learned how to assess the health status of a newborn—how to assess their neurodevelopment, how to take their vital signs, how to remove extra fingers (sometimes [black babies are] born with six fingers), how to draw blood, and other skills needed for a well-baby check. The other thing, too, is that it was on the postpartum floor. For the breast-feeding, I got to take the babies to the mothers at night. And I think with any midwife, you learn best from the women themselves. I would ask them, "How was the birth experience? How was the pregnancy? How would you want it different? Why are you breast-feeding?" I learned a lot from one year talking in the middle of the night and listening to their stories.

Between 18 and 21, I enrolled at [the] University of Massachusetts as a pre-med student, considering maybe getting into obstetrics, doing work at the hospital, and still running around trying to find midwives of color, which was really difficult. In 1972, you couldn't find many African-American midwives.

EW: In the North or Northeast?

SM: The ones whom I did find, who were from the South, they were old. Unfortunately, I think the system invalidated them. They didn't want to talk: "Oh, girl, that's an idea from a long time ago; you don't want to do that now, we got bottles, you don't have to do that now." And I was trying to tell them we did want to do that, that was positive. But I did get some information from them. Midwives from Africa and the West Indies also taught me a lot. I met a midwife from Zaire who went to my university, studying to be a doctor. And I met a midwife from Pakistan, who helped me catch a baby. And then I met a midwife who was from Alabama, an older woman. We did a few births together.

Then, at 21, I had my [first] baby, and I had a home birth. I couldn't find any midwives who would come into my area. There were no black midwives. So I ended up using a white male doctor, which I wasn't happy about. But since I wanted a home birth no matter what, I dealt with him. Two years later, I was pregnant again with my second child, and I went to this event and met a woman named Majeeda, who had just had a baby and had to use a white male doctor. We said we wished we could find a group and we said, "Let's get together and start a group!" And so we did.

We called it the Traditional Childbearing Group, because this is the traditional way. Hospital births are nontraditional. Bottle-feeding is nontraditional. I tell people that this is the right name. We are truly traditional in the sense of the history of birth, and because we use information passed on by word of mouth. I teach midwifery, and how to be a parent, how to give birth, by talking. We give information by paper, but we do most of our stuff hands-on, touching and talking. This is what we've always done as black women in this country—doing each other's hair, grabbing each other, hugging each other, slapping each other in jest or serious, whatever. So we choose that same approach within our framework, and it's very effective. It's completely opposite in hospitals. Doctors don't talk to you. How can they in fifteen minutes? The nurse is the first twelve minutes. She does all the blood pressure, weight; you see the doctor a couple of minutes and you are out.

When I was pregnant with my five children, I went to clinics for all my prenatal care though I was having home-births. I did that as an investigator. So I knew first-hand what women had to go through. I sat there for many hours and walked into very impersonal care. I don't think I ever had a doctor who was black or a midwife who was black. They were always not of my community, not of my ethnicity, usually middle-class, didn't understand my lingo. One thing I noticed was that they didn't touch you. They would say to you, "Oh, Shafia, how are you feeling?" I'd say, "I'm okay, but my back is killing me." They'd say, "Okay, let's get on the scale now." Not even acknowledge it.

EW: But not even touch your back.

SM: That's right. And with me, if your back hurts, "Well, take off that shirt, lay down and let's get the coconut oil out—or olive oil?" and we get into it. People call up and say, "My back hurts." I say, "Come on in." To me, that's what midwives do.

I used to go out to people. I did all my visits in people's homes. You learn more in someone else's environment. This [TCBG office] is not their home, even though it's warm. It's still not their house. I can't really see what their needs are here. We have pride. If we're poor, we don't say, "Well, I have no food in my house." If I make a home visit and they offer me tea, I can see that their cupboard is low, or it's cold, they don't have heat. I can say, "Hey, sis"—I'll say it in calm way, a sisterly way—"we can get you vouchers for some food, we can call ABCD [a community assistance organization in Boston] and get you some heat."

A doctor will never know that. They don't know what people are going through on an everyday basis. And when they do know, it's very scrutinizing: "You don't have enough, we're going to get you services or we're going to file a 51A [a form filed with the state accusing a parent of neglecting or abusing a child] and take your baby out." We've never had to file a 51A in twelve years. I don't believe in that. Unless you're throwing kids out the window, literally. If there isn't a way to work it out, well then let's talk to your mother, let's talk to the baby's father; we have to be able to do something about this before we resort to having to bring in the outside, the authorities.

EW: What's the difference between a lay midwife and a nurse midwife? Do you need to be certified? What is your official status?

SM: Well, the lay midwife was first. We are the original midwife. It was a calling, or someone in the community appointed you because of your behavior or your personality. It was an honored position. But then in Europe—not in Africa and not in the South—they went through that whole witch-burning. [Midwives] didn't get burned as witches in Africa; we were always honored, and we still are very respected today.

A nurse midwife means you become a nurse first in a two- or four-year program, and then decide to continue on with midwifery studies, so you come out with the degree C.N.M. [certified nurse midwife]. For the traditional [lay] midwife, we are taught by other midwives; we use the apprenticeship program. Even though you have a calling, you still have to find another midwife who knows more than you. I try to practice what I call Afrocentric midwifery. That, and the Southern experience of midwifery—of black midwives—are much different from the experience of middle-class white women who become midwives.

In this state we have the Massachusetts Midwives Alliance, which is an organization of lay midwives statewide, a racially mixed organization. We have our own code of ethics, protocols, and an optional test to see if you're at a certain level. So if someone calls up and says, "I want Shafia Monroe as a midwife, what do you know about her?" they can run her name on the computer and say well, she took the test, she's certified, we know her, she is qualified. The disadvantage [of being a lay midwife] is we can't get third-party reimbursements. We can't get Medicaid to pay for us or Blue Cross/Blue Shield. Though we're not always liked by the physicians, they respect us. We work with some type of collaboration. At this point, Boston and the country's getting desperate for solutions to the high cost of health care, and infant mortality is a problem for black people across the country.

EW: Speaking of the high infant mortality rate, what's going on in Boston? Second in the nation?

SM: I think third. Mississippi first, maybe Chicago and Detroit. . . . But it's high enough. I always tell women who come through here, if my father had a sixth-grade education and his mother had no education and she was able to birth healthy children that got through the first year of life, what's our excuse? We have to take some responsibility. You can control what you put in your mouth. I don't care if it's beans and rice and corn bread, it has got to be better than chips and Coca-cola. In a bad relationship? Get up, and get out of it. Things you can control, let's start with that and then we can challenge the system.

At the same time, we don't want the system to get off the hook. Even if you're an educated, middle-class black woman making over $30,000 per year, you're still at risk for infant mortality as opposed to a white woman of the same economic and educational background. It's the racism. I don't care how well you eat or how many herb teas you drink, you're going to have to fight racism on your job, in your neighborhood, and in your school system on a daily basis, and that's going to affect you. Why do you have higher blood pressure among black women? Because we're angry.

EW: That's what Toni Morrison talks about. The anger and the sadness from slavery, and I think that's part of the chronic depression among so many black people in general.

SM: Yeah, we have to figure out among ourselves, how can we get rid of it? Any time you're oppressed it comes out through the lives of your children—premature births, etc. Infant mortality is not so much the baby dying, but how many babies who are born live are sick forever, because they were born too soon or their mothers carried them to full term but they were born too small? The baby can't thrive inside, because the mother's not thriving. A lot of women don't know that we're the highest death rate in the country. And I let them know we're the highest death rate because our babies get fewer health options; we have more parenting struggles, earlier exposure to drugs; and we have more diabetes, hypertension, strokes, obesity . . . I say, we have got to start working on ourselves; we have to be sisters.

EW: What's the response like?

SM: Very positive. I let them see things and tell them, "You're not being paranoid. What you're telling about is true. Yes, they are giving too many tests, and right, your visit was too short and the doctor was unfriendly, and you're right, he doesn't really care about you." These are teaching hospitals. They put teaching hospitals in black areas, poor areas, and oppressed areas because we don't ask questions. We sign on the dotted line. We feel so grateful that they're even looking at us, with a fifteen-hour wait.

I hug them. [I say] ask your great-grandmother, how does she eat? Look at her teeth. Look at her skin. Look at our sisters and brothers in Africa. They can see that . . . "Oh, yes, my grandmother did say she didn't have a cavity." I tell them, because they were breast-fed and they eat vegetables. I say, "See, that was our history, but the white man took it off the books so we don't know. So we have to bring her back and ask them how."

EW: Why are black women so hesitant to breast-feed? I remember my mother breast-feeding my baby sister, but I also remember her specifically sitting us all down and explaining to us what she was doing, and not to be ashamed of it.

SM: You're one of the more blessed ones. The system did a very good job. They took away midwifery, home birth, and breast-feeding. In the '50s, we were still breast-feeding and white America had stopped. They stopped in the '40s and went to bottles. So you're poor, you're black, and here comes the white man who says, "Oh my god, not only are you poor and black and ignorant, you're still breast-feeding! You're outdated."

EW: No progress. Still no progress.

SM: Yes. I talked to a black physician and said, "I'm a homebirth midwife and I want you to help me with backup." And she went off, "Are you crazy? I'm against it. You know how long we fought to get in a hospital, and you're going to try to take us back out." I said, "We don't have rights in a hospital yet." We should have the right to birth where we want, that's all I'm saying. Why is it that only white middle-class America has homebirths, midwives, and breast-feeding support, and we don't? And childbirth classes? Boston City Hospital offers them, and another place offers them all in Spanish. Otherwise you can go to major white institutions—Beth Israel and Brigham and Women's. The class is probably taught by a white nurse.

EW: What's the importance of having these services provided in the community by women from the community?

SM: Most nurse midwives, even if they come to the community, are not of color. They're white women, and they're serving black people. Which is fine. Anyone can help anyone have a baby. Obviously, the doctors have been doing it for years. What's unique about having the community midwife is that when I see the mother at her home and help her, I'm going to see her again—we go to the same food store and I see them shopping or I go to a party or I'm at someone's house and we know the same people, so there's that continuity. But when you have to commute in and then go out, you don't see people. . . . You only see them 9 a.m. to 5 p.m., usually in the clinic setting. You don't see them just walking down the street. . . .

Any midwife and any woman can teach people about empowerment of women, but I think for black women, we need black empowerment. We have a crisis right now. Our boys are killing each other and our babies are dying and we're having real hard times as a people. What is unique about the Traditional Childbearing Group is that we use an African perspective. You have to be political. I can take all the blood pressures I want, but it won't do anything if I don't teach folks, "Hey, genocide is alive and well in America." I don't care what they say, I believe that. The system does not want us, doesn't need us anymore. My kids get after me, "why are you like this?" They don't understand why I am so fanatical about this. I say, "Because I believe that until we define ourselves, and fight for ourselves, we're not going anywhere." I always tell my son, "You have to look at the system, brother. The white man wants you to go up and kill black men because he doesn't want you to live either. That's why you can get a gun, but you can't get a job. You can get crack, but you can't get an education." I say, "Look outside, what do you see? Can you go out? Can you ride your bike? Do you feel safe?"

EW: Can't go outside, live, and do normal things like we did as kids.

SM: Every time you go out, you hope you get back in one piece. That's a reality. My sons go out, I always hug them, because I don't know if I'll ever see them again. That's not paranoia, that's reality. Every day is like another blessing if your children come back home. As a midwife, that's part of it. A midwife doesn't just catch babies. A midwife is an educator as well. I can say to a father some things that a male doctor could never say. "Now, I know you don't want to talk about this, but I know that you beat your wife. She didn't tell me. I saw her face. We have to talk about it. And I still like you and you love your woman, but you cannot handle this this way, brother." And they'll open up because I've been in their house. I've used their toilet and a lot of times before I got this office, they used to come to my house. We were equal. I'm poor like them, and they know it. I have a commitment to their children, to their women, so they care about me. And I care about them. I can call them and ask for a favor and get it: I need a ride, a jump, I need a car, I need a baby-sitter. So that's the difference between traditional midwives who live in the community, as opposed to those who commute in and out.

Now I have to include gang violence in my parenting. Informally. I don't do things real formally. I just meet someone [with kids, and] I just start talking, 'cause I know what they're going through. I make them aware. "Are you keeping track of him? You know where he's going? Is he having sex? Does he use condoms? Do you talk to him about sex?" 'Cause if you ain't, who's going to talk to them? . . . you don't tell him he's going to get AIDS, then you aren't going to have a son.

EW: That's the end of the story.

SM: So that's all part of midwifery. It's not just checking the mother. It's the whole family, because the whole family affects this woman's life. If her son is out all night getting shot at or shooting somebody, she cannot grow a healthy baby. If her boyfriend is unemployed and strung out on crack or he has HIV or is getting laid up, that's going to affect her pregnancy. If her teen daughter is pregnant and not coming home at night, everything is going to affect her pregnancy.

EW: Who pays for all this, especially if you can't get third-party payments?

SM: Our first support came from the Boston Women's Fund. Since then, we have been getting great support from the Boston Foundation. We call them our Mother Group, our Mother Source. They make sure we stay intact. They've been giving us funding since 1987, $25,000 to $35,000. And we just got a state contract for the first time. This is very important for us, since we're the first group that's not associated with a clinic or a teaching hospital. They gave us a contract for $69,000. We can hire two people [to do outreach], knock on doors and stand at the bus stops and find pregnant women.

We have to rely on the grants because folks who come through, they can't afford it. The visit should cost $65 to $200. They get a complete history, blood work, Pap smear, gonorrhea culture, the massage with blood pressure, baby's heartbeat, the whole bit. We only charge $3, if they can pay, and of course, they can't pay . . . so we do it anyway. And we give childbirth classes and a lot of folks can't afford to do those either. So we do it for free. My thing now is I'm trying to get more women in the community to be midwives.

EW: How many have you trained so far? How many apprentices?

SM: Five have come through here in twelve years.

EW: That's not a big number.

SM: And only two are part-time active. I think the main thing is because of money. You can't make a lot of money. What I had to do was develop the Traditional Childbearing Group so I could write grants, so we get paid for education. But we need the state to legalize traditional midwives and let us get third-party reimbursements so we can help people who need to be helped.

EW: So you have the doctors standing in your way right, 'cause they see you as a threat to their business.

SM: Right. In the state of Massachusetts, to get any third-party reimbursements, you have to be licensed. And we don't have any way of being licensed in this state. There's no school for us to be licensed without becoming a nurse first. I don't want to be a nurse. In Africa, in Asia, and even Europe, midwives are not nurses—they are two separate professions. Nurses are taught to work with sick people and they're taught to be subordinate to male physicians as a rule. Midwives are independent, strong women who run a practice autonomously. They don't have to work for anyone, and they see pregnancy as a normal state.

EW: Not a disease.

SM: Right.

EW: Now, concluding things. What do you want people to know? Why should black women come here? People always say, "What happens if there's a problem with my baby? You don't have any machines. What are you going to do?" That sort of thing.

SM: I want to say that with the Traditional Childbearing Group, and myself, we don't try to force people to have their babies at home. What I see as the most powerful aspect of our program is that we teach black empowerment, black woman empowerment. No matter where you give birth—at home or in the hospital—we want you to know that you're somebody, you have rights in the hospital, you have rights with your own birth midwife, you need to know how to interview her. You have to love yourself, you have to love your unborn baby. It already has something against it. You're all it's got and you have to get yourself empowered to keep this baby alive. You have to honor yourself and be proud, so that you can maintain your pregnancy and do it with dignity by taking care of yourself. You have to reach out to your pregnant sister and give her birth information and encourage her and rub her back and love her and make her feel good about her new spirit coming into the world. Everything's against that child when it comes out. It's been born probably in a teaching hospital, by a white person probably, that really doesn't have any connection to it. So you're all it's got right now. Go back to our history. Find out and try to live by it and do what you can do. You can read. You can eat right. You can breast-feed. And you can call us.

NOTE

This chapter is reprinted from Evelyn C. White, *Sojourner: The Women's Forum* (Second Annual Health Supplement), Volume 16, No. 7 (March 1991):1H–4H.

Commentary by Alison Jaggar

Second-wave feminists of my generation have always been concerned about health care. We are the generation who challenged the authority of what we called the male medical establishment in a wide variety of arenas. One major battlefront was the birthing room where we resisted many procedures perceived as instituted primarily for the convenience or profit of our physicians. Such procedures included barring our family and friends from delivery rooms, strapping us to delivery tables, shaving our pubic hair, giving us enemas and episiotomies, inducing our labor, performing caesarian sections, and removing our babies immediately after birth. We insisted that birth was a "natural" process rather than a medical crisis, and to prove this we remained active throughout our pregnancies, made do with minimum medical intervention, and employed midwives whenever we could.

As a white professional-class feminist, I attended prenatal childbirth classes and delivered all my three children with the help of their father and without anaesthetic. At the birth of my youngest child, I was attended by a midwife, and those present included my 13-year-old daughter and a close friend. I breastfed each child immediately after birth and for a long time afterward. I regarded each birth as a triumph achieved in defiance of the male medical establishment and made possible by my rebellious feminist consciousness. I did not think much about what else made possible those triumphs, additional factors that obviously included my race and my class—not to mention the race- and class-related fact that my births were covered by health insurance.

Reading Evelyn C. White's interview with lay midwife Shafia Mawushi Monroe led me to reconsider the meanings I had assigned to my own experiences of giving birth. Although White's interview focuses on lay midwifery and home birth, it raises wider questions concerning the nature of health care and the responsibility of health care providers—not to mention how such providers may be compensated. The richness of Monroe's conceptions of health care and of the appropriate relation between birthing women and those attending them may be illustrated by comparing her views with those that I held when I gave birth.

Basic Conceptions of Pregnancy and Birth

AJ: I regarded pregnancy and birth as joyful adventures, rather than medical emergencies. I did not consider them in financial terms at all.

SM: Monroe is certainly aware of the joyful potential of pregnancy and birth, but she also recognizes that these processes may be health- and even life-threatening crises for some women and their infants. In addition, for some women and their families, they may precipitate economic crises.

Conceptions of Health Hazards to Mothers and Infants

AJ: I saw most hazards to my babies and myself as originating primarily in unwanted medical interventions such as anaesthetic, silver nitrate eye drops, and hospital-imposed obstacles to breast-feeding. While I thought of these interventions as undermining optimal health, it never occurred to me that they might threaten my baby's or my own life. The only non-iatrogenic health hazards that I worried about at all were genetic conditions such as Down's syndrome and spina bifida.

SM: Monroe is conscious of many more factors threatening not only the health but even the lives of mothers and infants. Some of these factors may stem from medical interventions, but others are rooted in the life situations of African-American women. They include inadequate nutrition or heat, drugs, domestic abuse, and guns, as well as the daily emotional toll of surviving in a racist society.

Conceptions of Healthy Birth

AJ: My conception of birth was, in the jargon of the time, "holistic." This meant that I regarded birth not just as a matter of getting the baby out undamaged but as a significant emotional and physical event involving not only the infant and myself but also our circle of family and friends. So I was concerned not only with my strictly reproductive capacities or even with caring for my body as a whole organism, but also with creating an atmosphere in the delivery room supportive to me and welcoming to my baby.

SM: Following from her more inclusive conception of possible health hazards to mothers and babies, Monroe has a much broader conception of the requirements for healthy birth. Like me, she recognizes the need for mothers to eat healthy food and breast-feed their babies—but she is also concerned that mothers and babies have sufficient warmth and shelter and be free from domestic and street violence, as well as the emotional violence of institutionalized racism. Monroe's conception of healthy birth is thus far more "holistic" than mine. While we both see the bodies of birthing women and their babies in a social context, I focused primarily on my own intimate circle while Monroe takes into consideration the mothers' relations not only with their families but also with the larger society.

Conceptions of the Birth Attendant's Responsibilities

AJ: Reacting against the sexist authoritarianism of official U.S. medicine, I wanted to take charge of my birthing and to relegate the birth attendant to the position of assistant. I was preoccupied with preserving my autonomy, in collaboration with my partner, to decide such things as the timing, place, and method of the birth as well as who should be present. I took if for granted that I had expert help available, and my main concern was not to be subordinated to it. I regarded as intrusive any questions not related directly to the birth, such as whether the pregnancy was intentional and what kind of contraception I planned to use in the future. My anxieties about autonomy were symbolized in my resistance to my white male physicians' practice of addressing me by my given name while reserving the title of "doctor" for themselves; I wanted them to recognize that I was a doctor too! Because I saw the threat to my autonomy primarily in gendered terms, I did not feel similarly defensive with my white female midwife and was very comfortable with each of us calling the other by our given names.

SM: As a midwife, Monroe clearly regards herself as an assistant to birthing women, but she has a much more extensive conception of the kinds of help she may be called on to provide. So she may intervene in her clients' life situations in a variety of ways, from helping them meet their basic needs for heat and food to counseling their male partners and teenage children. She states explicitly that her job is more than catching babies, even more than providing mothers and babies with material aid. For Monroe, Afrocentric midwifery also involves offering an overtly political education to entire families. Monroe's primary concern is for her clients' health and survival rather than for their autonomy in any individualistic sense. Ensuring the health and survival of mother and infant is seen as a responsibility to be shared by the client, her family, and Monroe.

I suspect that I would agree with Monroe on many issues going far beyond our shared enthusiasm for minimally medicated childbearing. Nevertheless, the foregoing comparisons clearly reveal how each of our perspectives has been shaped by our respective class and race. My point in making the comparisons is not to elevate one model over the other. I do not wish to idealize or universalize Monroe's vision, which she herself probably would not recommend for all birthing women. Neither do I wish to join the popular pastime of bashing white middle-class feminism, since my own views certainly do not represent those of all white middle-class feminists. Finally, I am not interested in personal breast-beating; at the times when I gave birth, I was thinking primarily about my own situation, not developing a comprehensive philosophy of health care.

One reason for offering these comparisons is to provide a context for the ethical questions raised for me by White's article. Some of these questions cluster around the issue of patient–client autonomy. If I were one of Monroe's clients, I imagine that her interventions might make me feel ambivalent, simultaneously appreciative and resentful of her help. I realize that such feelings may be products of my specific class and race consciousness, but I wonder if they might be shared by some African American women. That Monroe had my own and my baby's best interests at heart might not be enough to prevent me from regarding her talks with my mother, my older children, and my male partner as interfering in my life. The fact that she was a full member of my community, sharing my gender, race, class, and neighborhood, might alleviate my resentment—but it could also intensify it. Monroe notes the advantages of health care providers being personally acquainted with their clients, and I do not dispute these. On the other side, however, I think there are also reasons for keeping social and professional relationships separate.

Monroe's lack of formal credentials raises further questions. These are not at all questions about her competence; many highly credentialed health care providers are incompetent or even abusive, and I have no doubt that Monroe makes a unique contribution to the health of her clients and their babies. Instead, my questions are about getting lay midwifery covered by health insurance. How can we make "alternative" medical therapies available to poor as well as wealthy people without simultaneously opening the door to unqualified practitioners, quacks, and charlatans?

Regardless of these uncertainties, I think my comparisons do point toward one definite conclusion. Since they clearly illustrate how occupying certain social positions encourages us to perceive certain things rather than others as problematic—and certain solutions rather than others as satisfactory, my comparisons demonstrate that developing an adequate U.S. perspective on health care needs the insights not simply of women in general but of working-class women of color in particular.

20 Grandparents Who Care: An Empowerment Model of Health Care

Margo Okazawa-Rey

INTRODUCTION

The crack cocaine epidemic affects practically every aspect of life in poor, urban, African-American communities throughout the nation. The more dramatic effects of the epidemic are clearly visible: infants inhale their first breaths and experience withdrawal from drugs; youngsters "run" illegal substances for their older peers and "mentors"; men murder one another over deals gone sour; women sell themselves for a smoke of dope.[1] A less dramatic consequence of the crack cocaine plague, one that is often invisible to the public eye, is the increasing number of grandparents who are now assuming the primary responsibility of caring for their grandchildren because their adult children cannot provide adequate care (Kell 1990; Minkler and Roe 1993).

Although the extended family's care of children is not a new phenomenon in African-American communities, the current trend defies traditional arrangements. Historically, grandparents have always played an active role in childrearing. Because crack-using parents of this generation of children and infants participate erratically and are often completely absent, however, grandparents have assumed a far greater role in the care of their grandchildren than they ever have.

Health care providers in urban areas were among the first professionals to identify this wave of grandparents suddenly becoming parents to their grandchildren and to associate the change in their roles with the grandparents' worsening health problems. For instance, health care providers in the outpatient clinics at San Francisco General Hospital and in community health centers observed a dramatic increase in the number of missed appointments and acute aggravation of previously controlled chronic physical illnesses, such as diabetes and high blood pressure. It seemed that the added day-to-day child care and homemaking responsibilities often prevented the grandparents from keeping medical appointments, and the stress related to their new roles aggravated their illnesses.

Stress mounts when a person consciously or unconsciously determines that his or her personal and environmental resources are inadequate to meet the demands (stressors) he or she faces. According to Germaine, "As a consequence of an appraisal that the demand exceeds coping resources, the individual experiences the subjective state of emotional stress. The subjective experience then evokes physiological and psychological responses or coping efforts" (Germaine 1984, p. 61). The aggravation of controlled illnesses was a signal that the grandparents had reached the limits of their coping resources.

According to the providers at San Francisco General Hospital, these grandparents identified the increased stress as a direct outgrowth of complicated family arrangements, violence associated with the drug-using lifestyles of their adult children, and assumption of primary or sole responsibility for their grandchildren. "These patients expressed feelings of anger, isolation, . . . intense frustration at their inability to negotiate complex legal, child welfare, and [criminal] justice systems" (Miller and Trupin 1990, p. 1). The experiences of these grandparents are borne out by research which shows that the health risks of low-income women are increased by stressful life conditions and events (Greywolf 1982).

In this chapter I describe one way that health care providers at community-based health centers, in partnership with their patients, are responding to the multiple needs of grandparents: the Grandparents Who Care Support Network of San Francisco. I argue that health care providers must acknowledge and address connections between medical and nonmedical issues in the overall health of their patients. I show that a powerful and empowering alliance can result when professionals and patients collaborate as knowledgeable and capable partners.

NATURE OF THE PROBLEM

Poor and working-class, middle-aged, and elderly black women constitute a significant proportion of grandparents who have assumed the responsibility for raising their grandchildren. These women range in age from their mid-forties to early seventies. Contrary to stereotype, most of the grandmothers were not welfare mothers themselves; many are single through either divorce or the death of spouses. Many were employed full or part time in traditional female service occupations and professional occupations, until they were forced to quit due to difficult-to-resolve conditions such as unaffordable child care (Kell 1990). The most commonly cited reasons for the women to assume the care of the grandchildren were:

1. Involvement of adult children with crack cocaine or alcohol and the resultant neglect of their children.

2. Incarceration of adult children on drug- or alcohol-related charges.

3. Reluctance to surrender their grandchildren to the state foster care system. (Miller and Trupin 1990, p. 1)

After having raised their own children, often under difficult circumstances and sometimes recently, the grandmothers are ambivalent about their new role as active parents to their grandchildren. On the one hand, they believe they are fully capable, they are willing to fulfill their obligations to family, and they are satisfied knowing that they can provide their grandchildren with safe, comfortable, and loving surroundings. On the other hand, they are also frustrated and angry about losing their independence—even on the most basic level such as having private bathroom time—and their hopes of fulfilling personal dreams. As one grandmother exclaimed, "I was ready to go on a two-week cruise before I got these grandchildren!"

It is important to emphasize that many grandparents, despite their ambivalence about their new role, are willing to take on the responsibility of parenting because of their strong belief in the importance of keeping the family intact—not surrendering the children to state social services officials—and because of their faith that their adult children eventually will be able to resume fully functional lives. Their unfaltering commitment and faith are reflected in repeated comments such as "I will never let the state take these kids!" and "when my daughter straightens herself out. . . . "

While the initial contact between the grandparents and health care providers is health-related, the problems experienced by the grandparents extend far beyond particular health concerns: they desperately need day care, special education services, transportation, respite care, and money; they must learn to negotiate complicated and sometimes resistant social services, educational, and criminal justice bureaucracies; and they must address the intrafamilial issues related to the problems, such as dealing with the erratic behaviors of their drug-using adult children or the emotional injuries experienced by the grandchildren.

The needs of grandparents who are served by urban community health centers, therefore, seriously challenge the existing modes of health care delivery and tax the already meager resources of the centers. Given the changing nature of social problems in poor African-American communities, health care organizations can no longer simply address health concerns as isolated phenomena, just as schools in those communities can no longer focus only on the "Three 'Rs" (see Young, Chapter 22, in this volume).

HEALTH AND ILLNESS: THE CONTEXT FOR THE GRANDPARENTS' GROUP

In the 1940s the World Health Organization defined health as a "state of complete physical, mental, and social well-being" (Germaine 1984, p. 34).

This holistic view contrasted with prevailing Western biomedicine, and it was criticized as an unrealistic goal for individuals and society. The Western model still dominates, with health defined almost exclusively in biomedical terms and considered to be the absence of disease. "Disease," from the biomedical perspective, is explained as a departure from the norm of biochemical variables (Engel 1977). This definition "inhibits the view of the patient as a total person in a total environment by overlooking the personal and environmental dimensions in health" (Germaine 1984, p. 34).

Some health care professionals are moving away from the Western biomedical model. Paul Ahmed, Aliza Kolker, and George Coelho, for example, define health as "*a multidimensional process* involving the well-being of the whole person in the context of his [*sic*] . . . environment" (Ahmed et al. 1979, p. 9; emphasis in original). C. B. Germaine also includes the concept of "illness" in the "disease" model.

"Illness" is a sociopsychological concept [that] includes the cultural meaning of the discomfort or pain to the patient and her family. . . . When disease is the only focus of treatment, the care given to patients will be less than satisfactory and less effective clinically than in situations where both "disease" and "illness" are treated together. (Germaine 1984, p. 35)

During the past two decades, the writings of David Mechanic have also contributed to the concept of illness. He identifies two important aspects of illness behavior. One is the nature and quality of the symptoms of the disease and illness and how they make an impact on the daily function of the person. The other is the interconnection between the symptoms and environmental factors such as the culture of the individual and the community, the individual's life circumstances of age, gender, and accessibility—both geographic and social—of the health care facility (Mechanic 1976a, 1976b). Other medical sociology literature also suggests the need to consider the social and economic conditions surrounding patients' lives if they are to be served effectively (Fox 1989).

PHILOSOPHY OF THE GRANDPARENTS' GROUP

Two health care providers, Doriane Miller, MD, and Sue Trupin, RN, observed at firsthand the physical, social, economic, and emotional toll exacted on grandparents. They took seriously the need to address the entire complex of issues—biomedical, social, cultural, and economic—that surround the lives of grandparenting patients at San Francisco General Hospital. In 1989 they founded a formal support network—Grandparents Who Care—to help address these needs and to take over where the health care services ended.

Ms. Johnson,[2] a typical participant of Grandparents Who Care, is a middle-aged, working-class, African-American woman. She recently shouldered the responsibility for her three grandchildren after she saw that they were being neglected by her adult son and his wife, who were actively using crack cocaine. Her "babies" are ages 3, 2, and 6 months. At her first meeting, she described her reason for attending: "I started havin' a lot of problems after the babies came to live with me. I tried to talk to the doctor about it but you know how they are. [She waves her arms above her head as she speaks.] They're kind of up there with it. I'm glad he told me about this meeting though...."

Ms. Johnson feels a desire to confide in her physician, yet she feels a sense of distance and alienation in relation to him. Patients like Ms. Johnson often disclose, or wish to disclose, to "The Doctor" problems they would not disclose to anyone else, because physicians may be perceived as godlike. However, chances are that the physician, trained in mainstream medicine and working in an already overutilized health center, lacks the time and inclination to discuss in detail problems unrelated directly to a patient's "physical" condition. Fortunately, however, in this case Ms. Johnson's physician had heard of Grandparents Who Care and referred her there.

The philosophy of Grandparents Who Care rests on the following assumptions:

1. The health problems of individuals relate closely to their family, home, and community situations,
2. Cultural and institutional barriers often impede access to needed health care and other services.
3. Professional health care services alone are inadequate or inappropriate in meeting all the needs.
4. Individual and collective empowerment of African Americans, grandparents, and community members is essential to maintaining health.

Currently, the organization comprises five support groups. Each group meets for one and a half hours weekly and is attended by two to twenty-five grandparents; an overwhelming majority are women. One group was established especially for adolescents who are in the care of their grandparents.

The groups are based on a social support intervention model that provides emotional, informational, and practical aid. Each is co-facilitated by two health care professionals—nurses, doctors, or social workers. Although the social support intervention model is the basic design, each group has unique features depending on the perspectives, skills, and personalities of the facilitators and the needs of the participants. A volunteer board, made up of grandparents, community members, and professional health care providers, advises the organization in matters such as policy formulation. Two neighborhood health centers and San Francisco General Hospital provide the rooms where the meetings take place. Following is a detailed description of one group within the network that I co-facilitate with another female African-American social worker, whose roots are in the community where the group is run.

Our group was formed in March 1991, although active outreach and recruitment efforts began in early winter. Our membership includes approximately twenty women and one man, who has attended only sporadically. In an active core group of approximately eight women, three of the longest enrolled members have emerged as leaders within our group and within the larger network. Two features of this group make it particularly appropriate for meeting the needs of poor and working-class African-American women. First is the implicitly Afrocentric feminist content and approach used in the group. Second is the explicit commitment to empowerment.

The content and process of the group are rooted in Afrocentric feminist epistemology: we confront, resist, and redefine Western male conceptions of legitimate knowledge and notions of leadership and expertise. Participants control the criteria used for determining expertise, the power of decision making, and the "text" for the discussions and exchanges in the groups (Collins 1990). We validate and attempt to deepen the belief in the grandmothers as experts about their lives and the communities where they live. This expertise includes their knowledge of the numerous institutions (the city and county social services departments, the school, and criminal justice systems) derived from negotiating them in their daily lives.

The grandmothers' knowledge base is discovered both deliberately and inadvertently. For example, when one woman is facing a particular problem with her grandchild in the school system, another will describe her dealings with it and offer suggestions concerning the most effective ways of interceding. Or, in telling of her personal experiences, a grandmother will display the range of information, knowledge, and skills she has obtained through negotiating the system. For example, one grandmother may refer another to a physician who is adept at obtaining social services for children.

Equal participation in the dialogue is emphasized within the groups. This type of dialogue has "long [been] extant in Afrocentric . . . tradition whereby power dynamics are fluid, everyone has a voice, but everyone must listen and respond to other voices in order to be allowed to remain in the community" (Collins 1990, p. 237). It is a modified version of the "call-and-response" mode of communication. Any member, not just the designated facilitators, can call; any and all members respond. Whoever knows about a subject or has information, from any source, especially personal experience, is encouraged to share it.

The meetings often assume the qualities of a conversation in the kitchen, on the porch, in the street, or in church. Each meeting begins as participants "check in" to inform each other of any significant problems and victories they experienced during the previous week, or simply to say "Hi." We also make a specific request for reports about acts of self-care and self-love by asking the question, "What good thing did you do for yourselves. . . ?" Next, anyone with particularly pressing or significant concerns, as defined by the participant, takes the floor. At any point, other participants may ask for clarification, offer a suggestion, or add their own experiences to the story.

In our group, the professional facilitators assume two primary functions. One is to attend to the more technical aspects of a problem or an issue. For example, we use our contacts in the educational system to secure special services or to help grandmothers negotiate the bureaucratic labyrinth. Hence, we are technical consultants. The other function is to provide a long-term view and offer visions of hope for those who are engulfed in the immediate, often dire, situations confronting them. We use our personal experiences as illustrations of possibilities. For instance, we have shared our own stories of dealing with family members who are substance users. Here we serve as role models. It is important to stress that the facilitators serve primarily as consultant, reflector, and role model rather than as all-knowing "Leaders."

Following is an excerpt of a typical meeting:

Facilitator: Good morning, ladies. How is everyone this morning? And what good thing did you do for yourselves during the week?

The women slowly respond by briefly describing their condition and an act of self-care they performed during the previous week. Before everyone gets a chance to report, one grandmother is ready to share a problem she is facing.

Ms. Daniels: I have something I wanna talk about. My grandson is having a lot of problems with his teacher at school. . . . They've suspended [him] again. . . . They don't know what to do with him. You know he's smart, but he's not reading at his right level and he keeps having trouble with his teacher Ms. Anderson, a young white lady. . . . I'm not being prejudiced but I think it's somethin' racial. . . .

Ms. Jackson: Uh huh! These schools just don't know how to deal with these black children, especially them boys. When my son was in school, they used to call me all the time saying he's been suspended. . . .

Ms. Daniels: I've been thinking about taking him out of that school. . . .

Ms. Brown: Didn't he just get to that school this year? Why did they move him from that other one anyway? Remember you sayin' last year that he was doin' real good there?

Ms. Daniels: I don't know why they moved him. They just did. . . .

Ms. Brown: They can't do that without your permission, although they will try to slip stuff past you. You have rights as a parent. They can't do anything with your child without you knowin' it or you givin' permission. . . .

A chorus of "Amen," "Yes, that's right!" and other responses echoes throughout the room. A detailed and lively discussion concerning the rights of parents, the faults of the schools and school system, and the ill state of special education programs dominates the next forty-five minutes of group time. The facilitator stops the action when everyone talks at once or when one person begins to dominate the discussion.

> Ms. B: You know what we need is someone to come in and tell us how the whole thing around special ed works. We need a guest speaker who knows about all that to explain to us what's going on and what we can do. . . .
>
> Facilitator: That's a good idea. I will call [an advocacy group for children in special education] to see when someone could come talk to us. . . . Does anybody who didn't get a chance to check in yet want to do that now?

The group meeting ends with the facilitator making closing summary statements and asking someone to pray, which results in something unrehearsed or the Lord's Prayer being said, while most people hold hands. The ritual of closing with a prayer is an essential facet of the meeting because religion is one of the primary coping strategies utilized by the women in the group.

EMPOWERING "GRANDPARENTS WHO CARE"

The grandparents in our group face daily issues of powerlessness rooted in racial and economic inequality; the grandmothers experience the "triple jeopardy" of race-, class-, and gender-based oppression. Thus, a primary goal of Grandparents Who Care is empowerment: we work to have the grandparents recognize and harness their individual and collective agency—their capacity to take action and to be the actors, rather than the acted upon.

The Changing Definitions of Empowerment

The contemporary roots of empowerment are embedded in the context of the progressive social movements of the 1960s: the Black Power, women's, and welfare rights movements, all of which were founded to transform oppressive conditions in society. Originally, empowerment was based on the principle of self-determination: individuals and communities have the right to determine their own fates. From this perspective, "empowerment" denoted both micro (personal) and macro (institutional) interventions to effect changes in the lives of subordinated peoples as well as in their communities, with these interventions geared ultimately toward progressive societal transformation. The concept of empowerment had an explicitly political meaning. For example, in working with female rape victims, the physical and emotional traumas of the women were addressed immediately (micro). The asymmetrical power relations between men and women, and society's approval of men violating the rights and integrity of women (macro) were challenged in the courts and other public arenas.

Empowerment has become a basic organizing principle in addressing contemporary health issues and problems. Organizations working in the AIDS epidemic, such as ACT-UP, constitute one example. Another is the Atlanta-based National Black Women's Health Project started by Billye Avery to address health issues confronted by African-American women. It now has self-help-group affiliates throughout the nation. Recovery and support groups that deal with substance addictions, breast cancer, and incest have also been founded on the principles of empowerment.

The term *empowerment*, however, has recently been appropriated and its meaning diluted or otherwise altered to suit mainstream interests. For example, the so-called me generation of the 1980s has used the term to denote furthering individualistic self-interests. The term *empowerment* has also been appropriated by the "men's movement"—mostly white, middle-class men (who are typically already in power) who gather in support groups and at weekend retreats. The most extreme of these groups are working to "reclaim" their "rightful" place and role as the dominant members of this society (Faludi 1991). Among social service professionals, the term *empowerment* is sometimes used as the 1990s euphemism for "pull yourself up by the bootstraps."[3]

Realizing the Goal of Empowerment

As one means toward empowerment, Grandparents Who Care has implemented a project to train grandparents to become group facilitators. Our purpose is to enable participants to practice and formally assert their own leadership skills, and eventually for all the support groups to become self-sufficient and led by the grandparents themselves. Women who are seasoned members of a support group and interested in becoming formal leaders are trained by professional trainers in the basic skills of support group facilitation. After a four-week training series, each trainee works with a professional to establish a new group. The trainee collaborates with the professional facilitator regarding all the outreach and initial startup work, such as making individual contacts with prospective group members, speaking to church groups, and following up on referrals from physicians at health centers around the city.

Another critical way the women are empowered is through active participation in political advocacy and lobbying. The grandmothers collaborated with a state legislator to draft a bill that would make it easier for grandparents who are raising their grandchildren to receive payments and entitlements under the foster care system. The bill was important for the grandmothers because the foster care system meets the needs of the children better than does AFDC, but care providers who are family members are ineligible for foster care funds. Therefore, most grandparents receive assistance not through foster care, but through the Aid for Families with Dependent Children system, which is limited not only in the amounts of money available, but also in the services that are covered.

It is particularly crucial to make available the wider range of services covered by foster care, because many of the babies and children suffer from the combined effects of poor prenatal care and neglect and they require special medical, psychological, and educational help. For instance, one member of our support group is caring for a 4 year old who must live with a tracheotomy tube. This child requires trained medical technical assistance during many of his waking hours. Many of the other grandchildren require help with manifestations of developmental disorders. The bill, co-authored by the women and sponsored by the legislator, reached the desk of the governor, who, regrettably, vetoed it. However, the grandparents have used the experience of succeeding to the extent they did as a collective referent for empowerment.

A final example of empowerment relates directly to the health concerns facing the grandmothers. Through the education and support they find in the group, the women learn to connect their health status to the circumstances of their daily lives. For example, when Ms. Turner arrived at one meeting, it was evident from her "lookin' tired," which included puffy eyes and nasal tone to her speech, that she was not her usual self. During check-in time, she stated that she almost did not attend the meeting because she had "sinus problems" over the weekend, and she described her symptoms in detail. When members probed her about her weekend, she disclosed that her grandchildren had been extremely distressed by an unexpected visit from their mother. They had become unruly, and Ms. Turner had to exert added emotional and physical energy to quiet and comfort the children.

Initially, Ms. Turner talked of her physical symptoms and the family crisis as two unrelated incidents. During the course of the meeting, however, as the other women in the group told similar stories relating family crisis to physical symptoms, she herself began to make the connections. In subsequent meetings, Ms. Turner has been able to better articulate her understanding of the connections between physical illness and emotional distress.

The examples above describe some specific ways that Grandparents Who

Care attempts to implement the goal of empowerment. As the current membership gains confidence and skills and the network becomes stronger and more formal, the possibilities for expanding the practice of empowerment multiply. For instance, in the future it might be possible for grandparents to organize in their neighborhoods around the issue of drugs.

The empowerment model also raises important questions: What are the limits of empowerment? How do we address the contradictions created when members of two bodies holding unequal power—patients and professionals—attempt to relate as equals? How do the effects of internalized racism, sexism, and classism prevent us from even seeing some of those contradictions? What role can groups like Grandparents Who Care play in bringing about the transformation of neighborhoods, communities, and society as a whole?

CONCLUSION

I have tried to show the necessity of expanding prevailing biomedical perspectives on health in order to recognize as central issues the social, economic, and cultural factors that shape overall health, particularly for both poor people and African Americans. From this perspective, not only are physical diseases at issue, but also the social problems that indirectly affect how individuals deal, or do not deal, with their physical conditions. Thus, health care systems and providers must address health concerns in the totality of individuals' and communities' circumstances. To address the problems in their totality, we must understand that they are rooted deeply in economic, social, and political inequality based on racism, sexism, and classism. Thus, economic, social, and political empowerment provides an important avenue to health and well-being.

In an era of diminishing economic resources for health care specifically, and human services generally, one creative way to help offset the shortage is to view community members as resources. During the Reagan and Bush administrations in the 1980s, cutbacks in government-sponsored human services and a conservative backlash against civil rights opposed the efforts of oppressed populations, such as people of color and women, to bring about equality. The extent to which we will progress will depend on our ability and willingness both to care for ourselves and to organize as communities to bring about the necessary societal changes. The empowerment model of health care is a way to do both.

NOTES

1. Crack is a smokable form of cocaine that is highly addictive and inexpensive. It is available in most states, and its principal users are black people living in urban areas. Since its introduction, crack has been associated with substantial increases in

drug-related arrests, adolescent gang violence, and incidence of neonatal cocaine addiction and syphilis, gonorrhea, and other sexually transmitted diseases. For more detailed information, see, for example, Nobles et al. 1987.

2. Pseudonyms are used to ensure patient confidentiality.

3. Efforts to promote empowerment are often confused with blaming the victim or with promoting the self-interests of those in the dominant group.

Commentary by Simona J. Hill

Confronting the massive effects of the crack cocaine epidemic as it rends the central fibers of U.S. social institutions will be of primary national concern well into the next century. In the inner cities, particularly in poor, urban African-American communities, the explosion of crack as the inexpensive, readily available drug of choice rages through the "social fabric of the ghetto like a nuclear bomb" (Koppleman and Jones 1989, p. 14). What remains in the aftermath of human suffering are families and professionals dealing not only with "crack" babies fetally exposed to the drug derived from cocaine who suffer from a multitude of physical and neurological problems, but also other children of crack addicts who are repeatedly victimized by their parent's (or parents') neglect and addiction.

The single toughest issue for child welfare agencies is to find some viable means of caring for these children in the present climate of restricted adequate resources for clientele (Besharov 1989). "Who will care for these children?" is a critical societal (human) question with no easy answers. Within the African-American community a strong response is increasingly coming from parents of crack-addicted adolescents and adult children who are willing to assume primary or sole responsibility for the care and welfare of their grandchildren.

Although the extended family structure is a long-standing cultural tradition among African Americans, and not a new phenomenon by any consideration, this is the first time it has ever confronted such a fearsome enemy as crack cocaine abuse. There is a desperate need in academic disciplines for investigative research on coping strategies, self-help groups, and the interaction of these families within the health care system. Most current research excludes a careful examination of African-American grandparents operating within a health care system that may not welcome them because of economic scarcity of resources, social, racial, or classist issues. The ethical dilemmas emerging from the disassociation of these grandparents from our health care system have yet to be explored within an Afrocentric feminist context or within a commitment to empowerment of the individual framework.

Okazawa-Rey describes her work as a co-facilitator of a self-help group, Grandparents Who Care. These poor, working-class African-American grandmothers, ranging in age from their mid-forties to early seventies, are coping with the impact of crack cocaine addiction on their extended family systems. Okazawa-Rey emphasizes the often neglected connections between medical and nonmedical issues in the delivery of health care to these patients. The Grandparents Who Care Support Network of San Francisco has evolved into an empowerment model that highlights an alliance between health care professionals and their patients. This alliance could result in a powerful collaboration in the recovery process for these families.

Okazawa-Rey asks the health care provider to consider the multidimensional facets of these grandparents' adjustment to new and sometimes unexpected roles. Her chapter outlines the problem for this population of African Americans; how it is addressed on both personal and institutional levels; and the ambivalence and concerns of the grandparents. She also recounts some of the immediate successes of the network members. The example of a typical session will be especially helpful to those practitioners unfamiliar with the "call-response" mode of communication utilized in many Afrocentric traditions.

Grandparents Who Care is based on techniques for empowering (mostly) African-American women on personal, interpersonal, and political levels. These techniques challenge practitioners to move beyond individual clients and problems to creating specific ways to engage these women in group efforts that decrease alienation and move toward change on individual, group, and community levels. The empowerment theme includes participation and concrete response to a sense of powerlessness over life circumstances. This process is clearly reflected in networking, shared leadership, facilitators who are "technical consultants" rather than omniscient experts, peer interchanges, and mutual aid which Okazawa-Rey observes.

By employing an empowerment model, we can consider matters that can be enigmatic at best and interpret mechanisms that these grandparents develop in conjunction with practitioners and among themselves. Such mechanisms allow otherwise oppressed patients to mobilize and maximize their resources to handle the complexities of the health care system and "gain new insights into forces that motivate and often threaten their lives and eventually expand their range of choices" (Stokes and Greenstone 1981, p. 770). Disclosure in dealing with crack addiction through self-help groups can be a liberating, yet painful, process, but ultimately one that can generate the impetus for political change and institutional transformation.

21 The Anatomy of a Black Community-Based Transplant Education Program: A Model for Community Empowerment

Clive O. Callender, Lannis E. Hall, Curtis L. Yeager, Ann Wood Washington, and Patti Grace Smith

INTRODUCTION

Between 1983 and 1989, the gap between organ donors and patients waiting for organs in the United States widened from approximately 1,000 to 10,000 people (Kusserow 1990). In June 1990, 20,828 people were waiting for organs for transplantation. The scarcity of organs is the major limiting factor in transplantation (Dechesser 1986) and contributes to the death of three people every day (United Network for Organ Sharing 1990).

Shortage of organs for transplantation is problematic for all groups, but as a result of unique medical predispositions, donor difficulties, and harsh socioeconomic conditions, the black community is more adversely affected than its white counterpart (Callender 1983, 1989). Despite a decline in deaths traceable to hypertensive heart disease and stroke, the incidence of end-stage renal disease in blacks with hypertension is still on the rise. The incidence of renal disease is almost seven times greater in blacks with hypertension than in whites. Furthermore, even though blacks represent only 12% of the U.S. population, they make up 30% of the patients on dialysis (National Institute of Diabetes and Digestive and Kidney Diseases 1989; United Network for Organ Sharing 1990).

Presently, patients who develop end-stage renal disease have three options: peritoneal dialysis, hemodialysis, and organ transplantation. Of these three, successful transplantation provides a better quality of life than does maintenance on dialysis. Unfortunately, however, no group, regardless of race, takes full advantage of transplantation; all groups overwhelmingly choose hemodialysis (80% whites versus 90% blacks) (National Institute of Diabetes and Digestive and Kidney Diseases 1989). These statistics are particularly striking considering the burdensome problems associated with dialysis. It is costly and requires attachment to a dialysis machine for twelve hours a week, constraining and altering the patient's lifestyle physically, socially, emotionally, professionally, and sexually.

Despite improved quality of life for successful organ recipients, certain restrictions on transplantation are relevant to blacks. Immunogenetic studies have indicated that mismatches for certain histocompatibility locus A (HL-A) molecules, such as DRW6, are found with greater frequency in blacks than in whites and are associated with a more intense graft rejection. Recovering more organs from black organ donors with similar antigens may, therefore, be crucial to increasing graft survival in black transplant recipients (Callender and Dunston 1987, 1988; Dunston et al. 1987).

In 1989 there were 16.1 donors per 1 million Americans. Blacks donated 8% of the available kidneys for transplantation but were recipients of 23% of the available donor kidneys. Consequently, in 1989 blacks received almost three times as many kidneys as they donated (United Network for Organ Sharing 1990).

The transplant community must focus its innovative and creative energies on addressing the general shortage as well as increasing black participation in organ donor programs. In the last ten years, the authors have made the shortage of organ and tissue donors one of their highest priorities, focusing on reasons for low donorship and on strategies for increasing participation in the black community (Callender 1983, 1987a, 1987b, 1989; Callender et al. 1982; Callender and Dunston 1987, 1988). This chapter discusses the origin and successes of a grassroots initiative, the District of Columbia Organ Donation Project (DCODP), and the development of subsequent programs to overcome obstacles to organ and tissue donation and transplantation among blacks.

THE WASHINGTON, D.C., ORGAN DONOR PROGRAM

In 1978 members of the Southeastern Organ Procurement Foundation (SEOPF) asked the authors to identify the reasons for the black community's reluctance to donate organs, considering the higher need for donor kidneys as a result of their high incidence of end-stage renal disease. In 1980, in response to the SEOPF initiative, Howard University Hospital sponsored a pilot study to identify primary factors that influence low black donorship. Using a grassroots approach, forty members of the black community were individually interviewed for two hours regarding their attitudes toward organ donation. Results suggested five primary reasons for the low black donorship: (1) lack of transplant awareness, (2) religious myths and superstitions, (3) distrust of the medical community, (4) fear of premature declaration of death after signing an organ donor card, and (5) black donor preference for assurance of black receivership (Callender et al. 1982). While only 10% of the participants agreed to sign organ donor cards before the interview, all participants did sign at the conclusion of the focus session. This grassroots approach appeared to be the key to changing attitudes about donation.

Drawing from the successes of this pilot study, we developed the District of Columbia Organ Donor Project (DCODP) in 1982 using the same grassroots approach employed in our pilot study. Under the auspices of the National Kidney Foundation (NKF) and with the support of Howard University Hospital, the DCODP worked with representatives from local medical, political, educational, business, and religious communities.

The DCODP steering committee met monthly from 1982 to 1984 to provide subcommittee progress reports, propose future initiatives, discuss strategies for raising funds, and suggest methods for educating and disseminating information into the black community. The funds raised paid for communication materials (videotapes, slide presentations, brochures, books, and posters), and the salary of a full-time program coordinator. Most importantly, our goal was to develop a strategic plan for increasing the number of black organ and tissue donors. This plan set up guidelines for educational presentations or messages, specifying the information to be delivered as well as who was to deliver it. The message consisted of facts explaining the problem and proposed solutions, and was to be delivered by ethnically appropriate or sensitive donors, recipients, transplant candidates, or family members as well as health care providers. The guidelines also specified that time be set aside for meaningful dialogue and for evolving answers to key questions.

We built our education program around the following facts: The incidence of all types of kidney disease is highest in black patients, and blacks with hypertension between ages 25 and 44 are twenty times more likely to have kidney failure as whites. While blacks make up 12% of the American population, they constitute 30% of kidney patients waiting for transplantation. Twenty percent of blacks have transplant genetic markers that are rarely found in whites; therefore, kidney transplantation is less successful in blacks than in whites, and hence, the pressing need for more black donors. In all, blacks receive 50% fewer organ transplantations than whites.

To address these problems, we proposed several general solutions in both prevention and treatment. We pointed out that the critical first step in prevention of kidney failure is the early treatment of hypertension. This not only decreases the incidence of kidney failure, but also reduces the number of deaths due to heart attack and stroke. We thus proposed that blacks should have semiannual blood pressure evaluations after the age of 12 (Rostand et al. 1982, 1989; Stamler et al. 1976; Voors et al. 1976). If a diagnosis of high blood pressure results, treatment should start as soon as possible.

While acknowledging the benefits of hypertension treatment for prevention of kidney disease, some of our male participants expressed concern about impotence or decreased sexual libido as a side effect of some antihypertensive medications. We pointed out that these effects can be avoided since not all such medications cause this side effect, and we encouraged patients to provide feedback regarding side effects to the health care provider. We stressed that the patient has the prerogative to request an alternative medication. The physician, in turn, must respond in a sensitive and caring fashion, keeping in mind that the patient's needs must be the most important part of the health care decision.

When hypertension is not treated, it may result in end-stage renal disease, requiring either dialysis or transplantation. Although transplantation allows a better quality of life than dialysis, histocompatibility factors may prevent a black recipient's acceptance of a white donor's organ. We therefore stressed that more black donors are needed to make kidney transplantation as successful for blacks as it has been for whites. We encouraged the black community to initiate open public discussions about organ donation and transplantation and to sign organ donor cards. In addition, we suggested that the black families involve their children in discussions about organ donation and transplantation.

OTHER INITIATIVES

In 1986 representatives of the Dow Chemical Company attended one of our DCODP presentations at the American Council on Transplantation Conference. Impressed by the project results, they inquired about possible participation in continuing or expanding this local initiative. As a result, the Dow-Take Initiative Program (Dow-TIP) took our donor education effort on tour to twenty-two U.S. cities with large black populations. This tour was completed in 1989. Then, in 1989–90, building on its previous successes, Dow joined the National Association for the Advancement of Colored People (NAACP) to develop National Black Donor Education Projects in New York, St. Louis, Memphis, Detroit, Baltimore, and Houston.

The success of Dow's initiative led to the development in 1988 of a joint effort between the National Medical Association (NMA) and the black clergy.[1] This project was directed at the clergy in an attempt to dispel widely held religious myths concerning organ donation.[2] In 1990 the NMA expanded its involvement by starting a National Black Physician Education Project with the National Institute for Allergy and Infectious Diseases (NIAID). Thus, the messages and the lessons regarding transplantation and organ tissue donation learned from lay communities were brought back into the hospitals and medical communities to the benefit of both. All of these groups relied on the grassroots approach that had proven successful in previous donor programs.

RESULTS

Since the development of the District of Columbia Organ Donor Project in 1982, our educational efforts have been greatly rewarded. Our message has been presented through schools, conferences, community groups, and the news media. Below we list some of the far-reaching results of our original outreach program.

We worked locally to bring organ donation information to the attention of our community. For example, in 1985 a curriculum on kidney disease was introduced and has been included in the District of Columbia Public School system at the high school level since then. In 1988 we developed two slide presentations for black audiences. One is targeted for the lay community and one for the medical community. We developed a list of experts who were available to speak to civic and social groups, including sororities, fraternities, Neighborhood Advisory Councils, funeral directors, lodges, women's organizations, and other community-based organizations. Presentations have been made to more than 100 black churches in the metropolitan D.C. area.

Our group developed a number of print publications and videos. More than 250 copies of our publication, *Organ Donation: A Minority Dilemma—Howard University Hospital*, have been distributed since 1988, and more than 10,000 copies of "Start a Family Tradition," a black organ/tissue donor-targeted brochure, have been distributed since 1988. A black donor awareness guidebook based on the DCODP experience was created in 1987 for the Dow/NAACP Black Donor Education Program, and Dow/NAACP also put together a Black Donor Question and Answer Brochure in 1989, with a distribution of 5,000. In addition, seven videos targeted at potential black organ donors were produced between 1987 and 1990.[3] Finally, we widely distributed the poster A Gift of Life featuring organ donor cards signed by basketball star Rick Mahorn and former Senator Edward Brooke.

We also worked to reach people through the national press, radio, and television. Information from the Dow/NAACP Black Donor Education Media program was featured in more than 275 national newspapers and magazines, including *USA Today*, the *St. Louis Post-Dispatch*, the *Detroit News*, the *New York Daily News*, the *Houston Post*, *Newsweek*, *Parade*, *Jet*, *Ebony*, and the *Journal of the National Medical Association*. In addition, information concerning blacks and organ donation has been included on sixty local and national television broadcasts and seventy local radio stations, reaching more than 300 million people.

Working with other organ donation programs around the country, we established collaboration or cooperative ventures between the DCODP and organ donor programs in Georgia, Florida, Illinois, California, New Jersey, and Pennsylvania. Educational materials produced by our program have been shared with at least forty cities and twenty states interested in initiating their own programs. In addition, the Dow/NAACP Black Donor Education program has been launched in six cities: New York, St. Louis, Memphis, Detroit, Baltimore, and Houston.

At the local level, we initiated a program within the District of Columbia Motor Vehicle Administration licensing unit whereby drivers could have a symbol placed on their licenses as an indication of their status as potential donors. This program increased the number of licensed drivers willing to donate organs or tissue from 25 per month in 1982 to 750 per month in

1989 (Callender et al. 1991). We heightened black awareness concerning the highly successful nature of organ transplantation, tripling the number of persons signing organ donor cards, as shown by a comparison of the Dow Gallup Polls of 1985 and 1990.

Finally, at a professional level, the First, Second and Third International Symposia on Renal Failure and Transplantation in Blacks were held in Washington, D.C., in 1985, 1989 and 1993, respectively. Those symposia were sponsored by the Howard University Hospital (HUH) and the National Institute of Diabetic and Digestive and Kidney Diseases (NIDDK).

WHY IT WORKED: THE GRASSROOTS APPROACH

When our pioneering work began, no education about organ donors and transplantations targeted the black community. Nor could efforts to enlist the black community in the solution of this problem be found in the literature. We used a grassroots approach because it has a unique meaning for the black population. It has been used throughout black history, but most prominently during the civil rights movement in the 1960s. For example, it was effective in mobilizing Mississippians to form the Mississippi Freedom Democratic party as well as in garnering support for the freedom bus rides throughout Alabama. A sense of community empowerment is generated because community organizers discuss the problem, consider the factors surrounding the issue, and, most importantly, illustrate each individual's ability to effect change (Blendon et al. 1989; Braithwaite and Lythcott 1989; Martin et al. 1988; Olson 1989).

The grassroots approach is not restricted to the political sphere, but can be appropriated to address the medical problems of the black community. The approach is not dependent on a large cadre of health care professionals. This is particularly important since access to large numbers of professionals is limited in black and other underserved communities. In addition, there is general mistrust of the medical profession by the black community. Such obstacles have been overcome using the grassroots method (Jones 1981). Our results have shown that the black community will respond to meet its needs when appropriately challenged by a method that is sympathetic to the style of the community (Callender 1987b, 1989; Callender et al. 1982; Callender and Dunston 1988).

Whether grassroots organizing is employed in research or education, an atmosphere of reciprocal learning is created which leads to more open communication between the medical and the lay communities. This openness is particularly crucial in the African-American community where economic factors have produced a more pronounced schism or social distance between the medical and lay communities (Blendon et al. 1989; Braithwaite and Lythcott 1989; Olson 1989). Coalitions are developed, and ethnically sensitive role models deliver the message to all areas of the African-American community. The coalitions emphasize that community and medical roles are equally important in increasing organ donations.

The Dow-TIP—as well as other programs modeled after the DCODP—was highly successful because it utilized several principles of grassroots mobilization. An ethnically oriented media campaign using magazines like *Ebony, Jet, Essence, Black Enterprise*, and *Black Health*, as well as community and national newspapers, played a crucial role in illuminating the urgency and necessity for black community involvement. Such articles, along with TV/radio broadcasts and numerous community discussions, laid the foundation for the dramatic increase in the number of blacks who signed donor cards from 7% in 1985 to 24% in 1990 (U.S. Gallup Organization 1990). Other grassroots donor organizations were just as impressive in their results. The Washington Regional Transplant Consortium data, for instance, demonstrate an increase in black organ donor consent rates from 10% in 1978 to 43% in 1989 (Rostand et al. 1982). For the first time it also reveals data that depict highly statistically significant differences between blacks and whites in medical unsuitability (9% whites, 30% blacks) and willingness to donate, at least in one locale (Callender et al. 1991). The most obvious benefit of these grassroots initiatives is an increase in the organ and tissue pool across the racial spectrum, which significantly increases the likelihood of a black transplant candidate having a successful transplantation. A report recently released from the Office of the Inspector General revealed that blacks must wait twice as long as whites to receive kidney transplants (Kusserow 1990). One factor in this discordance is the shortage of black organ donors. Consequently, an increase in the available black organ donor pool may help to reduce the long waiting times.

The message is important, but just as critical is who will carry it. Messengers need not be health care providers, but they must have certain characteristics. We have observed that the most effective and credible messengers are organ donor families, patients waiting for transplantable organs or tissues, and successful transplant recipients. Where possible, messengers should be of the same ethnicity as the community addressed. Since only 5% of transplant coordinators in the United States are black (Kusserow 1990), we must make maximum use of the expertise of these black coordinators. In their absence, however, we must be willing either to educate other black messengers, including psychologists, social workers, nurses, physician assistants, and community advocates, or to use ethnically sensitive nonblack transplant coordinators who have been trained to communicate with black families and communities. When delivered appropriately, these messages increase awareness about the transplant dilemma and the need for community participation in resolving it. In addition, by emphasizing frequent blood pressure evaluations and the importance of treatment for hypertension, they fulfill a community preventive health need.

CONCLUSION

Organ donation is the major limiting factor in transplantation today. Innovative and creative approaches to increasing the number of organ/tissue donors in all ethnic groups must be fostered and given a high priority. A successful grassroots approach in the black community has heightened transplant awareness, increased the number of blacks signing organ donor cards, the number of organ donors, and the number of black transplant recipients. This approach emphasizes a synergistic relationship between the public sector, the private sector, and the black community. It has been successful locally (DCODP), regionally (Dow-TIP), and nationally (Dow-TIP and Dow/NAACP). Its success requires the use of ethnically similar and sensitive community role models as effective transplant community educators. These principles are applicable across the racial spectrum and, when used with all races, may reduce the current acute shortage of transplantable organs and tissues. Our project's success demonstrates the importance of community education and empowerment in improving health care.

NOTES

1. This effort took place under the direction of Dr. Jesse Barber, chair of the religious subcommittee and former NMA president, and Dr. Frank Staggers, past NMA president.

2. Religious Myth #1: In that "Great getting up morning" if you are missing body parts you will be denied entrance to the Pearly Gates: with one kidney you'll get one wing; without eyes you won't be able to see great grandma in the hereafter.

Reality: It is spiritual rebirth that religion teaches. "In dying we are born to eternal life," and "it is in giving that we receive" (St. Francis of Assisi). Therefore, it is right and proper to leave organs and tissues behind after death.

Religious Myth #2: If you become an organ or tissue donor after death, you cannot have an open casket and a normal funeral.

Reality: Whatever organs or tissues you donate, you will be able to have a normal open casket funeral and the normal burial. If you leave behind eyes, skin, heart, liver, kidneys, etc., you can help forty different people live a better life: the deaf shall hear and the blind shall see.

3. A Gift of Life, August 1989; Organ Donation: A Dilemma of Black Americans, August 1990; Second Chance, October 1990; Organ Donation: Dilemmas in Long Island Transplants, December 1990; A Guide to Requesting Organs and Tissues from Black Families, December 1990; Organ Donation, My Brother's Keeper Program, Cable Network, 1989; Organ Donation, "The Today Show," October 1988.

Commentary by Wayne B. Arnason

Dr. Callender's chapter describes a successful and innovative grassroots approach to transplant education within the African-American community.

Beginning in 1982, the District of Columbia Organ Donor Project (DCODP) recruited community leaders and churches to assist in a transplant education effort involving a variety of media and role models designed to reach African Americans. Beginning in 1988, this donor education effort was expanded to twenty-two cities with large black populations, with assistance from the Dow Chemical Company, the NAACP, and the National Medical Association. These programs have laid the foundation for dramatic increases nationally in the number of blacks who have signed organ donor cards and, in some locations, black donor consent rates. This empowerment approach, involving the public sector, the private sector, and community leadership holds great promise for transplant education across the racial spectrum.

While a shortage of organs is a problem for all groups, education programs directed at African Americans are especially important because the black community is more harshly affected by this shortage. African Americans have a higher incidence of renal disease but a very low rate of organ donation. Blacks currently receive three times as many kidneys as they donate, although they receive proportionately fewer kidneys than whites. Blacks also have a smaller rate of graft survival than whites. The reasons for this pattern include some unique medical predispositions of African-American potential recipients and donors, socioeconomic factors, and cultural barriers involving religious beliefs and mistrust of a predominantly white medical establishment. The DCODP and its offspring programs, Dow-TIP and Dow/NAACP, have addressed these last two problems through an educational effort that has overcome the socioeconomic factors and the cultural barriers.

The success of these programs demonstrates that education towards the goal of greater access to health care is most effective when the target community is involved and empowered in the design and delivery of the message. The public/private partnership involved in funding these programs is an encouraging model for future efforts. Recalling the success of grassroots empowerment in organizing the voter registration movement in the South during the civil rights era, Callender and his colleagues suggest that such a model is appropriate for health care education as well. While people will respond to the messages conveyed by role models they admire, and with whom they can identify, an even more powerful response can be evoked by people perceived as neighbors who speak from personal experience of the suffering that a shortage of organs from black donors can cause.

The ethical dilemmas produced by the medical predispositions of African Americans with renal disease are not easily addressed by educational programs, however. It is widely known that blacks wait twice as long for organs as white potential recipients, that they receive fewer organ transplants than whites, and that these transplants are less successful for black recipients. The medical reasons for these facts are complex and not easily explainable to the general public. Consequently, distrust of the medical community, and black donor preference for assurance of black receivership have resulted in low black donorship.

A program of directed donation that privileges black-to-black transplant could further help ease the chronic shortage of organs. The United Network for Organ Sharing (UNOS) has resisted applying any "social criteria" alongside the objective medical criteria it has used to create its point system for kidney allocation. However, "directed donation" of organs to a particular class or group of prospective recipients is an ethically legitimate component of allocation policies already in use. This chapter demonstrates that marketing organ donations as an act of community solidarity and group self-interest has produced results in the black community. Would African-American families in the hospital being approached with the "required request" for donation be more receptive to a donation if told that their loved one's kidney would in all likelihood be able to benefit another black person in need from their community or a nearby city? Are there any ethically and politically viable approaches to allocation which could allow such a claim to be made as part of organ procurement practices?

We cannot say with certainty that instituting a program of directed donation would be an *incentive* to increased donation. However, this chapter demonstrates that tying appeals for organ donation to the needs of prospective black recipients has proved to be an incentive. Seeking ways to enhance the prospect of a black donor's kidney finding its way into the body of a black recipient would certainly remove a *disincentive* for black donors and deserves further exploration.

22 Toward an Ethic of Care and Community in Education and Medicine

Lauren Jones Young

INTRODUCTION

In 1950 Charles Richard Drew, the brilliant African-American physician who developed techniques for separating and preserving blood and who founded the world's first blood bank, lay bleeding in a "white" North Carolina hospital from injuries sustained in an automobile accident. Drew was denied medical attention and died before he could receive treatment at a "colored" hospital (Wesley 1968).

This familiar story, repeated in folk memories and in anthologies of notable African Americans, is false. Drew did in fact receive prompt medical attention for his fatal injuries (Logan and Winston 1982). Still it was the everyday perception and commonplace reality that Jim Crow statutes made no distinction between African Americans of note and common folk. Thousands of African-American men, women, and children—like other people of color—lived in the "other" America, behind the veil of a segregated system of health and human services. Vestiges of that tradition linger on. For many citizens, barriers today are as formidable as those created by Jim Crow laws.

Institutional practices have much to say about a society's regard for the needs of its most underserved populations. The purpose of this chapter is to show how the structure of human services systems affects the accessibility and quality of public services. Drawing on diverse literatures—research on school and health organizations and on children's health and poverty—I examine particular kinds of connections between institutions and clients, focusing on what we do in both health and education for those least able to do for themselves, poor children. I end by attacking the prevailing rational-bureaucratic and market design of the institutions of health and education, and argue that the design be replaced by a vision of "learning community."

The discussion is presented in two parts. The first sections examine the health and social welfare of poor children and society's obligation to intervene on behalf of them. The second part describes the consequences for health care of institutional practices organized around industrial models of service provision. Promising reforms in education informed by principles of learning community are examined to suggest a framework for a more just system of health care and schooling for everybody's children.

WHY CONSIDER EDUCATION AND HEALTH CARE TOGETHER?

I draw examples from education and schooling not just because I am an educator and because that is the arena I know best but because there is a much closer connection between education and medicine that transcends analogies of the two systems. The medical system is actually an educational system: fundamentally, the aim of both education and medicine is learning. Improving the nation's health rests largely on educational measures that transform people's ways of thinking, their habits, and their environments. Combating AIDS, for example, is a vast public education enterprise that requires changing people's habits. Intimate behavior, however, is steeped in culture, and each community has its own obstacles to overcome. To advise women infected with the HIV virus not to conceive is to challenge deeply held beliefs in cultures where children are prized; health education efforts must be shaped by cultures and communities. Such an educational under- taking, currently the only course for stemming transmission of the HIV virus, challenges the best of what we know about good teaching. There are other examples: washing hands after defecating, adequate nutrition, exercise, breast self-examinations, and reducing consumption of alcohol, cigarettes, and animal fat. Learning and living and health are closely bound.

WHY FOCUS ON URBAN POOR CHILDREN?

Most of us live longer and healthier lives as a result of advances in tech- nology, medical knowledge, and greater understandings of personal actions that promote better health. Improvements in the health and longevity of most Americans, however, cannot mask abysmal differences—greater suffer- ing and shorter life spans—in the health status of some groups. Among the poor, disparities in health status extend to every life-cycle phase, every racial and ethnic group, and every corner of the nation (see Schensul and Guest, chapter 3, this volume). Each racial, ethnic, and age group experiences the tragedy of pain, pathology, and "early" deaths that are preventable, treatable, or curable. Quality health care remains a public good that is largely una- vailable to impoverished segments of this wealthy nation. Quality medical care is unavailable to many in the middle class and working poor. However, my focus is on the children of the urban poor.

I choose this group for several reasons. First, I choose children because they have no voice as to which families they are born into; they do not choose their parents. They share a dependence on the adults of society to fulfill their needs. While some families are able to muster vast and varied resources, children of many other families are left shortchanged. They are more vulnerable in the face of homelessness, hunger, and hurt. Although conditions may be worse for children of poor farmers, migrant workers, and Native Americans in particular, the status of poor children residing in central cities is my focus. I also choose this group because it is widely assumed that city kids have access to care. I draw the reader's attention to conditions for urban poor children in order to examine what does not happen for these children even when medical care is close by. While a major theme is the relationship of poverty and health status, the salience of race and racism demands closer attention to urban poor children who also are children of color.

THE GORDIAN KNOT: POVERTY AND HEALTH

Health status differences between poor and nonpoor, whites and people of color—adults and children alike—can be linked to differences in available services, the nature and quality of those services, and the ways people are helped to make use of them. Family income often distinguishes good experiences from bad. The National Research Council (Jaynes and Williams 1989), reporting on the health status of African Americans, reminds us of the marriage between family income and family well-being: "Who will live and who will die and how much handicap and disability will burden their lives depend in large part on conditions of education, environment, and employment as well as on access to adequate medical services. Health is not only an important 'good' in itself, but it is also a determinant of life options during the entire life span" (p. 393).

Causal relationships remain a mire. Yet, the pernicious links between poverty and living conditions, health, and early death are real for millions of citizens. The poor are more likely to be sick, and the sick are more likely to be poor. The Gordian knot of poverty and health is not easily untangled.

The magnitude of poverty among children does not reflect a healthy nation. One of every five children in this country—13 million in all—is growing up poor; children of color are grossly overrepresented in this group (Children's Defense Fund 1991). While African-American and Latino children comprise about one-quarter of the 0- to 17-year-old population, they account for more than half of the children in poverty (Pallas et al. 1989). Forty-eight percent of African-American and 42% of Latino children under the age of 6 were poor in 1987, in sharp contrast to 13% of young white children who were poor (National Center for Children in Poverty 1990). That younger children (those under the age of 6) are more likely to be poor than older children (those aged 6 to 17), especially among children of color, does not bode well for stemming these socioeconomic trends any time soon.

Poor children are trapped in the crossfire of poverty and ill health. They will know more pain, suffering, needless disability, and early death than their financially secure peers. Data from the Children's Defense Fund (1991) underscore this relationship: poor 5 to 17 year olds are almost half as likely to be in excellent health as children in more affluent families; poor children are twice as likely as affluent children to have physical or mental disabilities or other chronic health conditions that impair daily activity.[1] L. V. Klerman's study of health programs and policies for poor young children reports the all-too-familiar:

Poor children are more likely than nonpoor children to be born too soon or too small; to die in the first year of life or during early childhood; to experience acute illnesses, injuries, lead poisoning, or child abuse or neglect; and to suffer from nutrition-related problems and chronic illnesses, and handicapping conditions. . . . Certainly a large part of the problem is economic. (Klerman 1991, p. 3)

Her detailed portrait of poor children's health problems—whether present at birth or acquired later on—leads to one disturbing verdict: one's chances of being healthy increase with one's income.

The United States leads the world in health care spending, but the return on this investment underscores the gross inequities in who gets care, what kind of care, and when (Bowsher 1991). Abundance and scarcity exist side by side. Those able to pay can purchase the best medical care in the world from U.S. practitioners, making use of high-tech procedures honed by heavy investments in medical research. Hours-long operations are performed by teams of specialists, while a few floors below low-income patients spend hours awaiting attention in drab emergency rooms. Medicine has triumphed over most childhood diseases, but the growing number of poor U.S. preschoolers without immunizations threatens the return of these same terrible diseases (Hodgkinson 1990).

Those same inequalities color the education system. Some schools are just as poor as the students they serve. They receive less money per pupil, pay lower salaries, and suffer the consequences of rapid staff turnover. They have fewer instructional resources and try to manage in downright unpleasant work environments—leaking roofs, backed-up toilets, and textbook shortages. To the scandal of the profession, beginning teachers are assigned to children most in need of the best teachers (Beckum et al. 1987; Young et al. 1990). Such gross disparities convey powerful messages to everybody about who is valued.

SOCIETY'S RESPONSIBILITY IN CARING FOR POOR CHILDREN

What is society's responsibility to children whose own families are financially or otherwise unable to provide the full complement of services necessary to sustain their healthy development? More than seventy-five years ago, philosopher and educator John Dewey addressed this question in relation to parents and their children's schooling. He challenged the broader community to enlarge its interests in the nation's children:

That which interests us most is naturally the progress made by the individual child of our acquaintance. . . . [I]t is from such standards as these that we judge the work of the school. And rightly so. Yet the range of the outlook needs to be enlarged. What the best and wisest parent wants for his own child, that must the community want for all of its children. (Dewey 1915, p. 7)

Dewey's call to move beyond self-interest to embrace the children of strangers has deep meaning for us today. Current interest in poor children has been sparked by three concerns: the need for a high-quality labor pool, cost containment of public dollars, and social justice.

Hope for the nation's future is tempered by fears that conditions left untreated in childhood will later take their toll. By prolonging life, reducing disability and morbidity, and alleviating pain, those born with little will be able to compete equally in the marketplace. A world-class labor force, reduced economic dependency, and future strength of the national economy are strapped to early investments in children. Our collective futures rest on the healthy development of every child.

This same alarm saturates calls for education reform. Good teaching and learning can no longer be rationed to a few. Despite little past evidence of doing so, public schools are challenged to negate inequalities in wealth by providing all a chance to achieve commensurate with their abilities, thereby supplying the country with a world-class workforce. The nation's future well-being hinges on quality education of all its children.

There is also concern about the longer term financial costs in delaying services to children. Physical and mental suffering that could have been prevented by cheaper, earlier interventions—prenatal checkups and nutrition programs in early childhood, for example—will haunt society later with even greater education, medical, welfare, and correctional costs. Two examples show the scope of these savings. One dollar invested in the prenatal component of the Special Supplemental Food Program for Women, Infants, and Children (WIC)—where program participants have higher birthweight babies with lower incidences of handicapping conditions—saves as much as $3 in short-term hospital costs (Select Committee on Children 1990). One dollar spent on the childhood immunization program saves $10 later in medical costs (Children's Defense Fund 1991). The possibilities for similar savings occur in education. One dollar invested in quality preschool education returns $6 because of lower costs of special education, public assistance, and correctional facilities (Committee for Economic Development 1987). Early investments in health care and education for poor children offset much greater expenses later on. This is "pay-now or pay-more-later" pragmatism.

Apart from cost-benefit analyses, issues of social justice must be considered. No one should die for lack of financial resources to obtain adequate medical care; no one should suffer pain, premature death, or loss of functioning for lack of health care available to the more affluent (President's Commission for the Study of Ethical Problems in Medicine and Biomedical and Behavioral Research 1983). That is the view of those who see human dignity as the root value underlying an equitable social system. Ethical arguments for decency, charity, empathy, compassion, and justice are persistent themes in Western thought and rhetoric. Immanuel Kant's sense of "duty" (Kant 1963), John Rawls's "distributive justice" (Rawls 1971), and Nell Noddings's "natural caring" (Noddings 1988) are examples that compel caring, beneficence, and duty in terms of what citizens, individually and collectively, are willing to do for strangers. All three themes—economic, financial, and moral—oblige public interest in investing in poor children's health and educational welfare.

BARRIERS TO ACCESS

The United States and the Republic of South Africa remain the only major industrialized nations lacking universal entitlement to basic medical care (Waitzkin 1991). In a wealthy country such as ours, entitlement to health care ought to extend to all children. Yet many never see a physician; they are locked out of the health care system by an inability to pay. The "safety net" intended by Medicaid fails millions; complex eligibility requirements leave many poor families among the estimated 37 million uninsured (Children's Defense Fund 1990). Millions more are underinsured. Children are major victims: they and young adults ages 18 to 24 made up 50% of the uninsured population in 1987. Among those younger than 18, an estimated 9 to 12 million are uninsured (Children's Defense Fund 1990). The mean irony is that those most in need tend to get the worst and the least (Schorr 1988).

Lack of insurance means receiving less care, less timely care, and lower quality care than that received by the insured (Bowsher 1991). Uninsured individuals have less frequent visits to physicians each year, are less likely to have a hospital stay, and, if hospitalized, tend to have a shorter stay than insured individuals. Of particular note is an in-hospital mortality rate 1.2 to 3.2 times higher among uninsured than insured patients with certain demographic characteristics (Hadley et al. 1991).

For those who have neither the income, savings, nor private insurance, regular visits to a physician are a fantasy. And yet, access to quality medical care will not be accomplished by increased funding alone. Barriers extend well beyond dollars. A major factor is the mismatch between where doctors practice and where most children live. In New York City, for example, by 1980 the ratio of physicians to population within the boundaries of East and Central Harlem was one physician per 15,000 residents. Individuals in these medically underserved areas were thirty-six times more underserved than individuals residing in New York City as a whole (Governor's Advisory Committee for Black Affairs 1987).

More than 20 million Americans who live in areas considered medically underserved by the U.S. Public Health Service are women of child-bearing age and children (Children's Defense Fund 1991). It is not unusual for the few doctors left in these medically underserved neighborhoods to refuse poor patients because they are uninsured or because of relatively low Medicaid reimbursement fees, in some cases as low as 40% of prevailing private insurance rates (Buchanan 1988). They also fear bad risks. Health problems are greatly exacerbated by undesirable socioeconomic conditions and require services far in excess of those needed by the greater community. Private insurance companies are reluctant to write comprehensive health insurance policies for the poor because they fear similar bad risks. Often there is a greater outpouring of resources compared to what they collect. The few policies that are written limit benefits and require premiums far in excess of family income (Davis and Schoen 1978).

Public policy has failed to develop the incentives necessary to redistribute health care resources more equitably among "people so close geographically and yet so distant in terms of their environmental conditions" (Rushmer 1976, p. 89). A case in point is prenatal care. The limited availability of maternity care providers and meager prenatal services makes insufficient the kinds of care often needed most (Schorr 1988). The need for early and continuous prenatal care, especially for young, poor mothers-to-be, is well documented: routine prenatal care beginning in the first three months of pregnancy remains the most effective strategy to stem low birthweight and to improve infant health. Low-birthweight babies (those weighing under 5.5 pounds) are twenty times more likely to die and forty times more likely to be disabled than other infants, owing to complications associated with low birthweight and no prenatal care. Still, in 1987, 13% of teen mothers received late or no prenatal care at all, accounting in large part for the poorer health of infants born to teen mothers in comparison to those born to adult women. One in four pregnant women (almost 900,000) in 1987 received no prenatal care during the critical first three months (Children's Defense Fund 1990, 1991).

Poor pregnant teenagers, however, typically do not reside in communities with wide access to gynecologists and obstetricians; the few who are there tend not to accept Medicaid clients for the reasons cited above. For teens who persevere, travel to the local health department is the next step, where long lists for appointments delay services. Mounds of forms and paperwork further confuse and frustrate these adolescents, who have learned neither to manage the "system" nor to be their own advocate. Expense, distance, inconvenient hours, long waits, and the prospect of unfriendly treatment construct a formidable barrier. Facing this bewildering and unpleasant set of circumstances, many abandon their original quest for prenatal care.

A recent incident involving a young woman highlights the discrepancy between good intentions and good deeds. Tamika (not her real name) is 17 years old, African American, unmarried, and one year from completing her high school diploma. On discovering that she was pregnant, she tried to do all the right things. She began early prenatal care and continued seeing her physician regularly throughout her pregnancy; she tried to improve her diet and take her vitamins. She participated in a parent education program geared for new young mothers. She was and continued to be drug-clean; she did not sleep around. Tamika enjoyed the support of a concerned and involved teacher and a community mentor. Tamika is insured on her father's medical policy, even though she hasn't lived with him for eleven years.

The weekend of her son's birth, Tamika and her mother traveled ninety miles to a large metropolitan area to visit family and friends. Late Saturday night Tamika's contractions began. At midnight, her aunt took her to the nearest medical facility, a private hospital, which brusquely refused to see this African-American pregnant young woman because she did not have proof of medical insurance. Tamika's insurance card was with her mother, who had not yet returned from visiting friends. Tamika was sent to the public hospital. They, too, sent her home.

Tamika's contractions became stronger and more frequent, so she returned to the public hospital about 3:00 A.M., They still refused to admit her. At 5:30 A.M., she returned once again and was reluctantly admitted. Johnelle was born thirty minutes later, weighing 7 pounds and 2 ounces. Not having time for an episiotomy, Tamika experienced considerable tearing. The whole experience left her frightened, confused, and upset. Had she the money or an insurance card, it is highly likely that her experience would have been different. This level-headed young woman was turned away because she was perceived as poor and uninsured.

Many of her peers will not share Tamika's fortunes—a community support group and a thriving infant. They might not have undertaken the precautions Tamika sought to nurture her baby's healthy beginnings. They, too, however, will be turned away by hospital gatekeepers. But without the personal and community resources that sustained Tamika, they might not fully understand their entitlement to care.

THE "CULT OF EFFICIENCY" AND QUALITY OF CARE

Many reformers argue that better quality health care and schooling for the poor and others will result from greater efficiency of current health and education systems. An industrializing capitalist society brought large numbers of people into urban centers, concentrated people and machines in large workplaces, and portrayed specialization and technical competence as its ideals (Starr 1982). School systems came to share a similar vision: they evolved from consolidating small schools and districts to large, centralized bureaucracies. Starr describes similar developments in the organization of medical care. He suggests that, with the increased internal organization of hospitals, the division of medical labor was intensified according to current conceptions of efficiency and rational organization. Although not exact matches—largely because hospitals and schools also have professional lines of authority sometimes distinct from administrative lines of authority—the organization of hospital-based care and school systems increasingly came to resemble modern versions of the old factory. Schools today faithfully mirror the early-twentieth-century search for one best system that could apply to all teachers and children, and the lock-step bureaucracy that ensued. The rise of a corporate ethos has also affected medical care (Krause 1977; Starr 1982).

Work in organizations such as education and medicine is framed by several common themes of practice: efficiency, rationality, continuity, precision, and impartiality (Bidwell 1965; Tyack 1974). An end product is splintered into different tasks and gradations of similar tasks, ostensibly simplifying the operations of each worker and improving efficiency. Specialization across and within occupations, and in knowledge and skill, develops around new technologies. "Objective" standards and bureaucratic norms based on adaptation and conformity define each role. Students and patients—the "raw products"—are measured, sorted, treated, and measured again for judging the value added before moving to the next step. The range in what is taught and treated is increasingly narrowed to what is measured; what is measured is increasingly limited to what is easily measurable. Regulation of uniform procedures is intended to ensure standard, quality parts.

A hierarchical organization with careful allocation of authority and functions keeps all the parts running efficiently. At the head of the system is the mind and power, a small, elite group who control the work. Those at the top have the power to diagnose, prescribe, envelop new knowledge and information, and to take initiative (Krause 1977; Tyack 1974). Others must follow their lead. Workers have little ownership or control over what they do; authorities must legitimate their work. Teachers and nurses, for example, are the individuals closest to students and patients but have the least formal authority to make final recommendations, compared with physicians, administrators, and board members (Mumford 1983; Starr 1982).

The system is portrayed as efficient and impartial; it is not. The tracking system in education and medicine controls who gets access. Racial, social class, and gender distinctions of the wider society are reflected in the divisions of labor in education and health work. Sifting and sorting block the advancement of some demographic groups. Untrained and unskilled people of color and women fill most of the lower rungs of the health care hierarchy, while middle-class white males have better chances for careers at the "top" (Krause 1977; Oakes 1985). Practices that further this end cross institutional boundaries. Young black women interested in nursing, for example, are counseled to pursue careers in practical nursing while their white counter-parts are steered toward RN degrees in college programs (Krause 1977).

Profound differences in curriculum, pedagogy, expectations, control, re-sources, and what counts as knowledge perpetuate rifts in learning along racial and social class lines (Anyon 1981; Goodlad 1984; Young and Melnick 1988). Disproportionate numbers of African-American, Latino, and Native American students are sorted and assigned to lower ability groups and to watered-down subject matter. Curricular tracking, courses available, quality of teaching, and courses students are counseled to take open and close future opportunities. Schools in poor communities typically do not enjoy the same financial, physical, or human support available to schools serving more af-fluent areas (Kozol 1991).

Other barriers to quality care persist. The extensive bureaucracy of most hospital-based care and most schooling reduces access to quality services and limits the organizations' responsiveness to children's needs. I focus on hos-pital-based care for two reasons. On the one hand, it has come to represent medical care in its most technically sophisticated form (Starr 1982). On the other hand, the hospital emergency room has become the family doctor for the sick, inner-city poor. In addition to being an expensive form of care, emergency room care is neither designed for nor adapted to preventive and comprehensive services. Rather, emergency room care is focused on acute problems of the most severely ill and injured. Those with less obvious or less urgent symptoms are turned away, delaying diagnoses and treatments of conditions that might otherwise be stemmed.

In other parts of the health system, children with multiple problems must make their way through a labyrinth of services. Because hospital-based care defines problems in the short term and single aspects of individual condi-tions, care typically is acute, episodic, and fragmented. Teams of specialists have replaced the general practitioner; the same is true in education with the replacement of the all-purpose school marm. Doctors often don't know what other doctors are doing to the same patient. Teachers are ill informed about the work of their students with Chapter I[2] and special education teach-ers. Children receive duplicative services for overlapping problems; little or no attention is paid to other difficulties (Bullough and Bullough 1982). In 1971 then HEW Secretary Elliot Richardson commented on the overlapping and duplicative nature of several HEW programs: " . . . more than 85 per-cent of all HEW clients have multiple problems, . . . single services provided independently of one another are unlikely to result in changes in client's dependency status, and . . . chances are less than 1 in 5 that a client referred from one service to another will ever get there, the present maze encourages fragmentation" (Richardson 1973, p. 19). These bureaucracies may satisfy professional and administrative requirements, but they do not consider the obstacles faced by many disfranchised poor (Schorr 1988). The poor seem to fare worst in negotiating the system to get the help they need. Ronald Corwin and Roy Edelfelt describe the losers in the current structure: "Low-income people, in particular, often have difficulty with large service organizations. They generally lack knowledge about how to manipulate bureaucratic rules and procedures to their advantage" (Corwin and Edelfelt 1976, p. 36).

To provide optimal preventive care, children must be seen early and frequently. Early screening and preventive medicine work; inoculations against polio, measles, and other childhood diseases matter as do reducing cigarette smoking and wearing condoms. Preventive interventions in education work, too. High-quality preschool education, for example, returns high social outcomes in terms of greater student self-esteem and rates of high school graduation, and reduced rates of teenage pregnancy and welfare dependency.

In emergency room care, however, there are no yesterdays or tomorrows. Few permanent records are kept; charts and histories are incomplete, misplaced, lost. Physicians see children they have never seen before and never expect to see again; they don't know the child or the family medical history. Even when there is a chart, little time is spent studying the child's past history and current social context to explore preventive strategies with the child and the family. There are few opportunities for continuity of care. In such settings, preventive and comprehensive prenatal and pediatric services are difficult and rare.

The pattern is not unlike the massive transitions of children in and out of urban schools where the vast majority of students who enter in September are gone by June. Others take their seats—a human river flowing in and out of schools in the cities. The most mobile are the poor. Like many on the move, they experience the anonymity, alienation, and aloneness of losing community membership. School records are slow to follow, if they ever arrive. Administrators and teachers have little background information on which to base placement and instructional decisions. Under such conditions, there are few opportunities to attend to the long-term well-being of these children.

Disrespect and inferior treatment—or the perception of inferior treatment—diminish the power of learning and combine to discourage many from any type of health care until it is too late. Doctor–patient encounters become what Howard Waitzkin describes as "micropolitical situations," reflecting broader social relations, including social class and political-economic power (Waitzkin 1991). Studies of health care utilization by poor women highlight the link between help-seeking behavior and interactions with hospital staff. In one study of more than 2,100 Mexican-born women in San Diego, for example, it was found that these women often form negative attitudes that affect future health care-seeking behaviors, based on unpleasant interactions with hospital staff (Chavez et al. 1986). The belittling experiences make those most in need of care disinclined to seek services. A recent experience related by "Helen" suggests the nature of these encounters:

Helen—African American, female, elderly, unrich—was concerned when her eyes began to "feel tight—like it's swollen in there." She is 68 years old, lives on a fixed income, and travels thirty miles each way for health services at a clinic world renowned for its medical care. On describing this discomfort to an eye neurologist and after tests indicating high eye pressures, she was referred to the clinic's "glaucoma expert" who wasn't available until 6:00 p.m. After a half-hour wait, the expert entered, glanced quickly at her chart, and "put drops in my eyes and left." An hour later he returned with no apology or explanation for the wait. He discontinued her previously prescribed medication and suggested her eye pressures be retested in two or three months to assess the effect of no medication. Helen is afraid to discontinue the medication and is "distrustful of this doctor because he has no respect for me and he is not interested in my case. He billed me for a comprehensive eye examination but he didn't do anything for my eyes."

While the expert may have followed professional standards of "good practice," his personal manner eroded Helen's confidence in him. Helen is not a teenager like Tamika. She is an experienced, articulate adult. She helps us to understand what encounters with medical practitioners may be like for poor children of color who are not fully able to define and describe their experiences. She is not alone in her dissatisfaction. A 1986 survey found that "blacks were more likely than whites to report that their physician did not inquire sufficiently about their pain, did not tell them how long it would take for prescribed medicine to work, did not explain the seriousness of their illness or injury, and did not discuss test and examination findings" (AMA Council on Ethical and Judicial Affairs 1990, p. 2345).

Racism remains an organizing principle in U.S. society. In health care, it does not end with unpleasant personal encounters but creeps into treatment decisions. The medical literature reports that blacks are less likely than whites to receive certain surgical or other therapies for similar ailments, even after differences in income and severity of disease are taken into account (AMA Council on Ethical and Judicial Affairs 1990). Disparities based on race, income, education, socioculture, and failures by the medical profession are unjustifiable and, according to the American Medical Association's Council on Ethical and Judicial Affairs (1990), "violate fundamental principles of fairness, justice, and medical ethics" (p. 2346).

What school and health care people do is shaped by images of what constitutes learning and quality medical care. Unity, coherence, and efficiency achieved through standardization and homogeneity of pedagogy and curricula will not sponsor an information-age education for everybody's children. Market and technological arrangements in the name of efficiency and choice make complex, deep learning next to impossible. They deny certain children equitable schooling experiences and overlook the human element for most. They ignore the kind of learning experience we want for children and what it takes to promote that kind of learning: cognitive engagement within a social context.

That same relationship is necessary for quality health care. Children and youth share membership in broad networks of family and community. A young patient brings to a physician not only a physical problem but also a social context—relationships at school, in the family, and in the wider community (Waitzkin 1991). When professional practice focuses on narrow views of commitment and intention, it dismisses the importance of social context and limits the capacity to respond appropriately. A biomedical focus on pathology almost exclusively concerned with the treatment of disease ignores the obscure but powerful interconnections between "personal troubles" and "social issues" (Mills 1959). As educators and health care professionals attempt to respond to illiteracy and dropping out, addiction and abuse, AIDS, and other ravages of the human mind and body, the social context becomes even more crucial. From that vantage, most interventions are not far-reaching enough, hampered by public policies that are too limited in scope to adequately respond to the multiple and interwoven needs of poor children today.

VISIONS OF CARE BASED ON LEARNING COMMUNITY

Education and medicine based on learning community embrace the concept of empowerment. Practices in both systems are informed by principles, embedded in an institutional structure and ethos that address common flaws of both health and education. My premise is this: The best ways of helping people think and act differently are within communities of learning.

Powerful thinking for a purpose requires participation and dialogue, essential qualities of "community." Social science abounds with definitions of community—about 100 descriptions at last count (Getzels 1979). By community I mean something particular—a set of relationships and a way of learning. Learning is fundamentally a communal experience, emerging from a sense of relationship and connection. Learning communities do not emerge spontaneously; they are carefully crafted to develop the habits and skills that sponsor much more than intellectual growth alone—they shape the person. It has been argued that essential qualities of one's true self arise only in interactions in some community; without community there are no selves (Kateb 1965; Schwab 1976).

All learning is a matter of participation in a dialogue, real or imagined. It requires continual interchange and negotiation; ideas interact and unite to foster growth. Reforms based on learning community explore the needs of individual learners within the context of a community. Teachers who create learning communities are students of their own students. They develop among their pupils a deep sense of belonging, engagement, and responsibility, collaborating in each other's learning and understanding. Reforms built on learning community connect children to powerful ways of thinking critically, of developing their voices, of learning to care for others.

Learning community gives "academic" knowledge purpose and meaning. Teaching reading as a technical skill, for example, is a much different experience than reading presented in the context of a learning community. Powerful reading programs, as good teachers know, embody the thick texture and uses and purposes of language in a real community of inquiry and discourse. Teachers readily attest to students' capacity to "tune out" when lessons taught in school isolate learners from their peers and from the dilemmas, meanings, and experiences outside of school (Newmann and Oliver 1967).

Just as young people are not reading and writing when that experience has no meaning, the health care system, too, is floundering. Thwarting the scourges of hunger and malnourishment, lead poisoning, sexually transmitted diseases, and the waste of minds and talent requires drastic changes in approaches to health services, toward a scheme that envelops the social context in which people live. It means quite different visions of patient care— involving people in deeper and wider networks of community.

Sponsoring this type of teaching and learning in education and health demands flexible structures. Genuine learning communities require the time and scale that allow participants to know each other and to be known. Better schools and hospitals will come when better structures are built—creating nurturing conditions that foster "deeper ties" among participants, with "the aim of establishing more committed learning communities" (Powell et al. 1985). Rigid modes of allocating time preclude deep discussions with patients about managing their health. They discourage profound conversations with students; teachers must move on before kids "get it."

Good teaching, like good nursing, does not flow from meager notions of role and authority. There are sound arguments for supervision, but excessive regulation along hierarchical divisions limits opportunities by practitioners to exercise clinical judgment and discourages optimal patient care (Mumford 1983). Where hierarchies are steep and expertise narrowly defined, nurses' opinions are muted; they become flunkies in places of cracker-jack medicine. The disparity between what nurses and teachers know and what they are allowed to do has oppressive consequences: it protects the professional dominance of physicians and administrators over conditions of practice; it reinforces white male privilege; it undermines rich resources for patient and student care; it drives thoughtful practitioners from the professions; and it demoralizes too many of those who remain. Teachers and nurses need room to take full advantage of the experience, talents, and knowledge among them.

In settings run more like learning communities, everyone participates in the conversation.

Empowerment will not be fostered by greater efficiency of present structures that focus on the shortcomings rather than the strengths of clients, or that reinforce compliance and dependence on those who control the knowledge. In a learning community, each learner is affirmed as capable of making sense of her experiences and of sharing in the power and authority for knowing. Just as we want schools to help students participate actively in learning, patients must be encouraged to take personal responsibility and initiative, and must be helped with the means and understanding to manage their own health. Teaching for understanding is not an advanced goal for a select few, but the basic aim of education for all. Accomplishing this will require breaking with false assumptions about what people can know and how they can affect their own lives. It will require changing assumptions that physicians' special knowledge and training allow them to control and solve alone other people's problems, and that patients are more easily managed if they are kept passive and in the dark. Changing these assumptions will not be easy: "Many analysts, policy makers, and even practitioners diminish—or worse, completely disregard—the assets and resources in the cultures of the people we intend to serve" (p. 179). Patients are much more likely to play a meaningful and active role in their own well-being if they understand the goals toward which they are moving (Mechanic 1968). "Nonmedical" activities (patient education for personal health management, respect, and community advocacy for healthful habits) may be just as important as the "treatment" itself.

In today's technological world of medical competence, it is hard to remember that caring relationships are entwined with learning and healing. Practices that meld technical competence and interpersonal skill—"curing" and "caring"—are central to high-quality care (Banta 1981). Listening is an important component of caring, just as the reverse is the case: "Concern and caring are indeed important parts of listening: concern for the other's integrity and dignity as an individual, caring for his unique efforts to make meaning and to communicate that meaning" (Morimoto 1973, p. 252). Caring not only sees doctor–patient encounters as human encounters embodying trust, respect, and empathy—elements of learning community—but it also underscores the importance of truly "seeing" clients, a view made difficult by racial, cultural, and class insularity that isolates practitioners from the worlds of the lower class, migrant, and poor (Pinderhughes 1989; see also Ferguson, Chapter 11, in this volume).

Entering the world of the patient is made difficult by practitioners who are unaware that their own subjective biases and lack of communication skills interfere with understanding the client (Bullough and Bullough 1982). Problems in human communication suggest that these difficulties arise from blinders on our own hearing and seeing: we interpret what we hear and see in terms of our own experiences, beliefs, values, and attitudes (Otto 1969). When language, literacy, and culture are not shared, the meanings others intend and receive are easily and often misinterpreted. Misunderstandings are further compounded when facial expressions, "extraneous" information, and voice tone are misread. Practitioners who make the effort to understand verbal and nonverbal cues can and do learn. That effort must become part of the professional education for all future practitioners.

Increasing the number of people from varied racial, ethnic, and socioeconomic communities in medical and education school faculties and student bodies will enhance the process, although alone it is insufficient. In true communities of learning, participants in service delivery would resemble the United States' rainbow of nations and peoples. The declining proportion of African-American and other students of color in medical schools over the last seventeen years—after rapid gains between 1968 and 1974—cannot be explained away by trends in applications and MCAT scores. Both increased as acceptance rates and need-based financial aid fell (Shea and Fullilove 1985). Countering the prevailing monochrome of the nation's practitioners will require political and social will—that is, affirmative action in admissions and hiring decisions and renewed commitment to recruit, finance, and retain students.

What are the implications for a caring, communal system? What would it look like to create settings in which care and community flourish in health and education? Examples in education abound around the country (Comer 1980; Meier 1991). Communities of caring are also found in health delivery, and they are deliberately built. The King/Drew Medical Center in Los Angeles, serving predominantly African-American and Latino communities, is one example. The pediatrics department there acknowledges the importance of the social antecedents of disease and death, particularly among youngsters growing up in the inner city (Schorr 1988). The following pages show the integration of the biological and social factors in a resident's training.

One resident recalls prescribing a course of home-based physical therapy for a handicapped child. The community worker pointed out to him that this child's family consisted of ten people in a two-bedroom home and that the parents couldn't possibly carry out his elaborate program. The community worker insisted that the resident come out to the house with her. "It wasn't until that visit," the resident explained, "that I began to understand who these people really were, where they lived, what they really thought, what they were saying about the hospital and the physicians and the nurses. It was only then that I fully realized that we had to take a different approach to meeting this child's needs" (Schorr 1988, p. 108).

King/Drew shares several features common to promising interventions on behalf of poor children: they think expansively about services children require, they view the child in the context of family and community, and practitioners are redefining their roles to better respond to children's needs.

A neonatologist reflects on aspects of this philosophy at King/Drew: "Is the job done when I have saved them here? Is the child simply a biological organism? We think otherwise. We think of health as not just providing health services. We think that over the years we have to care about what happens to these kids" (Schorr 1988, p. 110).

Learning community in health systems is as important as learning community in schools. Good teaching based on empowering individuals in learning communities is central to both. Adopting an ethic of caring and community requires scrapping efficiency, market, and individual choice assumptions about schools and health care. The broader issue is assuring every child easy access to a continuing relationship with a medical practitioner, to comprehensive primary care by practitioners familiar with the child and her family, and to opportunities to have an informed say about one's life and the lives of one's children. The organization of schools and hospitals as learning communities in and of the wider community facilitates that possibility.

TOWARD A JUST SYSTEM

Empowering individuals includes empowering their communities. No medicine can make up for the cumulative effects of poor nutrition, environmental pollution, lead poisoning, and drafty-cold housing. If the purpose of health care is to enhance health, services must be reoriented to the health promotion of communities as well as to serving immediate individual needs. The erosion of the tax base in central cities; structural economic changes wiping out good-paying jobs; the crack epidemic; and lack of decent housing are just a few examples of social phenomena ripping away the social fabric in poor urban neighborhoods. That is where these poor children live. The social, physical, and biological environments in these communities further constrain options for healthful living and reduce individual choices about good health habits. As Sol Levine states:

As we become alarmed by the smoking behavior of women, teenagers, and members of minority groups, we should address the intensified advertising and sales efforts of tobacco companies to target these groups. As we bewail the nutritional deficits in the diets of the poor, we should attend to whether, in the first place, they are able to obtain the green vegetables, fish, and poultry we are recommending. (Levine 1991, p. 44)

The entwined needs of poor children and their families demand responses that cross traditional professional and bureaucratic boundaries. They demand institutions and public policies that are broadly responsive to today's life circumstances. The problems of poor children in inner cities are not packaged in neat, single-issue boxes; they transcend narrow definitions of professional roles, services, and client-eligibility criteria. The long-term consequences of their mothers' addiction are seen in the increasing number of "crack" babies entering elementary schools, and neither physicians nor educators know much about the dilemmas posed by *in utero* addiction. Who helps substance-abusing pregnant dropouts understand what they are doing to their unborn children? Juvenile delinquency and school failure often have their origins in early physical problems that later balloon into antisocial activity (Schorr 1988). How do young mothers learn about nutrition when they have no access to fresh food?

Medical care is only a small part of health maintenance. The healthy community, the healthy school, the healthy home, the healthy family, and the healthy child are all parts of one mosaic. Single-strategy policies such as "Just Say No" ignore compounding factors that have lasting detrimental effects on the healthy development of poor children. Harold Hodgkinson reminds us that health, education, the economy, criminal justice, and social welfare are "all one system" (Hodgkinson 1985). Long-term improvements in community wellness will only be obtained by attention to the interconnections among poor children's multiple needs—housing, food, health, safety, child development, education, jobs, environment. A fragmented view will only exacerbate feelings of powerlessness, depersonalization, and fragmentation (Newmann and Oliver 1967), and undermine well-intentioned efforts to improve poor children's development and health.

Community—interdependence, acquaintance, communication, shared beliefs, an ethic of caring, a common ethos—performs functions that are important both to the development of the individual and to social cohesion and stability (Raywid 1988; Tonnies 1963). Empowering a community mobilizes residents toward a common vision, a shared dream of what the community can become. It merges community strengths and resources—churches, temples, social welfare agencies, community centers, businesses, fraternal and sororal organizations, and the power of individuals working collectively—toward social and political support for community wellness. Conceptions of learning communities may be a vehicle for unleashing that potential.

Learning communities are essential, but alone they are insufficient. It would be a sick joke to attempt to make community a reality without also paying attention to the resources necessary to extend accessible and quality learning and health care experiences to every child. One cannot celebrate trust, respect, and volunteerism in schools that have leaking roofs, or immunize children in clinics that have no vaccine. Adequate funding is just as vital as reconceptualizing what constitutes good teaching and quality health care and which organizational arrangements foster those ends. Each is a critical piece if schools and hospitals are to become empowering places for everybody's children. That is the essence of a true learning community—a place where everybody counts.

NOTES

I would like to thank Annette Dula for suggesting that I write this chapter and for her critical support and comments on various drafts. In their own special ways, Susan L. Melnick and Jay Featherstone also contributed invaluable insights and encouragement throughout the development of this chapter.

1. These data are based on the 1988 National Health Interview Survey, which defined "affluent" families as those with an annual income of more than $35,000 (Children's Defense Fund, 1991).

2. Chapter I, so named because it is authorized by Chapter I of the Education Consolidation and Improvement Act of 1981, has as its purpose "to provide financial assistance to State and local educational agencies to meet the special needs of educationally deprived children" (Section 552, Education Consolidation and Improvement Act, 1981). Chapter I programs provide compensatory educational services to children of low-income families.

Commentary by Joseph Featherstone

Lauren Young's analysis of some of the parallels between education and medicine as institutions is right on the mark. It may also be very timely as the country tries to move forward in real reform of both realms. It seems to me that she is inviting us to look at the ways in which classrooms and hospital services and wards sometimes become places where people participate in learning and healing, and that this participation is the heart of the matter, as is that much-abused word *community*. In schools and hospitals as well as clinics, two models of professionalism and science are contending for dominance. One model is a technical model in which practice consists of applying outside expertise to people. The other model looks more like dialogue or the creation of community. It says that healing and learning are the joint creation of people and the professionals trying to serve them. Both models have implications for how institutions define science. In one model, knowledge is primarily the creation of a research establishment. In the other, knowledge may draw on research, but in some fundamental sense knowledge as practice is local, grassroots, and site-based—above all, a joint creation of the people and the professionals. Each of these approaches has a very different agenda for reform and policy. Community models for health and education would look inward to the nurturing of places for conversations and sharing, and outward to the ways institutions could work with the aspirations of the communities they are serving.

In both fields, growing numbers of critics and practitioners are trying to move us away from the model of technical expertise (while still honoring research and inquiry) and to make hospital wards and school classrooms communities. Like *democracy* the word *community* will have to be dipped in acid to wash away sentimental and misleading encrustations, but it points us in medicine and education in some good directions for both research and practice. I would like to see something parallel in medicine to the Holmes Group report, *Tomorrow's Schools*.[1] In both medicine and education, the invocation of community and participation also points to the inescapably political and moral dimensions of the work, and that too is a good thing. Sooner or later we will start learning the wisdom of something Myles Horton[2] once said to me: "It's a hard truth, harder than the Golden Rule: The people that have the problem have the solution."

NOTES

1. Holmes Group, *Tomorrow's Schools: Principles for the Design of Professional Development Schools* (East Lansing, Mich.: Holmes Group, 1990).

2. Myles Horton, educator and civil rights activist, founded the Highlander Folk School in the 1930s and was its director for many years. One of the few places in the South where whites and blacks could meet under the same roof, Highlander at one time was the principal gathering place of the moving forces of the black revolution. Among those who came were Martin Luther King, Jr., Rosa Parks, Andrew Young, Julian Bond, Stokely Carmichael, and many others. (See Myles Horton with Judith Kohl and Herbert Kohl, *The Long Haul: An Autobiography* [New York: Doubleday, 1990].)

Epilogue

Leonard Harris

This anthology raises several questions of global significance—questions, I believe, that demand careful consideration: In a racist world, how can health care providers learn to respect the integrity of the individual and accord to each person honorable status as a member of the moral community of humanity? If various ethnic groups use health facilities in different ways, what is required to offer the best care? Along these lines, what differences in health care delivery are needed and could be implemented without seriously fragmenting health care? And finally, how can we avoid shuffling individuals between the public and private spheres of health care services?

Scientific racism, namely, the belief that races exist as fixed biological kinds that can be ranked as inferior or superior, has been defeated. However, it has been replaced by a symbolic racism in which deference is paid to "social merit," which translates nonetheless into racial exclusion. This shift from crude, overt forms of exclusion to sinister, covert forms is addressed by the authors, particularly in regard to its impact on health care: In what ways, and to what degree, are health care institutions responsible for ending preventable disease? Can the health care system reforms recommended by various contributors to this volume be implemented in a health care system that too often places profit over the care of indigent patients? What changes must occur in the relationship between marginalized populations and health care institutions? How are alienation, exclusion, sexism, and racism unintentionally promoted by health care providers? How should we conceive of patient consent and the patient–physician relationship, particularly when patients are under duress? The chapters in this volume explore the many effects of institutionalized racism on the health status and health care access of African Americans and address the questions that I have raised.

Several authors focus on African-American disenfranchisement from and distrust of the health care system. We normally feel helpless when we cannot provide adequate health care for our loved ones, and dishonored when we must humiliate ourselves in the pursuit of adequate health care. Although the World Medical Association notes that "a physician must recognize responsibility not only to patients (as individuals), but also to society," racial and ethnic oppression nevertheless constructs hierarchies of those who are deemed more or less worthy. In other words, "society" does not exist as a unified body. Our sense of self-worth is challenged when we cannot discern whether our health care provider perceives us as a person worthy of membership in the moral community. Although death is a specter that haunts all life, the possibility of an untimely and painful death haunts the oppressed unduly because the oppressed are always confronted with the possibility of being treated as inferior and receiving less than adequate care. Is it any wonder, then, as several of the authors suggest, that those disenfranchised from the health care system question the existence of systemic genocide in a racist world?

This anthology directly confronts the problems facing black people in particular and the oppressed in general, especially as African Americans and other oppressed peoples are demanding and taking full membership in the community of humanity, forcing a negation of stereotypes and a rethinking of the culture of modern civility. One of the groundbreaking features of this volume is that it requires the reader to consider respect and honor not simply as fundamental elements of the relationship between patient and physician, but as crucial values in the relationship between institutions and society, between the public and the private, and between the excluded and the privileged. African-American voices addressing issues of trust and respect in health care provide insights into ways in which society in general can improve its relationship with disenfranchised peoples.

Formulating new ideas often requires crossing disciplinary boundaries. The insights presented in this volume would not have been possible had the authors been confined to the intellectual strategies of morally bankrupt professional philosophy, the moral sensibilities of technocratic health care workers, or the decision theory formulas of medical ethicists looking for moral algorithms. Describing the experiences of those traditionally neglected by the world of letters requires words, expressions, and procedures that are not the property of segregated disciplines. The chapters in this book do not provide an algorithm that can be neatly applied to all possible problems. They do provide an understanding of the barriers that African Americans face in the health care system—barriers that may be cultural, economic, or attitudinal. The diverse disciplines represented here offer different perspectives on how these barriers negatively affect health status and create gross health disparities between blacks and whites.

The daunting realities presented here could be trivialized by focusing on the illusive notion of an "African-American perspective" as if it were an essence, essential quality, inborn racial trait, or an elixir made of racial poverty experiences that always produce an invariant conceptual scheme. This view fails to appreciate the book's moral force, acknowledge its distinctions, take seriously its suggestions, or ponder the debates—debates engaged in by persons of various backgrounds entering into and participating in the realities uncovered by African-American perspectives. A symphony of miseries affecting African Americans does not admit to a singular experience; rather, it offers an array of experiences. That array cannot be reduced to the life activities of one individual, nor can the life experiences of one individual constitute the basis for an account of all African Americans. Many voices are required to capture the range of African-American cultural experiences; many stories must be told; many voices make the choir. This volume brings together the voices of educators, social workers, philosophers, medical ethicists, medical students, and health care providers. All approach the same problem—the ethics of access—but each from a different angle. Each angle alone provides only a small part of the picture, but when we put them together, we see a bigger picture of shared experiences. Thus, as Bernard Boxill's *Blacks and Social Justice* painstakingly argues, there are morally compelling claims that all African Americans share, although not all have suffered the same miseries. Our sufferings, as a historical and contemporary cultural group, warrant collective entitlement, responses, and recognition.

Yet why should the health care profession acquiesce to the needs of various ethnic groups? The answer is clear: we are all members of the human community, regardless of our different ethnic identities. We all must share responsibility for preventing patterns of abuse that result from institutionalized racism. As this volume has shown, these patterns of racism and abuse are still common in health care institutions. Although these institutions may acknowledge and deal with specific individual cases of abuse such as consent violation, they must also recognize the more deeply engrained systemic abuse and racism. We do not need agreement on an appropriate conception of the distribution of health care to insist that institutions have a responsibility to combat these patterns of abuse. Even if the ideal for humanity is inherently contested, striving for bonds of mutual responsibility between individuals and groups is far more appealing than believing in an inherently fragmented, completely irreverent, and strictly disjointed conception of humankind.

It may take incurable romantics to invigorate interest in healing the wounds of racism. Engaging in dialogue in hopes of eliminating institutionalized racism and racial disparities in health status and health care access may be based on the romantic assumption that humanity is capable of improvement. It may take a belief in the power of moral suasion to prick the consciousness of technocrats and alienated, racist, and hedonistic egotists. The romanticism of *The American Evasion of Philosophy* by Cornel West,[1] which calls for "reinvigoration of a sane, sober, and sophisticated intellectual life in America and for regeneration of social forces empowering the disadvantaged, degraded, and dejected," may face a world of cynics and conservatives. Nonetheless, the *Faces at the Bottom of the Well* by Derrick Bell[2] are also the faces that rely on the success of incurable romantics.

It Just Ain't Fair appeals to an ethics of care enlivened by the African-American tradition of resistance against humiliation, degradation, and exclusion. It brings to the center of debate the moral force for preventing maltreatment, as well as a discussion of whether equity or need should be used to make moral judgments. It calls into question the use and misuse of medical technology, and whether and in what form ethnicity should be considered in the arrangement of health care resources. For too long concerns over patient consent, distribution and rationing of health care, and the patient–physician relationship have been subordinated to an array of humiliating treatments of individuals and groups. *It Just Ain't Fair* is a clarion call in an otherwise silent arena of discourse—calling on behalf of the voices that have been unjustly silenced.

Let us continue the struggle, loudly.

NOTES

1. Cornel West, *The American Evasion of Philosophy* (Madison, WI: University of Wisconsin Press, 1989).

2. Derrick Bell, *Faces at the Bottom of the Well* (New York: Basic Books, 1992). Also see Patricia Hill Collins, *Black Feminist Thought* (Boston: Unwin Hyman, 1992).

Bibliography

Abdul-Quades, A. S., S. R. Friedman, M. DesJarlais, M. M. Meslansky, and R. Barteleme. "Methadone Maintenance and Behavior by Intravenous Drug Users That Can Transmit AIDS." *Contemporary Drug Problems* 3 (1987):425–434.

Abramson, J. H., and S. L. Kark. "Community Oriented Primary Health Care: Meaning and Scope." In *Community Oriented Primary Care: New Directions for Health Services Delivery*, ed. E. Connor and F. Mullan, 21–59. Washington, D.C.: National Academy Press, 1983.

Achenbaum, W. A. "Historical Perspectives in Public Policy and Aging." *Generations*, Spring 1988, 27.

Aday, L. A., G. V. Fleming, and R. M. Anderson. *Access to Medical Care in the U.S.: Who Has It, Who Doesn't?* Chicago: Pluribus Press, 1984.

Ahmed, P. I., A. Kolker, and G. V. Coelho. "Toward a New Definition of Health: An Overview." In *Toward a New Definition of Health*, ed. G. V. Coelho and P. I. Ahmed, 7–22. New York: Plenum Press, 1979.

Alexander, G. R., M. E. Tomkins, J. M. Altekruse, and C. A. Hornung. "Racial Differences in the Relation of Birth Weight and Gestational Age to Neonatal Mortality." *Public Health Reports* (1985):539–547.

Alinsky, S. *Reveille for Radicals*. New York: Random House, 1969.

Allen, A. "Privacy, Surrogacy, and the Baby M Case." *Georgetown Law Journal* 76 (1988):1759.

———. "Surrogacy, Slavery, and the Ownership of Life." *Harvard Journal of Law and Public Policy* 13 (1990):139.

———. "The Black Surrogate Mother." *Harvard Blackletter Journal* 8 (1991):17.

Allen, J. R., and E. P. Setlow. "Heterosexual Transmission of HIV: A View of the Future." *Journal of the American Medical Association* 266 (1991):1695–1696.

Allen, L. "Otitis Media Among Puerto Ricans and Blacks: Ethnicity, Epidemiology and Family Health Cultures." Ph.D. Diss., University of Connecticut, 1988.

Alperstein, G., C. Rappaport, and J. M. Flanagan. "Health Problems of Homeless Children in New York City." *American Journal of Public Health* 78 (1988): 1232–1233.

Alter, M. J., S. C. Hadler, H. S. Margolis, W. J. Alexander, P. Y. Hu, F. N. Judson, A. Mares, J. K. Miller, and L. A. Moyer. "The Changing Epidemiology of

Hepatitis B in the United States: Need for Alternative Vaccination Strategies." *Journal of the American Medical Association* 263 (1990):1218–1222.

AMA Council on Ethical and Judicial Affairs. "Black-White Disparities in Health Care." *Journal of the American Medical Association* 263, no. 17 (1990):2344–2346.

American College Health Association. "Position Statement on Immunization Policy." *Journal of American College Health* 32 (1983):7–8.

American College of Physicians. "Access to Health Care." *Health* 78 (1988):1539–1545.

————. "Access to Health Care." *Annals of Internal Medicine* 112 (1990): 641–661.

American Public Health Association. *Illicit Drug Use and HIV Infection.* Report of the Special Initiative on AIDS of the American Public Health Association, 2nd ed., 1990.

————. *Women and HIV Disease.* Report of the Special Initiative on AIDS of the American Public Health Association, 1991.

Anastos, K., and C. Marte. "Women—The Missing Persons in the AIDS Epidemic." *Health/PAC Bulletin* 19, no. 4 (1989):6–13.

Anastos, K., and C. Marte. "Women—The Missing Persons in the AIDS Epidemic, Part II." *Health/PAC Bulletin* 20, no. 1 (1990):11–18.

Anderson, R. M., A. L. Giachello, and L. A. Aday. "Access of Hispanics to Health Care and Cuts in Services: A State of the Art Overview." *Public Health Reports* 101, no. 3 (May–June 1986):238–252.

Anderson, R. M., R. M. Mullner, and L. J. Cornelius. "Black-White Differences in Health Status: Methods or Substance." *Milbank Quarterly* 65 (Supplement 1) (1987):72–99.

Andrulis, D. "Patients with AIDS and Other HIV Infections: Examining and Estimating the Total Burden of Hospital Care." In *VII International Conference on AIDS in Florence, Italy, June, 1991,* abstract M.D. 113, 1991.

Andrulis, D. P., V. S. Beers, J. D. Bentley, and L. S. Gage. "The Provision and Financing of Medical Care for AIDS Patients in U.S. Public and Private Teaching Hospitals." *Journal of the American Medical Association* 258 (1987): 1343–1346.

Andrulis, D. P., V. B. Weslowski, and L. S. Gage. "The 1987 U.S. Hospital AIDS Survey." *Journal of the American Medical Association* 262 (1989):784–794.

Anyon, J. "Social Class and School Knowledge." *Curriculum Inquiry* 11 (1981):2–42.

Aptheker, H. "Sterilization, Experimentation and Imperialism." *Political Affairs* 53 (1974):37–48.

Arno, P. S., D. Shenson, N. F. Siegel, P. Franks, and P. R. Lee. "Economic and Policy Implications of Early Intervention in HIV Disease." *Journal of the American Medical Association* 262 (1989):1493–1498.

Ayers, W. "Thinking About Teachers and the Curriculum." *Harvard Educational Review* 56 (1986):49–51.

Baca-Zinn, M. "Family, Feminism, and Race in America." *Gender and Society* 4 (1990): 68–82.

Baldicci, L. "One Missing Check—And Her Family Is Homeless." *Chicago Sun Times,* November 21, 1990, 3.

Banner, W. A. "Is There an African-American Perspective on Biomedical Ethics? The View from Philosophy." In *African-American Perspectives on Biomedical*

Ethics, ed. H. E. Flack and E. D. Pellegrino, 188–191. Washington, D.C.: Georgetown University Press, 1992.

Banta, D. "What Is Health Care?" In *Health Care Delivery in the United States*, ed. S. Jonas, 12–36. New York: Springer Publishing Co., 1981.

Baquet, C. R., and T. Gibbs. "Cancer and Black Americans." In *Health Issues in the Black Community*, eds. R.L. Braithwaite and S. E. Taylor, 106–120. San Francisco: Jossey-Bass, 1992.

Barry, E. M. "Pregnant Prisoners." *Harvard Women's Law Journal* 12 (1989):189–205.

Bartlett, L. "Financing Health Care for Persons with AIDS: Balancing Public and Private Responsibilities." In *AIDS and the Health Care System*, ed. L. O. Gostin, 211–220. New Haven, Conn.: Yale University Press, 1990.

Bates, K. G. "AIDS: Is It Genocide?" *Essence* 21 (September 1990):77–116.

Bayer, R., D. Callahan, A. Caplan, and B. Jennings. "Toward Justice in Health Care." *Public Health and Law* 78, no. 5 (1988):583–588.

Bayer, R., A. L. Caplan, and N. Daniels, eds. *In Search of Equity: Health Needs and the Health Care System*. New York: Plenum Press, 1983.

Beauchamp, D. E. "Public Health as Social Justice." *Inquiry* 13 (1976):3–14.

———. *The Health of the Republic: Epidemics, Medicine, and Moralism as Challenges to Democracy*. Philadelphia: Temple University Press, 1988.

Beauchamp, T. F., and J. F. Childress. *Principles of Biomedical Ethics*. 3rd ed. New York: Oxford University Press, 1989.

Becker, M. E. "Can Employers Exclude Women to Protect Children." *Journal of the American Medical Association* 264, no. 16 (1990):2113–2117.

Beckum, L. C., S. Pflaum, and T. Minter. *Issues Which Impact on Teacher Education for the 21st Century*. A Report to the Exxon Foundation, 1987.

Belcher, J. R. "Are Jails Replacing the Mental Health System for the Homeless Mentally Ill?" *Community Mental Health Journal* 24 (1988):1985–1995.

Bell, D. *Faces at the Bottom of the Well*. New York: Basic Books, 1992.

Benenson, A. S. "Tuberculosis." In *Control of Communicable Diseases in Man*, ed. A. S. Benenson, 203–7. 15th ed., American Public Health Association, 1990.

Bernstein, A., and M. Berk. "Perceived Health Status and Selected Indicators of Access to Care Among the Minority Aged." Paper presented at the 110th Annual Meeting of the APHA, November 14–18 in Montreal, Canada, 1982.

Besharov, D. J. "The Children of Crack: Will We Protect Them?" *Public Welfare* 47, no. 4 (1989):6–11.

Bidwell, C. E. "The School as a Formal Organization." In *Handbook of Organizations*, ed. J. G. March, 972–1022. Chicago: Rand McNally, 1965.

Billingsley, A. *Black Families in White America*. Englewood Cliffs, N. J.: Prentice-Hall, 1968.

Blake, J. H. " "Doctor Can't Do Me No Good": Social Concomitants of Health Care Attitudes and Practices Among Elderly Blacks in Isolated Rural Populations." In *Black Folk Medicine: The Therapeutic Significance of Faith and Trust*, ed. W. H. Watson, 33–40. New Brunswick, N.J.: Transaction Books, 1983.

Blendon, R. J., L. H. Aiken, H. E. Freeman, and C. Corey. "Access to Medical Care for Black and White Americans: A Matter of Continuing Concern." *Journal of the American Medical Association* 261, no. 2 (1989):278–281.

Blendon, R. J., and K. Donelan. "Discrimination Against People with AIDS: The Public's Perspective." *New England Journal of Medicine* 319 (1988):1022–1026.

Bloom, B. R., and C. Murray. "Tuberculosis: Commentary on a Resurgent Killer." *Science* 257 (1992):1055.

Bogue, D. J. *Skid Row in American Cities*. Chicago: University of Chicago Press, 1963.

Bowman, J. E. "Genetic Screening Programs and Public Policy." *Phylon* 38 (1977): 117–142.

———. "Is a National Program to Prevent Sickle Cell Disease Possible?" *American Journal of Pediatric Hematology/Oncology* 5 (1983):367–372.

———. Invited Editorial: "Prenatal Screening for Hemoglobinopathies." *American Journal of Human Genetics* 48 (1991):433–438.

Bowman, J. E., and R. F. Murray, Jr. *Genetic Variation and Disorders in Peoples of African Origin*. Baltimore: Johns Hopkins University Press, 1990.

Bowsher, C. *Drug Exposed Infants: A Generation at Risk*. U.S. General Accounting Office Report to the U.S. Senate Committee on Finance, Washington, D.C., 1990.

———. *U.S. Health Care Spending: Trends, Contributing Factors, and Proposals for Reform*. Statement Submitted by U.S. Comptroller General Before the Committee on Ways and Means, House of Representatives, 1991.

Boxill, B. R. *Blacks and Social Justice*. Revised ed., Totowa, N.J.: Rowman and Littlefield Publishers, 1992.

Boyte, H. *CommonWealth*. London: Collier MacMillan, 1989.

Braithwaite, R. L., and N. Lythcott. "Community Empowerment as Strategy for Health Promotion for Black and Other Minority Populations." Letter to the Editor. *Journal of the American Medical Association* 261, no. 2 (1989):2282–2283.

Braithwaite, R. L., and S. E. Taylor, eds. *Health Issues in the Black Community*. San Francisco: Jossey-Bass, 1992.

Brickner, P. W. "Health Issues in the Care of the Homeless." In *Health Care of Homeless People*, eds. P. W. Brickner, L. K. Scharer, B. Conanan, A. Elvy, and M. Savarese, 3–18. New York: Springer, 1985.

Brickner, P. W., L. K. Scharer, B. A. Conanan, M. Savarese, and B. C. Scanlan, eds. *Under the Safety Net: The Health and Social Welfare of the Homeless in the United States*. New York: W. W. Norton., 1990.

Brickner, P. W., R. A. Torres, M. Barnes, R. G. Newman, D. C. DesJarlais, D. P. Whalen, and D. E. Rogers. "Recommendations for Control and Prevention of HIV Infection in Intravenous Drug Users." *Annals of Internal Medicine* 110 (1989):833–837.

Brodie, J. M. "In Locke's Footsteps: Black Philosophers Search for Wisdom and Validation." *Black Issues in Higher Education*, 1990, 1, 23–27.

Browlie, I., ed. *Basic Documents on Human Rights*. Oxford: Oxford University Press, 1981.

Brown, K., and A. Dula. "Sociocultural Reflections on the Case of Mr. W." *The Cambridge Quarterly* 62 (1992):256–258.

Buchanan, A. "An Ethical Evaluation of Health Care in the United States." In *Health Care Systems: Moral Conflicts in European and American Public Policy*, ed. H. M. Sass and R. U. Massey, 39–58. Boston: Kluwer Academic Publishers, 1988.

Budetti, P. "Achieving a Uniform Federal Primary Care Policy." *Journal of the American Medical Association* 269 (1993):498–501.

Bullard, R. D. *Dumping in Dixie: Race, Class and Environmental Quality.* Boulder, Colo.: Westview Press, 1990.

Bullough, B. L., and B. Bullough. *Health Care for the Other Americans.* New York: Appleton-Century-Crofts, 1982.

Buskin, S., S. G. Hopkins, E. H. Sohlberg, J. W. Ward, and K. M. Ferizio. "Are HIV-Infected Persons Receiving Care at an Emergency Facility Different from Those Using Outpatient Sites?" In *VII International Conference on AIDS in Florence, Italy,* abstract M.C. 3234, 1991.

Butler, P. A. *Too Poor to Be Sick: Access to Medical Care for the Uninsured.* Washington, D.C.: American Public Health Association, 1988.

Callahan, D. *What Kind of Life?* New York: Simon & Schuster, 1990.

Callender, C. O. "Organ Transplantation: The Minority Perspective." In *Organ Transplantation Hearing Before the Committee on Labor and Human Resources.* U.S. Senate, 98th Congress, 1st Session, on Examination of the Problems Involved in Obtaining Organs for Transplant Surgery, 1983, 183–187.

———. "Organ Donation in Blacks: A Community Approach." *Transplant Proceedings* 19, no. 1 (1987a):1551–1554.

———. "Organ Donation in Blacks: Where Do We Go from Here?" *Transplant Proceedings* 2 (Supplement 2) (1987b):36–40.

———. "The Results of Transplantation in Blacks: Just the Tip of the Iceberg." *Transplant Proceedings* 21, no. 3 (1989):3407–3410.

Callender, C. O., J. A. Bayton, C. L. Yeager, and J. C. Clark. "Attitudes Among Blacks Toward Donating Kidneys for Transplantation: A Pilot Project." *Journal of the National Medical Association* 74 (1982):807–809.

Callender, C. O., and G. M. Dunston. "Kidney Transplantation: A Dilemma for Black Americans." *Renal Life,* February/March 1987, 11–12.

Callender, C. O., and G. M. Dunston. "Organ Donation in Blacks: Once a Dilemma, Now a National Commitment." *Black Health* 1 (1988):22–25.

Callender, C. O., L. E. Hall, C. L. Yeager, J. B. Barber, G. M. Dunston, and V. W. Pinn-Higgins. "Organ Donation and Blacks: A Critical Frontier." *New England Journal of Medicine* 325 (1991):442–444.

Capitman, J. "Diversity Assessments in Aging Services." *Generations,* Fall/Winter 1991, 73–77.

Caplan, A. L. "Professional Arrogance and Public Misunderstanding." *Hastings Center Report* 19, no. 3 (1988):34–37.

Capron, A. M. "Tort Liability in Genetics." *Columbia Law Review* 79 (1979):619–684.

Carovano, K. "More Than Mothers and Whores: Redefining the AIDS Prevention Needs of Women." *International Journal of Health Services* 21 (1991):131–142.

Carter, J. H. "Chronic Mental Illness and Homelessness in Black Populations: Prologue and Prospects." *Journal of the National Medical Association* 83, no. 4 (1991):313–317.

Cassidy, J. "Access to Health Care: A Clinician's Opinion about an Ethical Issue." *American Journal of Occupational Therapy* 42, no. 5 (1988):295–299.

Castaner, A., B. E. Simmons, M. Mar, and R. Cooper. "Myocardial Infarction Among Black Patients: Poorer Prognosis After Hospital Discharge." *Annals of Internal Medicine* 109 (1988):33–35.

Cauley, K. *Testimony Before the National Commission on AIDS: State Legislation Related to HIV Testing.* Washington, D.C., 1990.

Centers for Disease Control (CDC). "Pneumococcal Polysaccharide Vaccine." *Morbidity & Mortality Weekly Report* 38, no. 64–8 (1989):73–76.

———. "Progress in Chronic Disease Prevention Mortality Trends—U.S. 1981–1988." *Morbidity & Mortality Weekly Report* 38 (1989):117–123.

———. "Health Beliefs and Compliance with Prescribed Medication for Hypertension Among Black Women—New Orleans 1985–1986." *Morbidity and Mortality Weekly Report* 39, no. 40 (1990a):701–704.

———. "HIV/AIDS in Racial/Ethnic Communities." *CDC HIV/AIDS Prevention Newsletter* 1, no. 1 (1990b):3–6.

———. "Prevention and Control of Influenza: Recommendations of the Immunization Practices Advisory Committee (ACIP)." *Morbidity & Mortality Weekly Report* 39(RR-7) (1990c).

———. "Protection Against Viral Hepatitis: Recommendation of Immunization Practices Advisory Committee (ACIP)." *Morbidity & Mortality Weekly Report* 39 (No. RR-2) (1990d):1–26.

———. "Public Health Burdens of Vaccine-Preventable Diseases Among Adults: Standards for Adult Immunization Practice." *Morbidity & Mortality Weekly Report* 39, no. 41 (1990e):725–729 (published erratum in MMWR 39 [42]: 7711).

———. *CDC HIV/AIDS Prevention: Special Report on Evaluation.* 1991a.

———. *The HIV/AIDS Epidemic: The First 10 Years.* 1991b.

———. "1993 Revised Classification System for HIV Infection and Expanded Surveillance Case Definition for AIDS Among Adolescents and Adults." *Morbidity & Mortality Weekly Report* 41 (No. RR-17) (1992a):1–3.

———. *HIV/AIDS Surveillance Report.* 1992b.

———. "Measles Surveillance—United States, 1991." *Morbidity & Mortality Weekly Report* 41 (SS-6 1992c):1–12.

———. "National Coalition for Adult Immunization: Activities to Increase Influenza Vaccination Levels, 1989–1991." *Morbidity & Mortality Weekly Report* 41, no. 41 (1992d):772–775 (published erratum in MMWR 41 [49]:930).

———. "Prevention and Control of Tuberculosis in the U.S. Communities with At-Risk Minority Populations: Recommendations for the Elimination of Tuberculosis." *Morbidity & Mortality Weekly Report* 41 (No. RR-5) (1992e):1–11.

———. *Infant Mortality—United States, 1990.* 1993a.

———. "Technical Guidance on HIV Counseling." *Morbidity and Mortality Weekly Report* 42 (RR-2) (1993b):11–17.

Chasnoff, I. "Maternal Drug Use." In *Crack and Other Addictions: Old Realities and New Challenges for Child Welfare,* 10–20. Child Welfare League of America, 1990.

Chavez, L. R., W. A. Cornelius, and O. W. Jones. "Utilization of Health Services by Mexican Immigrant Women in San Diego." *Women & Health* 11 (1986): 3–20.

Chavkin, W. "Preventing AIDS, Targeting Women." *Health/PAC Bulletin* 20, no. 1 (1990):19–23.

Chicago and Cook County Health Care Action Plan. *Executive Summary.* 1990.

Chicago and Cook County Title I Planning Council. *Unpublished Data.* 1991.

Chicago Department of Health. *AIDS Chicago: HIV/AIDS Surveillance Program.* 1991a.

———. *Sexually Transmitted Disease Surveillance Report.* 1991b.

Chicago Institute on Urban Poverty. *Promises Made, Promises Broken . . . The Crisis and Challenge: Homeless Families in Chicago. A Traveler's and Immigrant's Aid.* 1990.

"The Chicago Institute on Urban Poverty's Homelessness Prevention Project." *In Transition,* 1990.

Children's Defense Fund. *S.O.S. America!: A Children's Defense Budget.* Washington, D.C.: 1990.

———. *The State of America's Children.* Washington, D.C.: 1991.

Chu, S., J. Buehler, and R. Berkelman. "Impact of the Human Immunodeficiency Virus Epidemic on Mortality in Women of Reproductive Age, United States." *Journal of the American Medical Association* 264, no. 2 (1990):225–229.

Ciesielski, C., P. L. Fleming, and R. L. Berkelman. "Changing Trends in AIDS-Indicator Diseases in the United States." In *VII International Conference on AIDS in Florence, Italy,* abstract M.C. 3174, 1991.

Cloward, R. A., and L. Ohlin. *Delinquency and Opportunity: A Theory of Delinquent Gangs.* New York: Free Press, 1960.

Coates, T. J., R. D. Stall, S. M. Kegeles, B. Lo, S. Morin, and L. McKusick. "AIDS Antibody Testing: Will It Stop the AIDS Epidemic? Will It Help the People Infected with HIV?" *American Psychologist* 43 (1988): 859–864.

Cohen, J., and T. Rogers. "Secondary Associations and Democratic Governance." *Politics and Society* 20 (1992): 393–473.

Cohen, M. N. *Health and the Rise of Civilization.* New Haven, Conn.: Yale University Press, 1989.

Collins, J. W., and R. J. David. "The Differential Effect of Traditional Risk Factors on Infant Birthweight Among Blacks and Whites in Chicago." *American Journal of Public Health* 80 (1990): 679–681.

Collins, P. H. *Black Feminist Thought: Knowledge, Consciousness, and the Politics of Empowerment.* Boston: Unwyn Hyman, 1990.

Comer, J. P. *School Power: Implications of an Intervention Project.* New York: Free Press, 1980.

Committee for Economic Development. *Children in Need: Investment Strategies for the Educationally Disadvantaged.* Washington, D.C., 1987.

———. *The Unfinished Agenda: A New Vision for Child Development and Education.* Washington, D.C., 1991.

Committee to Study the Prevention of Low Birthweight. Institute of Medicine, Division of Health Promotion and Disease Prevention, Washington, D.C., National Academy Press, 1985.

Conference of Mayors. *The Impact of AIDS on American Cities: A 26 City Report for the U.S. Conference of Mayors Task Force on AIDS.* 1991.

Cooke, M., B. Koenig, N. Beery, and S. Folkman. "Which Physicians Will Provide AIDS Care?" In *VI International Conference on AIDS in San Francisco, CA,* abstract S.D. 50, 1990.

Cooper, E. B. "When Being Ill Is Illegal: Women and the Criminalization of HIV." *Health/PAC Bulletin* 22, no. 4 (1992): 10–14.

Corwin, R. G., and R. A. Edelfelt. *Perspectives on Organizations: Viewpoints for Teachers.*

American Association of Colleges for Teacher Education and Association of Teacher Educators, 1976.

Cotton, P. "Examples Abound of Gaps in Medical Knowledge Because of Groups Excluded from Scientific Study." *Journal of the American Medical Association* 263, no. 8 (1990a): 1051–1052.

———. "Is There Still Too Much Extrapolation from Data on Middle-aged White Men." *Journal of the American Medical Association* 263, no. 8 (1990b): 1049–1050.

Council on Ethical and Judicial Affairs. "Black White Disparities in Health Care." *Journal of the American Medical Association* 263, no. 17 (1990c): 2344–2348.

Council on Scientific Affairs. "Hispanic Health in the United States." *Journal of the American Medical Association* 265 (1991): 248–252.

Council on Scientific Affairs and the American Medical Association. "Health Care Needs of Homeless and Runaway Youths." *Journal of the American Medical Association* 262, no. 10 (1989): 1358–1361.

Crystal, S., and N. Schiller. "Outpatient Medical Care and the Course of AIDS." In *VII International Conference on AIDS in Florence, Italy*, abstract M.D. 115, 1991.

Curtis, J. L. "Civil Rights in Medicine." *Journal of Public Health Policy* (1980): 110–120.

Cutler, N. E. "Targeting and Means Testing Aging and Need." *Generations*, Fall/Winter 1991, 16.

D'Eramo, J. E., D. Z. Kirschenbaum, M. McCarthy, and T. Davis. "Women and Minorities Have Less Access to AIDS Drug Trials." In *VII International Conference on AIDS in Florence, Italy*, abstract W.D. 4291, 1991.

Dahl, R. A. *Democracy and Its Critics.* New Haven, Conn.: Yale University Press, 1989.

Dalton, H. L. "AIDS in Blackface." *Daedalus* 118, no. 3 (1989): 205–227.

Dandridge v. Williams. 397 U.S. 471, 485 (1970).

Daniels, N. "What Is the Obligation of the Medical Profession in the Distribution of Health Care?" *Social Science and Medicine* 15F (1981): 129–133.

———. "Health Care Needs and Distributive Justice." In *In Search of Equity: Health Needs and the Health Care System*, ed. R. Bayer, A. L. Caplan, and N. Daniels, 1–43. New York: Plenum Press, 1983.

———. *Just Health Care.* Cambridge: Cambridge University Press, 1985.

———. "Justice and Health Care." In *Health Care Ethics*, ed. D. Van De Veer and T. Regand, 290–335. Philadelphia: Temple University Press, 1987.

Davis, A. *Women, Race & Class.* New York: Vintage Books, 1981.

———. "Racism, Birth Control and Reproductive Rights." In *From Abortion to Reproductive Freedom: Transforming a Movement*, ed. M. G. Fried, 15–26. Boston: South End Press, 1990.

Davis, K., and C. Schoen. *Health and the War on Poverty: A Ten-Year Appraisal.* Washington, D.C.: Brookings Institution, 1978.

Dechesser, A. D. "The Supply/Demand Discrepancy." *Heart and Lung* 15, no. 6 (1986): 547–551.

Demkovich, L., ed. *Intergovernmental AIDS Reports: HIV Testing in the States.* George Washington University, Intergovernmental Health Policy Project, 1989.

Depalma, J. R. "Black Americans and the ESRD Program." *Contemporary Dialysis and Nephrology*, April 1989, 35–37.

Department of Health and Human Services. *Report of the Secretary's Task Force on Black and Minority Health.* 1985.

——. *Report of Secretary's Task Force on Black and Minority Health, Vol. III—Cancer.* U.S. Government Printing Office, 1986. No. 621–605: 00171.

——. *Secretary's Work Group on Pediatric HIV Infection and Disease.* Washington, D.C., 1987. NIH No. 89-3063.

——. *Council on Graduate Medical Education. First Report of the Council.* 1988.

——. *Health Status of the Disadvantaged Chartbook.* U.S. Public Health Service, Health Resources and Services Administration, 1990. (HRSA) HRS-P-DV 90-1.

——. *Healthy People 2000: National Health Promotion and Disease Prevention Objectives—Full Report with Commentary.* U.S. Government Printing Office, Department of Health and Human Services, 1990, 91–50212.

——. *Center on Budget and Policy Priorities Report.* U.S. Government Printing Office, 1991.

——, State of Connecticut. *AIDS in Connecticut.* Annual Surveillance Report, 1990.

DesJarlais, D., C. Casriel, B. Stephenson, and S. R. Friedman. "Expectations of Racial Prejudice in AIDS Research and Prevention Programs in the United States." In *AIDS and Alcohol/Drug Abuse: Psychosocial Research,* ed. D. G. Fisher, 1–8. New York: Haworth Press, 1991.

DesJarlais, D., M. Chamberland, S. Yancovitz, P. Weinberg, and S. Friedman. "Heterosexual Partners: A Large Risk Group for AIDS." *Lancet* 2 (1984): 1346–1347.

De Tocqueville, A. *Democracy in America.* New York: Alfred A. Knopf (first published in 1840), 1945.

Dewey, J. "The School and Social Progress." In *The School and Society,* 6–29. Chicago: University of Chicago Press, 1915.

Dickman, R. L. "Operationalizing Respect for Persons: A Qualitative Aspect of the Right to Health Care." In *In Search of Equity: Health Needs and the Health Care System,* ed. R. Bayer, A. L. Caplan, and N. Daniels, 161–182. New York: Plenum Press, 1981.

Dillingham, B. "Indian Women and IHS Sterilization Practices." *American Indian Journal* 3, no. 1 (1977): 27–28.

Dodson, J. "Conceptualizations of Black Families." In *Black Families, Second Edition,* ed. H. P. McAdoo, 77–90. Newbury Park, Calif.: Sage Publications, 1988.

Donabedian, A., S. Axelrod, and L. Wyszewianski. *Medical Care Chartbook.* Washington, D.C.: AUPHA Press, 1980.

Dooley, J. W., W. R. Jarvis, W. F. Martone, and D. E. Snider. "Multidrug Resistant Tuberculosis." *Annals of Internal Medicine* 117 (1992): 257–259.

Dowart, R. A. "A Ten-Year Follow-up Study of the Health Effects of Deinstitutionalization." *Hospital and Community Psychiatry* 39 (1988): 287–291.

Dowling, H. F. *City Hospitals: The Undercare of the Underprivileged.* Cambridge, Mass.: Harvard University Press, 1982.

Dresser, R. "Wanted: Single, White Male for Medical Research." *Hastings Center Report* 22, no. 1 (1992): 24.

Du Bois, W. E. B. *The Souls of Black Folk: Essays and Sketches.* Greenwich, Conn.: Fawcett Publications, 1961.

Dula, A. "Miz Mildred's Story: The PSDA." *Clinical Geriatrics.* Forthcoming (1994).

Dula, A., S. Kurtz, and M.L. Samper. "Occupational and Environmental Reproductive Hazards Education and Resources for Communities of Color." *Environmental Health Perspectives Supplement* 161, suppl. 2 (1993): 181–189.

Duncan, G. D. "Years of Poverty, Years of Plenty." Ann Arbor: University of Michigan Institute for Social Research, 1984.

Dunston, G. M., C. K. Hurley, R. T. Hartzman, and A. H. Johnson. "Unique HLA-D Region Heterogeneity in American Blacks." *Transplant Proceedings* 19, no. 1 (1987): 870–871.

Eddins, B. B., and E. A. Eddins. "Liberalism and Liberation." In *Philosophy Born of Struggle*, ed. L. Harris, 159–173. Dubuque, Iowa: Kendall/Hunt, 1983.

Edelman, M. W. *Families in Peril: An Agenda for Social Change.* Cambridge, Mass.: Harvard University Press, 1987.

El-Sadr, W., and L. Capps. "The Challenge of Minority Recruitment in Clinical Trials for AIDS." *Journal of the American Medical Association* 267, no. 7 (1992): 954–957.

Emanuel, I. "Maternal Health During Childhood and Later Reproductive Performance." *Annals of the New York Academy of Science* 477 (1986): 27–39.

Engel, G. L. "The Need for a New Medical Model: A Challenge for Biomedicine." *Science* 196 (1977): 129–36.

Engelhardt, H. T., Jr. *The Foundations of Bioethics.* New York: Oxford University Press, 1986.

Enthoven, A. C. "The History and Principles of Managed Competition." *Health Affairs* 12 (suppl.) (1993): 24–48.

Estes, C. "Health Care Policy in the Later Twentieth Century." *Generations*, Spring 1988, 44–47.

Fabrega, H. "An Ethnomedical Perspective of Medical Ethics." *Journal of Medicine and Philosophy* 15 (1990): 593–625.

Faludi, S. *Backlash: The Undeclared War on American Women.* New York: Crown Books, 1991.

Farfel, M. R., and N. A. Holtzman. "Education, Consent, and Counseling in Sickle Cell Screening Programs: Report of a Survey." *American Journal of Public Health* 74 (1984): 373–375.

Fein, R. "Health Care Reform." *Scientific American* 267, no. 5 (1992): 46–53.

Fife, D., and J. McAnaney. "Private Medical Insurance Among Philadelphia Residents Diagnosed with AIDS." *Journal of Acquired Immune Deficiency Syndrome* 6 (1993): 512–517.

Filardo, T. "Chronic Disease Management in the Homeless." In *Health Care of Homeless People*, eds. P. W. Brickner et al., 19–29. New York: Springer, 1985.

Flack, H. E., and E. D. Pellegrino, eds. *African American Perspectives on Biomedical Ethics.* Washington, D.C.: Georgetown University, 1992.

Flaskerud, J. H. "The Effects of Culture-Compatible Intervention on the Utilization of Mental Health Services by Minority Clients." *Community Mental Health Journal* 22, no. 2 (1986): 127–141.

Fordyce, E. J., S. Sambula, and R. Stoneburner. "Mandatory Reporting of Human Immunodeficiency Virus Testing Would Deter Blacks and Hispanics from Being Tested" (letter to the editor). *Journal of the American Medical Association* 262 (1989):349.

Fox, R. *The Sociology of Medicine.* Englewood Cliffs, N.J.: Prentice-Hall, 1989.

Freedman, E. "Introduction to Security Access to Health Care." In *Making Choices: Ethical Issues for Health Care Professionals,* ed. E. Freedman, 13–16. Chicago: American Hospital Publishing, 1986.

Freedman, H. E., R. J. Blendon, L. H. Aiden, S. Sudman, C. Mullinix, and C. Corey. "Americans Report on Their Access to Health Care." *Health Affairs* (1987): 6–18.

Freudenberg, N. *Preventing AIDS: A Guide to Effective Education for the Prevention of HIV Infection.* Washington D.C.: American Public Health Association, 1989.

Fried, C. "Equality and Rights in Medical Care." *Hastings Center Report* 6 (1976): 29–34.

Fried, M. G., ed. *From Abortion to Reproductive Freedom.* Boston: South End Press, 1990.

Friedman, E. *Professional Dominance: The Social Structure of Medical Care.* New York: Atherton Press, 1970.

———. "The Uninsured." *Journal of the American Medical Association* 265 (1991): 2491–2495.

Friedman, S. R., J. L. Sotheran, A. Abdul-Quader, B. J. Primm, D. C. DesJarlais, P. Kleinman, C. Mauge, D. S. Goldsmith, W. El-Sadr, and R. Maslansky. "The AIDS Epidemic Among Blacks and Hispanics." *Milbank Quarterly* 65 (Suppl. 2) (1987): 455–499.

Fullilove, R. *The Twin Epidemics of Substance Use and HIV.* Report of the National Commission on AIDS, 1991.

Gage, L. S., V. B. Weslowski, D. P. Andrulis, E. Hintz, and A. B. Camper. *America's Safety Net Hospitals: The Foundation of Our Nation's Health Care System.* Washington, D.C.: National Association of Public Hospitals, 1991.

Garcia, J. L. A. "African-American Perspectives, Cultural Relativism, and Normative Issues: Some Conceptual Questions." In *African-American Perspectives on Biomedical Ethics,* ed. H. E. Flack and E. D. Pellegrino, 11–66. Washington, D.C.: Georgetown University Press, 1992.

Garrett, R. B. *Famous First Facts about Negroes.* New York: Arno Press, 1972.

Gaston, M. H., J. I. Verter, G. Woods, C. Pegel, J. Kelleher, G. Presbury, and E. Zarkowsky. "Prophylaxis with Oral Penicillin in Children with Sickle Cell Anemia." *New England Journal of Medicine* 314 (1986): 1593–1599.

General Accounting Office. *Prenatal Care: Medicaid Recipients and Uninsured Women Obtain Insufficient Care.* 1978.

———. *WIC Evaluations Provide Some Favorable But No Conclusive Evidence on the Effects Expected for the Special Supplemental Program for Women, Infants and Children,* 1984. GAO/PEMD-84-4.

Germaine, C. B. *Social Work Practice in Health Care: An Ecological Perspective.* New York: Free Press, 1984.

Geronimus, A. T. "The Effects of Race, Residence, and Prenatal Care on the Relationship of Maternal Age to Neonatal Mortality." *American Journal of Public Health* 76 (1986): 1416–1421.

Getzels, J. W. "The Communities of Education." In *Families and Communities as*

Educators, ed. H. J. Leichter, 95–118. New York: Teachers College Press, 1979.

Giddings, P. *When and Where I Enter: The Impact of Black Women on Race and Sex in America.* Toronto: Bantam Books, 1984.

Ginzberg, E. "Access to Health Care for Hispanics." *Journal of the American Medical Association* 265, no. 2 (1991): 238–241.

Glass, L., H. Evans, D. Swartz, B. Rajegowda, and W. Leblanc. "Effects of Legalized Abortion on Neonatal Mortality and Obstetrical Morbidity at Harlem Hospital Center." *American Journal of Public Health* 64 (1974):717–718.

Goldenberg, R. L., K. G. Nelson, J. F. Koski, et al. "Neonatal Mortality in Infants Weighing 501 to 1000 Grams. The Influence of Changes in Birthweight Distribution and Birth Weight Specific Mortality Rates on Neonatal Survival." *American Journal of Obstetrics and Gynecology* 151, no. 5 (1985): 608–611.

Goodlad, J. I. *A Place Called School: Prospects for the Future.* New York: McGraw-Hill Book Co., 1984.

Gordon, L. *Woman's Body, Woman's Right: Birth Control in America.* Revised ed., New York: Penguin Books, 1990.

Gorovitz, S. *Doctors' Dilemmas: Moral Conflict and Medical Care.* New York: Oxford University Press, 1982.

Gortmaker, S. L. "The Effects of Prenatal Care upon the Health of the Newborn." *American Journal of Public Health* 69 (1979):653–660.

Gould, J. B., and S. LeRoy. "Socioeconomic Status and Low Birth Weight: A Racial Comparison." *Pediatrics* 82 (1988):896–904.

Gould, K. H. "Black Women in Double Jeopardy: A Perspective on Birth Control." *Health and Social Work* (1984):96–105.

Governor's Advisory Committee for Black Affairs. *Black Health Issues in New York State: Condition, Prognosis, Prescription.* Albany, N.Y.: 1987.

Green, J., and P. S. Arno. "The "Medicaidization" of AIDS: Trends in the Financing of HIV-Related Medical Care." *Journal of the American Medical Association* 264 (1990):1261–1266.

Greywolf, E. "The Politics of the Poor." In *Lives in Stress: Women and Depression,* ed. Deborah Belle, 120–130. Beverly Hills, Calif.: Sage Publications, 1982.

Griffiths, M., and M. Whitford, ed. *Feminist Perspectives in Philosophy.* Bloomington: Indiana University Press, 1988.

Grossman, M., and S. Jacobowitz. "Variations in Infant Mortality Rates Among Counties in the United States: The Roles of Public Policies and Programs." *Demography* 18 (1981):695–713.

Hack, M., and A. A. Fanaroff. "Outcome of Extremely Low Birthweight Infants Between 1982 and 1988." *New England Journal of Medicine* 321 (1989):1642–1647.

Hadley, J. *More Medical Care, Better Health?* Washington, D.C.: Urban Institute Press, 1982.

Hadley, J., E. P. Steinberg, and J. Feder. "Comparison of Uninsured and Privately Insured Hospital Patients." *Journal of the American Medical Association* 265, no. 3 (1991):374–379.

Hafner-Eaton, C. "Physician Utilization: Disparities Between the Uninsured and Insured." *Journal of the American Medical Association* 269 (1993):787–792.

Haller, M. H. *Eugenics: Hereditarian Attitudes in American Thought.* New Brunswick, N.J.: Rutgers University Press, 1984.

Hammell, J. R., and R. Sherer. "Health Care and AIDS Risks." *Chicago Tribune,* June 4 1991, 12.

Hanft, R. S., and C. C. White. "Constraining the Supply of Physicians: Effects on Black Physicians." *The Milbank Quarterly* 65 (Supplement 2) (1987):249–269.

Harris, L., ed. *Philosophy Born of Struggle.* Dubuque, Iowa: Kendall Hunt Publishing Co., 1983.

———. "Autonomy Under Duress." In *African-American Perspectives on Biomedical Ethics,* ed. H. E. Flack and E. D. Pellegrino, 133–149. Washington, D.C.: Georgetown University Press, 1992.

Harris v. McRae. 448 U.S. 297 (1980).

Hatziandreu, E., J. Sisk, R. Hughes, S. Hamilton, V. Cwalina, E. Murphy, C. Martin, and A. Dantzler. *The Effectiveness of Drug Abuse Treatment: Implications for Controlling AIDS/HIV Infection.* Background paper #6, Office of Technology Assessment, U.S. Congress, 1990.

Hawkins, C. A., and N. A. Handley. "HIV Disease and AIDS and Women: Current Knowledge and a Research Agenda." *Journal of Acquired Immune Deficiency Syndrome* 5 (1992):957–971.

Hawkins, J. B. W., and L. P. Higgins. *Nursing and the American Health Care Delivery System.* New York: Tiresias Press, 1982.

Haynes, M. N. "Tuskegee: A Deadly Experiment with African American Lives." *Positively Aware—Monthly Magazine of Test Positive Aware, Chicago IL,* 1992.

Haywood, L. J. "Hypertension in Minority Populations: Access to Care." *American Journal of Medicine* 88(3B) (1990):3B-18s–3B-20s.

Health Policy Advisory Center. *Managed Competition: Reform or Retreat?. Analysis, Critique, Alternatives.* Health/PAC Bulletin, 1993.

Health Services Amendments. Section 205 of Public Law 95-626 (1978).

Heckler, M. *Black and Minority Health: Report of the Secretary's Task Force.* U.S. Government Printing Office, Department of Health and Human Services, 1985.

Hein, K. "Commentary on Adolescent Acquired Immunodeficiency Syndrome: The Next Wave of the Human Immunodeficiency Virus Epidemic?" *Journal of Pediatrics* 114 (1989):144–149.

Held, P. J., R. Randall, J. D. Bovlbjerg, J. Newman, and O. Salvatierra. "Race, Income, and Kidney Transplantation." *Archives of Medicine* 148 (1988):2594–2600.

Henshaw, S. K. "Teenage Abortion, Birth and Pregnancy Statistics by State, 1988." *Family Planning Perspectives* 25, no. 3 (1993):122–126.

Herek, G. M., and E. K. Glunt. "An Epidemic of Stigma: Public Reactions to AIDS." *American Psychologist* 43 (1988):886–891.

Hidalgo, J., B. Sugland, R. Moore, and R. E. Chaisson. "Access, Equity, and Survival: Use of ZVD and Pentamidine by Persons with AIDS." In *VIth International Conference on AIDS in San Francisco, CA,* abstract Th.D. 59, 1990.

Hilfiker, D. "Unconscious on a Corner." *Journal of the American Medical Association* 258, no. 21 (1987):3155–3156.

Hill, P. J. "Demands to Fix U.S. Health Care Reach a Crescendo." *New York Times,* May 19, 1991, E1.

Hodgkinson, H. L. *All One System: Demographics on Education. Kindergarten Through*

Graduate School. Washington, D.C.: Institute for Educational Leadership, 1985.

———. *The Same Client: The Demographics of Education and Service Delivery Systems.* Washington, D.C.: Institute for Educational Leadership, Center for Demographic Policy, 1990.

Holmes, H. B. "Can Clinical Research Be Both Ethical and Scientific?" *Hypatia* 4, no. 2 (1989):156–168.

Holmes, K., J. Karon, and J. Kreiss. "The Increasing Frequency of Heterosexually Acquired AIDS in the United States." *American Journal of Public Health* 80, no. 7 (1990):858–862.

Holmes Group. *Tomorrow's Schools: Principles for Design of Professional Development Schools.* East Lansing, Mich.: Holmes Group, 1990.

"Homeless Need Humane Policies." *Chicago Sun Times,* November 22, 1990.

Hopkins, J. "Jail for Pregnant Cocaine Users in US." *News & Political Review, British Medical Journal* 303 (1991):873.

Horner, M. J., R. Schulman, J. Nelson, and G. S. Bowen. "Improving Access to AIDS Therapies: The Experience of the U.S. AIDS Drug Reimbursement Program." In *VII International Conference on AIDS in Florence, Italy,* abstract M.D. 4134, 1991.

Horton, M., with J. Kohl and H. Kohl. *The Long Haul: An Autobiography.* New York: Doubleday, 1990.

Howze, D. C. "Closing the Gap Between Black and White Infant Mortality Rates: An Analysis of Policy Options." In *Health Care Issues in Black America: Policies, Problems, and Prospects,* ed. W. Jones and M. F. Rice, 119–139. Westport, Conn.: Greenwood Press, 1987.

Illinois Department of Public Health. *Newborn Screening: An Overview of Newborn Screening Programs in the United States.* Chicago: 1990.

"The Importance of Dr. Sullivan." *New York Times,* December 23, 1988, A22.

Institute of Medicine, National Academy of Sciences. *Confronting AIDS: Update 1988.* Washington, D.C.: National Academy Press, 1988.

Jackson, J. S. "Health Status of Elderly Black Adults." Bethesda, Md.: National Institute on Aging Workshop, Development of Research Agendas in Minority Aging, 1990.

Jacobs, H. *Incidents in the Life of a Slave Girl.* ed. J. F. Yellin. Cambridge, Mass.: Harvard University Press (first published in 1861), 1987.

Jaynes, G. D., and R. M. Williams, Jr., eds. *A Common Destiny: Blacks and American Society.* Washington, D.C.: National Academy Press, 1989.

Jenkins, A. H. *The Psychology of the Afro-American: A Humanistic Approach.* New York: Pergamon Press, 1982.

Johnson, L. A. *The Devil, the Gargoyle, and the Buffoon: The Negro as Metaphor in Western Literature.* Port Washington, N.Y.: Kennikat Press, 1971.

Johnson v. Calvert No. X 63 31 90, consolidated with AD 57638 (1990).

Jonas, H. S., and S. I. Sylvia. "Undergraduate Medical Education." *Journal of the American Medical Association* 260, no. 8 (1988): 1063–1085.

Jones, J. H. *Bad Blood: The Tuskegee Syphilis Experiment: A Tragedy of Race and Medicine.* New York: Free Press, 1981.

Jones, R. *Black Psychology.* New York: Harper & Row, 1980.

Jones, W., and M. F. Rice. "Black Health Care." In *Health Care Issues in Black Amer-*

ica: Policies, Problems, and Prospects, ed. W. Jones and M. F. Rice, 3–20. Westport, Conn.: Greenwood Press, 1987.

Joyce, T., H. Corman, and M. Grossman. "A Cost-Effectiveness Analysis of Strategies to Reduce Infant Mortality." *Medical Care* 26 (1988):348–360.

Kaback, M., and J. S. O'Brien. "Tay-Sachs: Prototype for Prevention of Genetic Disease." *Hospital Practice* 8 (1973):107–116.

Kamikawa, L. "Public Entitlements: Exclusionary Beneficence." *Generations*, Fall/Winter 1991, 23.

Kane, S. "AIDS, Addiction, and Condom Use: Sources of Sexual Risk for Heterosexual Women." *Journal of Sex Research* 27, no. 3 (1990):427–444.

Kant, I. *The Groundwork of Metaphysic of Morals*. Translated by H. J. Paton. London: Hutchinson & Co. Ltd., 1963.

Karan, L. "AIDS Prevention and Chemical Dependence Treatment Needs of Women and Their Children." *Journal of Psychoactive Drugs* 21, 4 (1989):396–399.

Kass, L. R. "Practicing Ethics: Where's the Action?" *Hastings Center Report* 20, 1 (1990):5–12.

Kateb, G. "Utopia and the Good Life." *Daedalus*, 1965, 454–473.

Katz, W. L. *Eyewitness: The Negro in American History*. New York: Pitman Publishing Corp., 1967.

Kegeles, S. M., T. J. Coates, T. A. Christopher, and J. L. Lazarus. "Perceptions of AIDS: The Continuing Saga of AIDS-Related Stigma." *AIDS* 3(Supplement 2) (1989):S253–258.

Kell, G. "Raising Children of Addicts Taking Toll on Grandparents." *The Sacramento Bee*, August 14 1990, p. A1–A12.

Kelly, J. A., J. S. St. Lawrence, S. Smith, H. V. Hood, and D. J. Cook. "Stigmatization of AIDS Patients by Physicians." *American Journal of Public Health* 77 (1987):789–791.

Kevles, D. J. *In the Name of Eugenics*. New York: Alfred A. Knopf, 1985.

Keyserlingk, E. "Ethical Guidelines and Codes: Can They Be Universally Applicable in a Multi-Cultural Society?" In *Ethics in Medicine: Individual Integrity Versus Demands of Society*, ed. P. Allebeck and B. Jansson, 137–150. New York: Raven Press, 1990.

Kirn, T. F. "Research Seeks to Reduce Toll of Hypertension and Other Cardiovascular Diseases in Black Population." *Journal of the American Medical Association* 261, no. 2 (1989):195.

Kirp, D., and R. Bayer. *AIDS in the Industrialized Democracies: Passions, Politics, and Policies*. New Brunswick, N.J.: Rutgers University Press, 1992.

Kleinman, J. C., and J. L. Kiely. "Postneonatal Mortality in the United States: An International Perspective." *Pediatrics* 86 (1990):1091–1097.

Kleinman, L. C. "Health Care in Crisis: A Proposed Role for the Individual Physician as Advocate." *Journal of the American Medical Association* 265, 15 (1991): 1991–92.

Klerman, L. V. *Alive and Well? A Research and Policy Review of Health Programs for Poor Young Children*. New York: National Center for Children in Poverty, 1991.

Kolbert, Z. "SRO Housing May Be Demolished, Court Rules." *New York Times*, July 7 1989, B–1.

Kolder, V., J. Gallagher, and M. T. Parsons. "Court-ordered Obstetrical Interventions." *New England Journal of Medicine* 316 (1987):1192–1196.

Koppleman, J. and J. M. Jones. "Crack: It's Destroying Fragile Low-Income Families." *Public Welfare* 47, 4 (1989):13–15.

Kotelchuck, M., J. B. Schwartz, M. T. Anderka, and K. S. Finison. "WIC Participation and Pregnancy Outcomes: Massachusetts Statewide Evaluation Project." *American Journal of Public Health* 74 (1984):1086–1092.

Kozol, J. *Savage Inequalities.* New York: Crown Publishers, 1991.

Kraus, S. F., S. Greenland, and M. Bulterys. "Risk Factors for Sudden Death Syndrome in the U.S. Collaborative Perinatal Project." *Journal of Epidemiology* 18 (1989):113–121.

Krause, E. A. *Power and Illness: The Political Sociology of Health and Medical Care.* New York: Elsevier, 1977.

Krause, N., and L. Wray. "Psychosocial Consulates of Health and Illness Among Minority Elders." *Generations*, 1991, 25.

Kreiss, J., J. M. Karon, and K. Holmes. "Rate of Heterosexually Acquired AIDS Increasing in the U.S." *American Journal of Public Health* 80 (1990):858–862.

Kusserow, R. P. *The Distribution of Organs for Transplantation: Expectations and Practices.* Office of the Inspector General, Office of Evaluation and Inspections, 1990.

Lackman, C., R. Sherer, T. Louis, L. Capps, L. Brown, M. Carlyn, C. Cohen, G. Collins, J. Korvick, and T. Mitchell. "The CPCRA Observational Data Base Project: Preliminary Clinical Findings." In *VII International Conference on AIDS in Florence, Italy*, abstract M.B. 2451, 1991.

Lamb, H. R. "Deinstitutionalization of the Homeless Mentally Ill." In *The Homeless Mentally Ill*, ed. H. R. Lamb, 55–74. Washington, D.C.: American Psychiatric Association, 1984.

Lamboi, S. E., and F. S. Sy. "The Impact of AIDS on State Public Health Legislation in the United States: A Critical Review." *AIDS Education and Prevention* 1 (1989):324–339.

Lanman, J., S. Kohl, and J. Bedell. "Changes in Pregnancy Outcome After Liberalization of the New York State Abortion Law." *American Journal of Obstetrics and Gynecology* (1974):485–492.

Lappé, M. "The Limits of Genetic Inquiry." *Hastings Center Report* 17, no. 4 (1987): 5–10.

LaVeist, T. A. "Simulating the Effects of Poverty on the Race Disparity in Postneonatal Mortality." *Journal of Public Health Policy* 11 (1990):463–473.

Leary, W. "Uneasy Doctors Add Race-Consciousness to Diagnostic Tools." *New York Times*, September 25, 1990, C1.

Lee, K. S., N. Paneth, L. M. Gartner, M. A. Pearlman, and L. Gruss. "Neonatal Mortality: An Analysis of the Recent Improvement in the United States." *American Journal of Public Health* 70 (1980):15–21.

Lee, P. R., and R. D. Lamm. "Europe's Medical Model." *New York Times*, March 3, 1993, Op-Ed.

Lemp, G. F., S. F. Payne, and G. W. Rutherford. "Projections of AIDS Morbidity and Mortality in San Francisco." *Journal of the American Medical Association* 263 (1990):1497–1501.

Leven, J. S., K. S. Markides, J. C. Richardson, and A. H. Lubin. "Exploring the

Persistent Black Risk of Low Birthweight: Findings from the GLOWBS Study." *Journal of the National Medical Association* 81 (1989):253–260.

Levine, C. "In and Out of the Hospital." In *AIDS and the Health Care System*, ed. L. O. Gostin, 45–61. New Haven, Conn.: Yale University Press, 1990a.

———. "Women and HIV/AIDS Research: The Barriers to Equity." *Evaluation Review* 14, no. 5 (1990b):447–463.

Levine, C., and N. Dubler. "Uncertain Risk and Bitter Realities: The Reproductive Choices of HIV-Infected Women." *Milbank Quarterly* 68, no. 3 (1990):321–351.

Levine, S. "A Response." *Social Policy* 22, no. 1 (1991):44–45.

Lewis, C. E., R. Fein, and D. Mechanic. *A Right to Health Care*. New York: John Wiley, 1976.

Lewis, I. J., and C. G. Sheps. *The Sick Citadel: The American Medical Center and Public Interest*. Cambridge, Mass.: Gelgeschatter, Gunn & Hail, 1983.

Littlewood, T. B. *The Politics of Population Control*. Notre Dame, Ind.: University of Notre Dame Press, 1977.

Loader, S., C. J. Suters, M. Walden, A. Kozyra, and P. T. Rowley. "Prenatal Screening for Hemoglobinopathies. II. Evaluation of Counseling." *American Journal of Human Genetics* 48 (1991):447–451.

Logan, R. W., and M. R. Winston, ed. *Dictionary of American Negro Biography*. New York: W. W. Norton., 1982.

Lundberg, G. D., and L. Bodine. "Fifty Hours for the Poor." *Journal of the American Medical Association* 258, no. 21 (1987):3157.

MacIntyre, A. *After Virtue: A Study in Moral Theory*. Notre Dame, Ind.: University of Notre Dame Press, 1981.

Maher v. Roe. 432 U.S. 464 (1973).

Malveaux, J. "The Economic Statuses of Black Families." In *Black Families*, ed. H. P. McAdoo, 133–147. Newbury Park, Calif.: Sage Publications, 1988.

Mandelblatt, J., H. Andres, J. Kerner, A. Zauber, and W. Burnett. "Determinants of Late Stage Diagnosis of Breast and Cervical Cancer: The Impact of Age, Race, Social Class and Hospital Type." *Public Health Briefs* 81, no. 5 (1991):646–649.

Mann, J. "Global AIDS: Revolution, Paradigm and Solidarity." *AIDS* 4, suppl. 1 (1990):S247–250.

———. "Global Health Problem, AIDS and Women." In *Women and AIDS Conference in Boston, MA*, 1991.

Mansell, P.W.A. "Anderson Hospital and Tumor Institute." In *AIDS: Public Policy Dimensions*, ed. J. Griggs, 131–137. New York: United Hospital Hospital Fund of New York, 1987.

Manton, K. G., C. H. Patrick, and K. W. Johnson. "Health Differentials Between Blacks and Whites: Recent Trends in Mortality and Morbidity." *Milbank Quarterly* 65, suppl. 1 (1987):129–199.

"Many Plan to Avoid AIDS Care in Practice." *Internal Medicine News* 23 (1990):1, 22.

Mariner, W. K. "Access to Health Care and Equal Protection of the Law: The Need for a New Heightened Scrutiny." *American Journal of Law and Medicine* 12, nos. 3 & 4 (1989):345–380.

Marshall, P. "Anthropology and Bioethics." *Medical Anthropology Quarterly* 6, no. 1 (1992):49–73.

Martin, S., R. Wright, and L. Clark. "Required Request for Organ Donation: Moral, Clinical and Legal Problems." *Hastings Center Report* 18, no. 3 (1988):27–34.

Maso, M. J., E. J. Gong, M. S. Jacobson, D. S. Bross, and F. P. Heald. "Anthropometric Predictors of Low Birth Weight Outcome in Teenage Pregnancy." *Journal of Adolescent Health Care* 9 (1988):188–193.

Mass, B. *Population Target: The Political Economy of Population Control in Latin America.* Toronto: Women's Press, 1976.

Mauer, M. *Young Black Men and the Criminal Justice System: A Growing National Problem.* Washington, D.C.: The Sentencing Project, 1990.

May, W. "Attitudes Toward the Newly Dead." *Hastings Center Report* 19, no. 2 (1989):3–13.

Mays, V. "AIDS Prevention in Black Populations: Methods of a Safer Kind." In *Primary Prevention of AIDS: Psychological Approaches,* ed. V. Mays, G. Albee, and S. Schneider, 264–279. Newbury Park, Calif.: Sage Publications, 1990.

McAdoo, H. P. "Black Mothers and the Extended Family Support Network." In *The Black Woman,* eds. Rodgers and Rose, 125–144. Beverly Hills, Calif.: Sage Publications, 1980.

McCarthy, S., and R. Soliz. "Establishment of a National Program of HIV-Related Grants for Home and Community Based Health Care: Federal Grants, State Management." In *VII International Conference on AIDS in Florence, Italy,* abstract W. D. 4071, 1991.

McCord, C., and H. P. Freeman. "Excess Mortality in Harlem." *New England Journal of Medicine* 322, no. 3 (1990):173–177.

McCullough, L. B. "Are Physicians Obligated to Treat Indigent Patients?" *Texas Medicine* 87 (1991):81–86.

McGinnis, J. M. "The Mary E. Switzer Lecture: Reaching the Underserved." *Journal of Allied Health* (November 1986):293–305.

McLaughlin, F. J., W. A. Altemeier, M. J. Christensen. "Randomized Trial of Comprehensive Prenatal Care for Low-Income Women: Effect of Infant Birth Weight." *Obstetrical & Gynecological Survey* 47, no. 7 (1992):473.

McNeill, W. *Plagues and People.* New York: Doubleday, 1977.

Mechanic, D. "Response Factors in Illness: The Study of Illness Behavior." *Social Psychiatry* 1 (1966):11–20.

———. *Medical Sociology: A Selective View.* New York: Free Press, 1968.

———. *The Bureaucratization of Medicine.* New York: John Wiley, 1970.

———. "Social Psychological Factors Affecting the Presentation of Bodily Complaints." *New England Journal of Medicine* 286 (1972):1132–1139.

———. *The Growth of Bureaucratic Medicine.* New York: John Wiley, 1976a.

———. "Stress, Illness, and Illness Behavior." *Journal of Human Stress* 2 (1976b):2–6.

———. "Illness Behavior, Social Adaptation, and the Illness of Illness: A Comparison of Educational and Medical Models." *Journal of Nervousness and Mental Disease* 165 (1977):79–87.

Mechanic, D., and E. H. Volkart. "Stress, Illness Behavior, and Medical Diagnoses." *American Sociological Review* 26 (1961):51–58.

Meier, A., and E. Rudwick. *From Plantation to Ghetto.* New York: Hill & Wang, 1970.

Meier, D. "The Kindergarten Tradition in High School." In *Progressive Education for the 1990s: Transforming Practice,* ed. K. Jervis and C. Montag, 135–148. New York: Teachers College Press, 1991.

Melnyk, K.A.M. "Barriers: A Critical Review of Recent Literature." *Nursing Research* 37, no. 4 (1988):198–201.

Menzel, P. T. *Strong Medicine: The Ethical Rationing of Health Care.* New York: Oxford University Press, 1990.

Merzel, C., U. Sambamoorthi, and S. Crystal. "Predictors of Inpatient Utilization in an HIV Medicaid Waiver Population." In *VII International Conference on AIDS in Florence, Italy,* abstract M.D. 4191, 1991.

Michaels, D., and C. Levine. "Projections of the Number of Motherless Youth Orphaned by AIDS in the United States." *Journal of the American Medical Association* 268, no. 24 (1992):3456–3461.

Michigan State Education Department. "Personnel Registry." Lansing, Mich., 1993.

Milano, M., I. Long, J. Eigo, D. Z. Kirschenbaum, J. D'Eramo, and T. Davis. "Access to AIDS Clinical Trials and Experimental Drugs in New York State." In *VII International Conference on AIDS in Florence, Italy,* abstract W.D. 4291, 1991.

Miles, S. H. "What Are We Teaching About Indigent Patients?" *Journal of the American Medical Association* 268 (1992):2561–2562.

Mill, J. S. *On Liberty.* Boston: Ticknor & Fields, 1859.

Miller, D., and S. Trupin. *Grandparents Who Care of San Francisco: A Program Summary.* San Francisco: published by the authors, 1990.

Miller, E. S. "Money, Politics and Democracy." *Boston Review* (March/April 1993): 5–8.

Miller, H., C. Turner, and L. Moses. *AIDS: The Second Decade.* Washington, D.C.: National Academy Press, 1990.

Miller, S. M. "Race in the Health of America." *The Milbank Quarterly* 65, suppl. 2 (1987):500–531.

Mills, C. W. *The Sociological Imagination.* New York: Oxford University Press, 1959.

Minkhoff, H. L., and J. A. Dehovitz. "Care of Women Infected with the Human Immunodeficiency Virus." *Journal of the American Medical Association* 266 (1991):2253–2258.

Minkler, M., and K. M. Roe. *Grandmothers as Caregivers: Raising Children of the Crack Cocaine Epidemic.* Beverly Hills, Calif.: Sage Publications, 1993.

Minow, M. "Critique of Pure Harmonization: Problems of Diversity and Federalism." Paper for the Georgetown University Law Center Conference on Federalism, 1989.

Mizrahi, T. *Getting Rid of Patients: Contradictions in the Socialization of Physicians.* New Brunswick, N. J.: Rutgers State University of New Jersey, 1986.

Moien, M., and L. J. Kozak. "Hospital Utilization for Patients with HIV Diagnoses: United States, 1984–1989." In *VII International Conference on AIDS in Florence, Italy,* abstract M.D. 4185, 1991.

Moore, P. A., and V. B. Weslowski. *The Care of HIV-Infected Patients in Public Hospitals: Models of Care.* National Association of Public Hospitals' AIDS Committee, 1992.

Morgan, M. *Skid Road: An Informal Portrait of Seattle.* New York: Viking Press, 1962.

Morimoto, K. "Notes on the Context for Learning." *Harvard Educational Review* 43, no. 2 (1973):245–257.

Morrison, J. L. "Illegitimacy, Sterilization, and Racism: A North Carolina Case History." *Social Science Review* 39 (1965):1–10.

Morrison, T. *Beloved.* New York: Alfred A. Knopf, 1987.

Mosner, M. "A Decade of Progress in the Management of Hypertension." *Hypertension* 5 (1983):808.

Moulder, P., A. Staal, and M. Grant. "Making the Interdisciplinary Team Approach Work." *Rehabilitation Nursing* 13, no. 6 (November/December 1988):338–339.

Moynihan, D. *The Negro Family: The Case for National Action.* U.S. Department of Labor, Office of Policy Planning and Research, 1965.

———. "The Negro Family: The Case for National Action." In *The Moynihan Report and the Politics of Controversy*, ed. L. Rainwater and W. L. Yancy, 39–132. Cambridge, Mass.: MIT Press, 1967.

Mullings, L. "Minority Women, Work, and Health." In *Double Exposure: Women's Health Hazards on the Job and at Home*, ed. Wendy Chavkin, 121–138. New York: Monthly Review Press, 1984.

Mumford, E. *Medical Sociology: Patients, Providers, and Policies.* New York: Random House, 1983.

Munn v. Illinois. 92 U.S. 124, (1876).

Murray, J. F. "The White Plague: Down and Out or Up and Going." *American Review of Respiratory Disorders* 140 (1989):1788–1795.

National Association for Sickle Cell Disease. *Position Paper on Prenatal Diagnosis of Sickle Cell Anemia.* Los Angeles, Calif., 1990.

National Center for Children in Poverty. *Five Million Children: A Statistical Profile of Our Poorest Young Citizens.* New York: Columbia University School of Public Health, 1990.

National Center for Health Statistics. *Health United States 1989.* Washington, D.C.: Department of Health and Human Services, U.S. Government Printing Office, 1990.

———. *Health United States, 1990.* Washington, D.C.: Department of Health and Human Services, 1990. PHS 91-1232.

National Commission for the Protection of Human Subjects of Biomedical and Behavioral Research. *The Belmont Report: Ethical Principles & Guidelines for the Protection of Human Subjects of Research.* Bethesda, Md., 1978. DHEW (OS) 78-0012-78-0014.

National Commission on AIDS. *Hearings on HIV Disease in African American Communities.* Washington, DC: U.S. Government Printing Office, 1990.

———. *America Living with AIDS: Transforming Anger, Fear, and Indifference into Action.* Washington, D.C.: National Commission on AIDS, U.S. Government Printing Office, 1991a.

———. *HIV Disease in Correctional Facilities.* Washington, D.C.: U.S. Government Printing Office, 1991b.

———. *The Twin Epidemics of Substance Abuse and HIV.* Washington, D.C.: U.S. Government Printing Office, 1991c.

National Commission on Excellence in Education. *A Nation at Risk: The Imperative for Educational Reform.* Washington, D.C.: U.S. Government Printing Office, 1983.

National Institute of Diabetes and Digestive and Kidney Diseases. *The United States Renal Data System (USRDS) Annual Report.* Bethesda, Md., 1989. A1-11.

National Institute of Drug Abuse. *The Homeless Intravenous Drug Users and the AIDS Epidemic.* 1989.

National Sickle Cell Anemia Control Act. (1972): Public Law 92-294.

New York Department of Health. *Mary Lasker Heart and Hypertension Program.* 1983–88.

New York Department of Public Health. Bureau of Health Statistics Analysis, 1986.

Newmann, F. M., and D. W. Oliver. "Education and Community." *Harvard Educational Review* 37, no. 1 (1967):61–106.

Nichter, M., and E. Cartwright. "Saving the Children for the Tobacco Industry." *Medical Anthropology Quarterly* 5, no. 3 (1991):236–256.

Nobles, W. W., L. Goddard, and W. E. Cavil. *The Culture of Drugs in the Black Community.* Oakland: Black Family Institute, 1987.

Noddings, N. "An Ethic of Caring and Its Implications for Instructional Arrangements." *American Journal of Education* 96, no. 2 (1988):215–230.

Nozick, R. *Anarchy, State and Utopia.* New York: Basic Books, 1974.

Oakes, J. *Keeping Track: How Schools Structure Inequality.* New Haven, Conn.: Yale University Press, 1985.

Ogbu, J. "Cultural Discontinuities and Schooling." *Anthropology and Education Quarterly* 13, no. 4 (1982):290–307.

Olds, D. L., C. R. Henderson, R. Tattelbaum, and R. Chamberlain. "Improving the Delivery of Prenatal Care and Outcomes of Pregnancy: A Randomized Trial of Nurse Home Visitation." *Pediatrics* 77 (1986):16–28.

Olson, C. M. "Health Educators Turn to Black Community Leaders, Organizations, Other Strengths" (letter to the editor). *Journal of the American Medical Association* 261, no. 2 (1989):194–195.

Omi, M., and H. Winant. *Racial Formation in the United States, from the 1960s to the 1980s.* New York: Routledge and Kegan Paul, 1986.

Omnibus Genetics Bill. "The National Sickle Cell Anemia, Cooley's Anemia, Tay-Sachs, and Genetic Diseases Act." *Title IV of Public Law 84-278,* 1976.

Osborn, J. "AIDS: Politics, and Science." *New England Journal of Medicine* 318 (1988): 444–447.

Osbourne, N., and M. D. Feit. "The Use of Race in Medical Research." *Journal of the American Medical Association* 267, no. 2 (1992):275–279.

Otto, H. J. "Communication Is the Key." In *Parents-Children-Teachers: Communication,* ed. Association for Childhood Education International—Bulletin No. 28-A. 1969.

Overall, C. *Ethics and Human Reproduction: A Feminist Analysis.* Boston: Allen & Unwin, 1987.

Palca, J. "NIH Unveils Plan for Women's Health Project." *Science* 254 (1991):792.

Pallas, A. M., G. Natriello, and E. L. McDill. "The Changing Nature of the Disadvantaged Population: Current Dimensions and Future Trends." *Educational Researcher* 18, no. 5 (1989):16–22.

Panos, D. *The 3rd Epidemic: Repercussions of the Fear of AIDS.* London: Panos Institute and the Norwegian Red Cross, 1990.

Park, R. "Graduating Students' Debt and Speciality Choices." *Academic Medicine* 65 (1990):485–486.

Payne, L. "Forced Sterilization for the Poor." *San Francisco Chronicle*, February 26, 1974.

Pellegrino, E. D. "Toward an Expanded Medical Ethics: The Hippocratic Ethic Revisited." In *In Search of the Modern Hippocrates*, ed. Roger J. Bulger, 45–64. Iowa City: University of Iowa Press, 1987.

———. "The Problems and Necessity of Transcultural Dialogue." In *African-American Perspectives on Biomedical Ethics*, ed. H. E. Flack and E. D. Pellegrino, v-ix. Washington, D.C.: Georgetown University Press, 1992.

Pepper, B. "A Public Policy for the Longterm Mentally Ill: A Positive Alternative to Reinstitutionalization." *American Journal of Orthopsychiatry* 57 (1987):452–457.

Perkins, K. A. "The Shortage of Cadaver Donor Organs for Transplantation: Can Psychology Help?" *American Psychologist* 42 (1987):921–930.

Perrow, C., and M. F. Guillen. *The AIDS Disaster: The Failure of Organizations in New York and the Nation.* New Haven, Conn.: Yale University Press, 1990.

Pinderhughes, E. *Understanding Race, Ethnicity, and Power: The Key to Efficacy in Clinical Practice.* New York: Free Press, 1989.

Planned Parenthood v. Casey 1125. Ct. 2791 (1992).

Poelker v. Doe 432 U.S. 519 (1977).

Politzer, R. M., D. L. Harris, M. H. Gaston, and F. Mullen. "Primary Care Physicians and the Medically Underserved." *Journal of the American Medical Association* 266 (1991):104–108.

Popenoe, P. *The Conservation of Family.* Baltimore: Williams & Wilkins Co., 1926.

Popkin, S. J., W. A. Johnson, M. Clatts, W. Wiebel, and S. Deren. "Homelessness and Risk Behaviors among IVDUs in Chicago and New York." In *VII International Conference on AIDS in Florence, Italy*, abstract M.D. 4004, 1991.

Porter, A. C., and M. Brophy. "Synthesis of Research on Good Teaching: Insights from the Work of the Institute for Research on Teaching." *Educational Leadership* 45, no. 8 (1988):74–85.

Potterat, J., N. Spencer, D. Woodhouse, and J. Muth. "Partner Notification in the Control of Human Immunodeficiency Virus Infection." *American Journal of Public Health* 79 (1989):874–876.

Powell, A. G., E. Farrar, and D. K. Cohen. *The Shopping Mall High School: Winners and Losers in the Educational Marketplace.* Boston: Houghton Mifflin Co., 1985.

Pratt, J. H., J. J. Jones, J. Z. Miller, M. A. Wagner, and N. S. Fineberg. "Racial Differences in Aldosterone Secretion and Plasma Aldosterone Concentration in Children." *New England Journal of Medcine* 321, no. 17 (1989):1152–1157.

President's Commission for the Study of Ethical Problems in Medicine and Biomedical and Behavioral Research. *Making Health Care Decisions.* Washington, D.C.: U.S. Government Printing Office, 1982.

———. *Final Report: Summing Up.* Washington, D.C.: U.S. Government Printing Office, 1983.

———. "Patterns of Access to Health Care." In *Securing Access to Health Care*, 49–108. 1. Washington, D.C.: U.S. Government Printing Office, 1983.

———. *Securing Access to Health Care: A Report on the Ethical Implications of Differences in the Availability of Health Services.* Vol. 1. Washington, D.C.: U.S. Government Printing Office, 1983.

President's Commission on the Health Care Needs of the Nation, 14–16. Washington, D.C.: U.S. Government Printing Office, 1953.

Presser, H. B. *Sterilization and Fertility: Decline in Puerto Rico.* Berkeley, Calif.: Institute of International Studies, 1973.

Public Health Service. *Final Report of the Tuskegee Syphilis Study Ad Hoc Advisory Panel.* 1973.

Public Health Service. *Healthy People 2000: National Health Promotion and Disease Prevention.* 1990.

Purvis, A. "A Perilous Gap." *Time—Special Issue on Women,* Fall 1990, 67.

Quinn, S. "AIDS and HIV Testing: Implications for Health Education." *Journal of Health Education* 23, no. 2 (1992):95–100.

———. "AIDS and the African-American Woman: The Triple Burden of Race, Class and Gender." *Health Education Quarterly* 20, no. 3 (1993):305.

Rawls, J. *A Theory of Justice.* Cambridge, Mass.: Harvard University Press, 1971.

———. "Social Unity and the Primary Goods." In *Utilitarianism and Beyond,* ed. A. K. Sen and B. Williams. Cambridge: Cambridge University Press, 1982.

Raywid, M. S. "Community and Schools: A Prolegomenon." *Teachers College Record* 90, no. 2 (1988):197–210.

Reichman, L. B., C. P. Felton, and J. R. Edsall. "Drug Dependence: A Possible New Risk Factor for Tuberculosis Disease." *Archives of Internal Medicine* 139 (1979): 337–339.

Reider, H. L., G. M. Cauthen, G. W. Comstock, and D. E. Snider. "Epidemiology of Tuberculosis in the United States." *Epidemiology Review* 11 (1989):79–98.

Reillo, M., and M. J. McMahon. "The Economic Impact of AIDS on the Health Care System in the United States." In *VII International Conference on AIDS in Florence, Italy,* abstract M.D. 4290, 1991.

Reilly, P. R. *Genetics, Law, and Social Policy.* Cambridge, Mass.: Harvard University Press, 1977.

———. *The Final Solution.* Baltimore: Johns Hopkins University Press, 1991.

Rene, A. A. "Racial Differences in Mortality: Blacks and Whites." In *Health Care Issues in Black America: Policies, Problems, and Prospects,* ed. W. Jones and M. F. Rice, 20–41. Westport, Conn.: Greenwood Press, 1987.

Rhame, F. S., and D. G. Maki. "The Case for Wider Use of Testing for HIV Infection." *New England Journal of Medicine* 320 (1989):1248–1254.

Richardson, E. *Responsibility and Responsiveness (II): A Report on the HEW Potential for the Seventies.* Washington, D.C.: U.S. Secretary of Health, Education, and Welfare, 1973.

Robinson, J. C. "Trends in Racial Inequality and in Exposure to Work-Related Hazards, 1968–1986." *The Milbank Quarterly* 65 (Supplement 2) (1987):404–420.

Rodrique, J. M. "The Black Community and the Birth Control Movement." In *Unequal Sisters: A Multi-Cultural Reader in U. S. Women's History,* ed. E. C. Du Bois and V. L. Ruiz, 333–344. New York: Routledge, 1990.

Roe v. Wade. 410 U.S. 113 (1973).

Rolfs, R. T., M. Goldberg, and R. G. Sharrar. "Risk Factors for Syphilis: Cocaine Use and Prostitution." *American Journal of Public Health* 80, no. 7 (1990):853–857.

Rosen, G. *Preventive Medicine in the U.S.: 1890–1975.* New York: Prodist, 1977.

Rostand, S. G., G. Brown, K. A. Kirk, E. A. Rutsky, and H. P. Dustan. "Renal Insufficiency in Treated Essential Hypertension." *New England Journal of Medicine* 320 (1989):684–688.

Rostand, S. G., K. A. Kirk, and E. A. Rutsky. "Racial Differences in the Incidence of Treatment for End Stage Renal Disease." *New England Journal of Medicine* 306 (1982):1276–1279.

Rowan, B. "Commitment and Control: Alternative Strategies for the Organizational Design of Schools." In *Review of Research in Education,* ed. C. Cazden, 353–389. Vol. 16. Washington, D.C.: American Educational Research Association, 1990.

Rowley, P. T. "Prenatal Diagnosis for Sickle Cell Disease: A Survey of the United States and Canada." *Annals of the New York Academy of Sciences* 565 (1989):48–52.

Rowley, P. T., S. Loader, C. J. Sutera, M. Walden, and A. Kozyra. "Prenatal Screening for Hemoglobinopathies. I. A. Prospective Regional Trial." *American Journal of Human Genetics* 48 (1991a):439–446.

———. "Prenatal Screening for Hemoglobinopathies. III. Applicability of the Health Belief Model." *American Journal of Human Genetics* 48 (1991b):452–459.

Rubin, A. J. "Abortion Funding Rebuff Shows House Divided." *Congressional Quarterly Weekly Report* 51, no. 27 (1993):1735–1739.

Rush, D., N. L. Sloan, J. Leighton, J. M. Alvir, D. G. Horvitz, W. B. Searer, G. C. Garbowski, S. S. Johnson, K. A. Kulka, and M. Holt. "The National WIC Evaluation: Evaluation of the Special Supplemental Food Program for Women, Infants, and Children. V. Longitudinal Study of Pregnant Women." *American Journal of Clinical Nutrition* 48 (Supplement 2) (1988):439–483.

Rushmer, R. F. *Humanizing Health Care: Alternative Futures for Medicine.* Cambridge, Mass.: MIT Press, 1976.

Rust v. Sullivan. 59 U.S.L.W. 4451, (1991).

Ryan White CARE Act. *Amendment to the United States Public Health Services Act, Title XXVI—"HIV Health Care Services Program."* 1990.

Sabatier, R. *Blaming Others.* London: Panos Publications, 1988.

Sadd, S., and D. Young. "Non-medical Treatment of Indigent Alcoholics: A Review of Recent Findings." *Alcohol Health and Research World* 11, no. 3 (1987):48–49.

Salem, E., and P. Lenihan. "Financing HIV-Related Health Care in Chicago and Cook County." In *VII International Conference on AIDS in Florence, Italy,* abstract M.D. 4278, 1991.

Salvo, J. J., M. G. Powers, and R. S. Cooney. "Contraceptive Use and Sterilization Among Puerto Rican Women." *Family Planning Perspectives* 24, no. 5 (1992): 219–223.

Sanders, C. J. "Problems and Limitations of an African-American Perspective in Biomedical Ethics: A Theological View." In *African-American Perspectives on Biomedical Ethics,* ed. H. E. Flack and E. D. Pellegrino, 165–172. Washington, D.C.: Georgetown University Press, 1992.

Sanger, M. *Autobiography.* New York: W. W. Norton, 1938.

Saunders, E. "Higher Black Cancer Rates Related to Socioeconomics." *National Medical Association News*, March/April 1991, 6.

Savitt, T. L. *Medicine and Slavery—Disease and Health Care of Blacks in Antebellum Virginia*. Urbana: University of Illinois Press, 1978.

Scarborough, D. *On the Trail of Negro Folk-songs*. Hatboro, Penn.: Folklore Associates [Original edition published by Cambridge, Mass.: Harvard University Press, 1925], 1963.

Schensul, J., and L. Allen. *Pediatric Impairments in Hispanic Children*. Final report for the Pediatric Research and Training Center of the University of Connecticut, 1985.

Schensul, J., D. Donelli-Hess, R. Martinez, and M. Borrero. "Urban Comadronas." In *Collaborative Research and Social Policy: Anthropology in Action*, ed. D. Stull and J. J. Schensul, 9–32. Boulder, Colo.: Westview Press, 1987.

Schensul, J., and S. Schensul. "Collaborative Research: Methods of Inquiry for Social Change." In *The Handbook of Qualitative Research in Education*, ed. M. D. LeCompte, W. L. Millroy, and J. Goetz, 161–199. New York: Academic Press, 1992.

Schensul, J., T. Wetle, and M. Torres. *Educational Materials and Innovative Dissemination Strategies: Alzheimer's Disease among Puerto Rican Elderly*. The Puerto Rican Alzheimer's Education Project—Curriculum and visual materials prepared for the national dissemination under contract with the Administration on Aging, Hartford, Conn.: Institute for Community Research, 1992.

Schensul, S. L., and J. Schensul. "Helping Resource Use in a Puerto Rican Community." *Urban Anthropology* 11, no. 1 (1982):59–80.

Schiff, R. L., D. Goldberg, and D. A. Ansell. "Access to Health Care." In *Assessing Quality Care: Perspectives for Clinicians*, ed. R. P. Wenzel, 139–156. Baltimore: Williams & Wilkins, 1991.

Schlesinger, M. "Paying the Price: Medical Care, Minorities and the Newly Competitive Health Care System." *Milbank Quarterly* 65, suppl. 2 (1987):270–298.

Schmidt, R. M., and E. M. Brosius. *Basic Laboratory Methods of Hemoglobinopathy Detection*. U.S. Department of Health, Education and Welfare, Public Health Service, Centers for Disease Control, 1972. CDC 76-8266.

Schorr, L. B. *Within Our Reach: Breaking the Cycle of Disadvantage*. New York: Anchor Press, 1988.

Schroeder, S. A., J. S. Zones, and J. A. Showstach. "Academic Medical as a Public Trust." *Journal of the American Medical Association* 262 (1989):803–812.

Schumpeter, J. *Capitalism, Socialism and Democracy*. New York: Harper Torchbooks, 1989.

Schwab, J. J. "Education and the State: Learning Community." In *The Great Ideas Today, 1976*, 234–271. Chicago: Encyclopaedia Britannica, 1976.

Secundy, M. G., with L. L. Nixon, ed. *Trials, Tribulations, and Celebrations: African American Perspectives on Health, Illness, Aging and Loss*. Yarmouth, Me.: Intercultural Press, 1992.

Select Committee on Children, Youth and Families of the United States House of Representatives. *Opportunities for Success: Cost-Effective Programs for Children, Update 1990*. Washington, D.C.: U.S. Government Printing Office, 1990.

Shannon, C., and D. Saleebey. "Training Child Welfare Workers to Cope with Burnout." *Child Welfare* 59 (1980):463–468.

Shaw, M. W. "Conditional Prospective Rights of the Fetus." *Journal of Legal Medicine* 5 (1984):63–115.

Shea, S., and M. T. Fullilove. "Entry of Black and Other Minority Students into U.S. Medical Schools: Historical Perspective and Recent Trends." *New England Journal of Medicine* 313, no. 15 (1985):933–940.

Sherer, R. "AIDS Policy into the 1990s." *Journal of the American Medical Association* 263 (1990):1972–1974.

Shilts, R. *And the Band Played On.* New York: St. Martin's Press, 1987.

Shklar, J. N. *The Faces of Injustice.* New Haven, Conn.: Yale University Press, 1990.

Shor, I. "Equality Is Excellence: Transforming Teacher Education and the Learning Process." *Harvard Educational Review* 56, no. 4 (1986):406–426.

Short, P., A. Monheit, and K. Beuregard. *A Profile of Uninsured Americans, National Medical Expenditures Survey Research Findings 1.* National Center for Health Services Research and Health Care Technology Assessment, Department of Health and Human Services, Rockville, Md., Public Health Service, 1989. PHS 89-3442.

Simon, B. L. "Rethinking Empowerment." *Journal of Progressive Human Services* 1, 1(1990):27–39.

Simonds, R. J., and M. F. Rogers. "Epidemiology of HIV in Children and Other Populations." In *HIV Infection and Developmental Disabilities: A Resource for Service Providers,* ed. A. C. Crocker, H. J. Cohen, and T. A. Kastner, 3–13. Baltimore: Paul H. Brooks Publishing, 1992.

Singer, M. "Cure, Care and Control: An Ectopic Encounter with Biomedical Obstetrics." In *Encounters with Biomedicine: Case Studies in Medical Anthropology,* ed. H. Baer, 249–265. New York: Gordon & Breach Science Publishers, 1987.

Singer, M., L. Davison, and G. Gerdes. "Culture, Critical Theory and Reproductive Illness Behavior in Haiti." *Medical Anthropology Quarterly* 2 (1988):370–385.

Singer, M., Z. Jia, J. Schensul, M. Weeks, and J. B. Page. "AIDS and the IV Drug User: The Local Context in Prevention Efforts." *Medical Anthropology* 14, 1 (1992a):1–22.

Singer, S., J. Restrepo, J. Zhongke, M. Weeks, and J. J. Schensul. "Culturally Specific AIDS Prevention for IV Drug Users: It Works!" In *NIDA: Third Annual National AIDS Demonstration Research Projects Conference and Annual Publication,* 1992b.

Sirgio, M. A., C. A. Cook, and J. B. Modrak. "Hypertensive Therapy in Blacks: Significance of Pathophysiologic Observations." *Journal of Clinical Hypertension* 1 (1986):1–6.

Sloan, F. A., M. A. Morrisey, and J. Valvona. "Case Shifting and the Medicare Prospective Payment System." *American Journal of Public Health* 78 (1988):553–556.

Small, C. B., G. Laper, and L. Ricci. "Homelessness in Patients with the Acquired Immune Deficiency Syndrome." In *IV International Conference on AIDS in Stockholm, Sweden,* abstract 197, 1988.

Smith, R. "Muhammad Warns Blacks to Beware: Social AIDS." *Eclipse: The Black Student News Magazine of the University of Maryland* 21 (1988):6.

Snider, D. E., and W. L. Roper. "The New Tuberculosis." *New England Journal of Medicine* 326 (1992):703–705.

Stamler, J., W. F. Redlinger, G. D. Algera, and R. H. Roberts. "Hypertension

Screening of One Million Americans: Community Hypertension Evaluation Clinic (CHEC) Program: 1973–1975." *Journal of the American Medical Association* 235 (1976):2299–2305.

Stanworth, M. "Reproductive Technologies and the Deconstruction of Motherhood." In *Reproductive Technologies: Gender, Motherhood and Medicine*, ed. M. Stanworth, 10–35. Minneapolis: University of Minnesota Press, 1987.

Starfield, B. *The Effectiveness of Medical Care: Validating Clinical Wisdom.* Baltimore and London: Johns Hopkins University Press, 1985.

———. "Primary Care and Health." *Journal of the American Medical Association* 266 (1991):2268–2271.

———. *Primary Care.* New York: Oxford University Press, 1992.

Stark, L. "A Century of Alcohol and Homelessness." *Alcohol and Health Research World II* 3 (Spring 1987).

Starr, P. "Medical Care and the Pursuit of Equality in America." In *Security Access to Health Care*, ed. President's Commission for the Study of Ethical Problems in Medicine and Biomedical and Behavioral Research. 2 (Appendix A). Washington, D.C.: U.S. Government Printing Office, 1982.

———. *The Social Transformation of American Medicine.* New York: Basic Books, 1982.

Stein, M. D., J. Piette, V. Mor, T. J. Wachtel, J. Fleishman, K. H. Mayer, and C. C. Carpenter. "Differences in Access to Zidovudine (AZT) Among Symptomatic HIV-Infected Persons." *Journal of General Internal Medicine* 6 (1991): 35–40.

Stell, L. K. In *Troubling Problems in Medical Ethics*, ed. M. D. Basson, R. E. Lipson, and D. L. Ganos, 213–225. New York: Alan R. Liss, 1982.

Sternberg, C., R. Sherer, G. Cohen, M. Cohen, M. Williamson, and M. Driscoll. "The Cook County HIV Primary Care Center: Integrated Service Delivery in a Model HIV Primary Care Center." In *International Conference on AIDS*, abstract P.O. D21-4020, 1993.

Stevens, R. A., and R. Stevens. *Welfare Medicine in America: A Case Study of Medicaid.* New York: Free Press, 1974.

Stockbauer, J. W. "WIC Prenatal Participation and Its Relation to Pregnancy Outcomes in Missouri: A Second Look." *American Journal of Public Health* 77 (1987):813–818.

Stoddard, T. B. and W. Reiman. "AIDS and the Rights of the Individual: Toward a More Sophisticated Understanding of Discrimination." *The Milbank Quarterly* 68 (Supplement 1) (1990):143–174.

Stokes, J., and J. Greenstone. "Helping Black Grandparents and Older Parents Cope with Child Rearing: A Group Method." *Child Welfare* 60, no. 10 (1981):691–701.

Svensson, C. K. "Representation of American Blacks in Clinical Trials of New Drugs." *Journal of the American Medical Association* 261, no. 2 (1989):263–265.

Swinton, D. "The Economic Status of African Americans: 'Permanent' Poverty and Inequality." In *The State of Black America 1991*, ed. J. Dewart, 53–63. New York: National Urban League, 1991.

Tapper, M. "Tuberculosis." In *Burroughs Wellcome Conference on Clinical Management of HIV Disease in Chicago IL.* 1992.

Tavris, C. *The Mismeasure of Woman.* New York: Simon & Schuster, 1992.

Taylor, J. "Toward a Philosophy of Recovery: A Prolegomenon to Any Future African American Ethic." *American Philosophical Association Newsletters* 191 (Fall 1992):14–18.

Thomas, S. "Evaluation of Community Based AIDS Education and Risk Reduction Projects in the Black Community." *Journal of Health Education* 22 (1991):24–29.

Thomas, S., and B. Hodges. "Assessing AIDS Knowledge, Attitudes, and Risk Behaviors Among Black and Hispanic Homosexual and Bisexual Men." *Journal of Sex Education and Therapy* 17, no. 2 (1991):116–124.

Thomas, S., and C. H. Morgan. "Evaluation of Community Based AIDS Education and Risk Reduction Projects in Ethnic and Racial Minority Communities: A Survey of Projects Funded by the U.S. Public Health Service." *Evaluation and Program Planning* 14, no. 4 (1991):247–255.

———. "The Burdens of Race and History on Black Americans' Attitudes Toward Needle Exchange Policy to Prevent HIV Disease." *Journal of Public Health Policy* 14 (1993):320–347.

Thomas, S., and S. Quinn. "The Tuskegee Syphilis Study 1932–1972: Implications for HIV Education and AIDS Risk Education Programs in the Black Community." *American Journal of Public Health* 81, no. 11 (1991):1498–1505.

Thomas, S. B. "Community Health Advocacy for Racial and Ethnic Minorities in the United States: Issues and Challenges for Health Education." *Health Education Quarterly* 17 (1990):13–19.

Thompson, L. H. *Within-School Discrimination: Inadequate Title VI Enforcement by the Office for Civil Rights.* Washington, D.C.: General Accounting Office, 1991.

Titmuss, R. M. *The Gift Relationship: From Human Blood to Social Policy.* New York: Vintage Books, 1971.

Tonnies, F. *Community and Society.* Ed. C. P. Loomis. New York: Harper and Row, 1963.

Treichler, P. A. "AIDS, Gender and Biomedical Discourse: Current Contests for Meaning." In *AIDS: The Burden of History*, ed. E. Fee and D. M. Fox, 190–266. Berkeley: University of California Press, 1988.

Trevino, F. M., and A. J. Moss. *Health Indicators for Hispanic, Black and White Americans.* Vital and Health Statistics, Series 10, No. 148, ed. U.S. Department of Health and Human Services. Washington, D.C.: U.S. Government Printing Office, 1984.

Trevino, F. M., M. E. Moyer, R. Burciaga Valdez, and C. A. Stroup-Benham. "Health Insurance Coverage and Utilization of Health Services by Mexican Americans, Mainland Puerto Ricans, and Cuban Americans." *Journal of the American Medical Association* 265, no. 2 (1991):233–237.

Tribe, L. H. *Abortion: The Clash of Absolutes.* New York: W. W. Norton., 1990.

Tyack, D. B. *The One Best System: A History of American Urban Education.* Cambridge, Mass.: Harvard University Press, 1974.

U.S. Bureau of the Census. *Money Income and Poverty Status of Families and Persons in the United States: 1988.* Washington, D.C.: U.S. Government Printing Office, 1989.

U.S. Gallup Organization. *Public Attitudes Toward Organ Donation.* 1990.

Unger, R. M. "The Critical Legal Issues Movement." *Harvard Law Review* 96 (1983): 561–675.

United Network for Organ Sharing. *Cadaveric Donor Demographics Transplant Recipients by Race and Organ.* Table of Race by Censor, 1990.

Vanderkooi, R. "A Harbor Light for Chicago's Skid Row." Unpublished paper for the Salvation Army Historical Writing Contest, 1982.

Veatch, R. M. *A Theory of Medical Ethics.* New York: Basic Books, 1981.

———. *Medical Ethics.* Boston: Jones & Bartlett, 1989.

Verby, J. E., J. P. Newell, S. A. Anderson, and W. M. Swentko. "Changing the Medical School Curriculum to Improve Patient Access to Primary Care." *Journal of the American Medical Association* 266 (1991):110–113.

Vermund, S. "Personal Communication." Epidemiology Branch, National Institute of Health, October 1991.

Voors, A. W., T. A. Foster, R. R. Frerichs, L. S. Webber, and G. S. Berensoon. "Studies of Blood Pressure in Children Ages 5–14 in a Total Biracial Community: The Boagulusa Heart Study." *Circulation* 54 (1976):319–327.

Waitzkin, H. *The Politics of Medical Encounters: How Patients and Doctors Deal with Social Problems.* New Haven, Conn.: Yale University Press, 1991.

Wakeford, R. E., and R. Stephney. "Obstacles to Organ Donation." *British Journal of Surgery* 76, no. 5 (1989):435–439.

Walle, T. W., R. P. Byington, C. D. Furberg, K. M. McIntyre, and P. S. Vokonas. "Biological Determinants of Propranolol Disposition: Results from 1308 Patients in the Beta-Blocker Heart Attack Trial." *Clinical Pharmacology and Therapeutics* 38 (1985):509–518.

Watson, W. H., ed. *Black Folk Medicine: The Therapeutic Significance of Faith and Trust.* New Brunswick, N.J.: Transaction Books, 1984.

Webster v. Reproductive Health Service. 492 U.S. 490 (1989).

Weeks, M., ed. *Community Outreach Prevention Effort: Designs in Culturally Appropriate AIDS Intervention.* Hartford, Conn.: Institute for Community Research, 1991.

Wegman, M. E. "Annual Summary of Vital Statistics." *Pediatrics* 86 (1990):835–847.

———. "Annual Summary of Vital Statistics." *Pediatrics* 90 (1992):835–845.

Weinberg, D. S., and H. W. Murray. "Coping with AIDS: The Special Problems of New York City." *New England Journal of Medicine* 317 (1987):1469–1473.

Weisz, G., ed. *Social Science Perspectives on Medical Ethics.* Dordrecht: Kluwer Academic Publishers, 1990.

Welter, B. "The Cult of True Womanhood: 1820–1860." *American Quarterly* 18 (1966):152.

Wennecker, M. B., and A. M. Epstein. "Racial Inequalities in the Use of Procedures for Patients with Ischemic Heart Disease in Massachusetts." *Journal of American Medical Association* 261 (1989):253–257.

Wesley, C. H. *International Library of Negro Life and History. The Quest for Equality, From Civil War to Civil Rights.* New York: Publishers Co., 1968.

West, C. *American Evasion of Philosophy: A Genealogy of Pragmatism.* Madison, Wisc.: University of Wisconsin Press, 1989.

Wetle, T., J. J. Schensul, M. Torres, and M. Mayen. "Identifying Symptoms of Alzheimer's Disease Among Elderly Puerto Ricans and Their Family Caregivers." *Newsletter of the University of Connecticut Travelers Center on Aging,* 1989.

White, J. L. *The Psychology of Blacks: An Afro-American Perspective.* Englewood Cliffs, N.J.: Prentice-Hall, 1984.

Wilcox, S. K., P. Schram, G. Lappan, and P. Lanier. *The Role of a Learning Community in Changing Preservice Teachers' Knowledge and Beliefs About Mathematics Education.* East Lansing, Mich.: National Center for Research on Teacher Education, 1991, 91–1.

Wilkin, G., M. Mukenge, M. Guttman, A. Moncrieff-Arrarte, K. Glastris, B. Burgower, and A. L. Stern. "The Men Who Created Crack." *U.S. News and World Report* 11, no. 8 (1991):44–53.

Wilkinson, J. H. *From Brown to Bakke.* New York: Oxford University Press, 1981.

Williams, B. *Ethics and the Limits of Philosophy.* Cambridge, Mass.: Harvard University Press, 1985.

Willis, D. P., ed. *Health Policies and Black Americans.* New Brunswick, N.J.: Transaction Publishers, 1987.

Wilson, C., and L. Wright. "Enhancing Access to Knowledge Through School and District Organization." In *Access to Knowledge: An Agenda for Our Nation's Schools,* eds. J. I. Goodlad and P. Keating, 223–236. New York: College Entrance Examination Board, 1990.

Wilson, W. J. *The Truly Disadvantaged: The Inner City, the Underclass, and Public Policy.* Chicago: University of Chicago Press, 1987.

Winter, G. *Caring for the Uninsured and the Underinsured—A Communication from the Front Lines* (in press).

Wise, P. H., M. Kotelchuck, M. L. Wilson, and M. Mills. "Racial and Socioeconomic Disparity in Childhood Mortality in Boston." *New England Journal of Medicine* 313 (1985):360–366.

Wofsy, C. B. "Prevention of HIV Transmission." In *The Medical Management of AIDS,* ed. M. A. Sande and P. A. Volberding, 38–56. Philadelphia: W. B. Saunders Co., 1990.

Woolhander, S., and D. Himmelstein. "Reverse Targeting of Preventive Care Due to Lack of Health Insurance." *Journal of the American Medical Association* 259 (1989):2572–2575.

Woolhandler, S., and D. U. Himmelstein. "Militarism and Mortality: An International Analysis of Arms Spending and Infant Death Rates." *Lancet* (June 1985): 1375–1378.

Woolhandler, S., and D. U. Himmelstein. "Resolving the Cost/Access Conflict: The Case for a National Health Program." *Journal of General Internal Medicine* 4 (1989):54–60.

World Health Organization. *World AIDS Day Newsletter,* No. 7, June/July 1991.

Wright, J. D., and E. Weber. *Homelessness and Health.* Washington D.C.: McGraw-Hill, 1987.

Yankauer, A. "What Infant Mortality Tells Us." *American Journal of Public Health* 80 (1990):653–654.

Yanker, G., ed. *Prop Art: Over 1000 Contemporary Political Posters.* New York: Darien House, 1972.

Yates, G. L. "Health-Risk Profile Comparisons of Runaway and Non-runaway Youths." *American Journal of Public Health* 78, 37 (1988):820–821.

Yelin, E. H., R. M. Greenblatt, H. Hollander, and J. R. McMaster. "The Impact of HIV-Related Illness on Employment." *American Journal of Public Health* 81 (1991):79–84.

Young, L. S., and S. L. Melnick. "Forsaken Lives, Abandoned Dreams: What Will Compel Us to Act?" *Harvard Educational Review* 58, no. 3 (1988):380–394.

Young, L. S., G. Sykes, J. Featherstone, R. F. Elmore, and K. Devaney. *Tomorrow's Schools: Principles for the Design of Professional Development Schools.* East Lansing, Mich.: Holmes Group, 1990.

Zhou, H-H. "Racial Differences in Drug Response—Altered Sensitivity to and Clearance of Propranolol in Men of Chinese Descent as Compared to American Whites." *New England Journal of Medicine* 320, no. 9 (1989):565–570.

Zusman, J., R. M. Freidman, and B. L. Levin. "Moving Treatment into the Community. Implications for Psychiatry." *Psychiatric Quarterly* 59 (1988):140–149.

Index

About the Editors and Contributors

ANITA L. ALLEN-CASTELLITO is a professor of law at Georgetown University Law Center.

WAYNE B. ARNASON is minister of Thomas Jefferson Memorial Church (Unitarian Universalist) in Charlottesville, Virginia.

NEAL BAER is a medical student at Harvard University and plans to specialize in pediatrics.

JAMES E. BOWMAN is professor in the Departments of Pathology and Medicine, Committees on Genetics, and African and African-American Studies, and senior scholar at the Center for Clinical Medical Ethics at the University of Chicago.

HOWARD BRODY is professor of family practice and professor of philosophy, as well as director of the Center for Ethics and Humanities in the Life Sciences, at Michigan State University.

KATE BROWN is the assistant director for health policy at the Creighton University Center for Health Policy and Ethics, and Assistant Professor in Creighton University School of Medicine.

CLIVE O. CALLENDER is the Transplant Center director at Howard University Hospital.

CHRISTINE K. CASSEL is a professor of medicine, a professor of public policy, and chief, section of General Internal Medicine at the University of Chicago, Pritzker School of Medicine.

ANGELA Y. DAVIS is a professor in the History of Consciousness program at the University of California, Santa Cruz.

PATRICK DOWLING is chairman of the Department of Family Medicine at L.A. County Harbor-UCLA Medical Center and associate clinical professor at the UCLA School of Medicine.

ANNETTE DULA is a research associate at the Center for the Study of Ethnicity and Race in America (CSERA) at the University of Colorado. She was a fellow at the University of Chicago Center for Clinical Medical Ethics. At the University of Massachusetts Medical Center she taught everyday ethics to interns and residents in neighborhood clinics. She has participated in numerous conferences on the teaching and practice of health care ethics from a cultural perspective, including the Society for the Teachers of Family Practice Medicine, the Society for Bioethics Consultations, the American Public Health Association, and the American Association for the Advancement of Science. Most recently, Dula served on the bioethics committee of the President's Health Task Force in Washington, D.C.

JOSEPH FEATHERSTONE is in charge of one of the new teacher education programs at Michigan State University.

WARREN J. FERGUSON is vice president of medical services at the Family Health and Social Service Center, Worcester, Massachusetts, and assistant professor in the Department of Family and Community Medicine at the University of Massachusetts Medical Center.

J.L.A. GARCIA is professor of philosophy at Rutgers University.

SARA GOERING is a doctoral candidate in philosophy and is affiliated with the Center for Values and Social Policy at the University of Colorado at Boulder. She is past editor of *From the Center*, a newsletter produced by the Philosophy Department at Boulder. She has previously done work in neuropsychology and is currently specializing in medical ethics.

DAVID GOLDBERG is an attending physician in the Division of General Medicine at Cook County Hospital in Chicago.

BARBARA H. GUEST is a senior project manager for Macro International Inc. of Silver Spring, Maryland, where she writes guidelines for the standardization of substance abuse treatment for Macro Inc., Washington, D.C.

LANNIS E. HALL is currently a second-year postgraduate surgical trainee at the Howard University Hospital. Previously, Hall was a Dow-Callender fellow at Howard University Hospital.

LEONARD HARRIS is professor of philosophy at Purdue University, West Lafayette, Indiana.

MICHAEL HEBRARD is a medical student at Creighton University, Omaha, Nebraska.

BRIAN HERTZ is a family physician at Provident Cook County Hospital and Claretian Medical Center.

SIMONA J. HILL is an assistant professor of sociology at Chestnut Hill College, Philadelphia, and a lecturer in sociology at the University of Pennsylvania.

ALISON JAGGAR is professor of philosophy and women's studies at the University of Colorado at Boulder.

WILLIAM M. KING is associate professor and coordinator of Afro-American Studies at the University of Colorado at Boulder.

JOHN D. LANTOS is assistant professor of pediatrics and associate director of the Center for Clinical Medical Ethics at the University of Chicago. He is also chief of the Medical Staff at La Rabida Children's Hospital and Research Center in Chicago.

DAVID MCBRIDE is associate professor in African and African-American Studies at Penn State University, University Park, Pennsylvania.

STEPHEN MILES is associate professor of medicine at the University of Minnesota and Hennepin County Medical Center, and also an associate faculty at the Center for Biomedical Ethics.

SHAFIA MAWUSHI MONROE heads the Traditional Childbearing Group in Jamaica Plain, Massachusetts.

KATHRYN MOSELEY is clinical medical ethics consultant for Henry Ford Hospital and a fellow at the University of Chicago Center for Clinical Medical Ethics.

ROBERT MURRAY, JR., is chief, Division of Medical Genetics at Howard University's College of Medicine.

LAURENCE J. O'CONNELL is president and CEO of the Park Ridge Center for the Study of Health, Faith and Ethics in Chicago. He also holds an appointment in the Department of Medicine, Stritch School of Medicine, Loyola University.

MARGO OKAZAWA-REY is associate professor in the Department of Social Work Education at San Francisco State University.

CHESTER PIERCE is professor of education and psychiatry in the Faculty of Medicine, the Graduate School of Education, and the Faculty of Public Health at Harvard University.

RUTH PURTILO is professor of clinical ethics at Creighton University's Center for Health Policy and Ethics, and is also a fellow of the Hastings Center.

SANDRA CROUSE QUINN is a research associate at Westat Inc., where she specializes in health promotion and disease prevention projects. Previously, she was research associate in the Minority Health Research Laboratory, Department of Health Education at the University of Maryland, College Park.

ALMA ROBERTS is vice president of corporate development for Liberty Medical Center.

JEAN J. SCHENSUL is executive director of the Institute for Community Research, an applied health research institution in Connecticut, and associate professor of anthropology and community medicine, University of Connecticut.

RICHARD SCHMITT is professor of philosophy at Brown University, Providence, Rhode Island.

MARIAN GRAY SECUNDY is a professor and director of the program in medical ethics at Howard University College of Medicine, Department of Community Health and Family Practice. She recently served as co-chair of the ethics working group of Hillary Rodham Clinton's Health Care Task Force. She has been a visiting scholar at the University of San Francisco Health Policy Institute, the University of Chicago program in Clinical Medical Ethics, Michigan State University, and Hiram College.

RENSLOW SHERER is the director of the Cook County HIV Primary Care Center in Chicago.

MARK SIEGLER is a general internist who is a professor of medicine and the director of the Center for Clinical Medical Ethics at the University of Chicago Pritzker School of Medicine.

PATTI GRACE SMITH is a deputy director of policy for the Federal Communication Commission in Washington, D.C.

STEPHEN B. THOMAS is an associate professor of health education in the School of Public Health at Emory University. Previously, he was director of the Minority Health Research Laboratory at the University of Maryland in College Park.

STEPHEN TOULMIN is Henry R. Luce Professor at the Center for Multiethnic and Transnational Studies at the University of California, Los Angeles.

ANN WOOD WASHINGTON is a psychologist at the University of Illinois and is currently a doctoral candidate there.

NATHANIEL WESLEY, JR., is director of planning at Howard University Hospital.

BRUCE DAVID WHITE is pediatrician at the Children and Youth Health Center, clinical ethics consultant at Saint Thomas Hospital, and adjunct associate professor of medicine (Health Law and Ethics) and assistant director of the Center for Clinical and Research Ethics at Vanderbilt University Medical Center.

EVELYN C. WHITE is a reporter for the *San Francisco Chronicle*.

SEPTEMBER WILLIAMS is a critical care specialist who trained at Creighton University, Chicago's Cook County Hospital, and the University of Chicago's Center for Clinical Medical Ethics. She is currently pursuing a long-time interest in film and considering its application for ethical problems in patient care.

MILDRED WILLIAMSON is the administrator for the Women and Children HIV Program at Cook County Hospital in Chicago and a doctoral student in social welfare policy at the University of Chicago School of Social Services Administration.

KRISTY WOODS is an assistant professor of clinical medicine at the University of Chicago, Pritzker School of Medicine.

CURTIS L. YEAGER is the transplant coordinator at Howard University Hospital and was the first coordinator for the DC Organ Donor Program

LAUREN JONES YOUNG is associate professor in the Departments of Teacher Education and Educational Administration, Michigan State University, as well as senior researcher at the National Center for Research on Teacher Learning.